ARTICULATORY AND PHONOLOGICAL IMPAIRMENTS

ARTICULATORY AND PHONOLOGICAL IMPAIRMENTS
A CLINICAL FOCUS

JACQUELINE BAUMAN-WAENGLER

Clarion University

ALLYN AND BACON

Boston   London   Toronto   Sydney   Tokyo   Singapore

Executive Editor: Stephen D. Dragin
Vice President and Editor-in-Chief: Paul A. Smith
Series Editorial Assistant: Bridget McSweeney
Director of Education Programs: Ellen Mann Dolberg
Senior Marketing Manager: Brad Parkins
Production Editor: Christopher H. Rawlings
Editorial-Production Service: Omegatype Typography, Inc.
Composition and Prepress Buyer: Linda Cox
Manufacturing Buyer: David Repetto
Cover Administrator: Jennifer Hart
Electronic Composition: Omegatype Typography, Inc.

Library of Congress Cataloging-in-Publication Data

Bauman-Waengler, Jacqueline Ann.
    Articulatory and phonological impairments : a clinical focus / Jacqueline Bauman-Waengler.
       p.   cm.
    Includes bibliographical references and index.
    ISBN 0-205-28064-1
    1. Articulation disorders.   2. English language—Phonetics.   I. Title.

  RC424.7 .B378 2000
  616.85'5 21—dc21
                                                                                99-044138

Printed in the United States of America

10   9   8   7   6   5   4   3   2   04   03   02   01   00

CONTENTS

PREFACE

Throughout my years of university teaching and clinical supervision, I became increasingly aware of a growing gap between classroom instruction and clinical knowledge. For many students, there was no smooth transition between principles and foundations taught in the classroom and their applicability to clinical practice. Although they had acquired a fine knowledge of the subject matter, they often could not apply this knowledge. In addition, the multitude of assessment and remediation possibilities led to confusion and overdependency on a single procedure. This book is an attempt to integrate strong academic foundations directly with clinical applications. The rationale behind this attempt is that a clearer understanding of basic principles and their application to specific clinical decision-making strategies will produce more knowledgeable clinicians who are goal-directed and efficient in assessment and remediation procedures.

Two principles guided my efforts from the beginning: First, the textbook had to provide solid, up-to-date information about the subject matter. Second, this information always had to be linked to clinical application; it had to make clinical sense. This translated into some time-honored discussions on the one hand and into their important implications for everyday clinical practice on the other. Therefore, clinical applications are built into each chapter to demonstrate certain principles, and clinical case studies are used to promote the transfer of knowledge.

This text offers a broad range of topics, from phonetic transcription and the use of diacritics to the assessment and treatment of children with emerging phonological systems, the dialect speaker, and individuals with English as a second language.

In addition, it provides an up-to-date treatment of both articulatory and phonological impairments. Although newer contemporary topics such as phonological assessment, phonemic-based therapy, and nonlinear phonologies are covered in detail, there is also a comprehensive discussion of phonetic principles applied to the diagnosis and treatment of motor-based disorders, that is, articulatory impairments. Individuals with articulatory and phonological impairments compose the largest percentage of clients who come to us for services. Therefore, most clinicians will have to deal with clients displaying these disorders. It is important that we have a broad-based understanding of the dimensions of both of these speech disorders.

ACKNOWLEDGMENTS

First and foremost, I would like to thank my husband, who has had a tremendous impact both on my life and, subsequently, on the development of this book. Without his generous input, untiring devotion, and hard work, this project would never have begun and most certainly would not be anywhere near completion. To him, my deepest love and gratitude. His many years of being my mentor have broadened and deepened my perspective on phonetics, on phonology, and on being a

Mensch. I would also like to acknowledge my colleagues Kathy Linnan, who read several versions of this manuscript and who contributed many ideas about how to present the subject matter in a more clinically and pedagogically efficient manner, and Judy Janes, who provided helpful suggestions on organization. In the last few months, the help of my graduate students, the 1998 class of Articulation and Phonological Disorders in Children, proved extremely beneficial. They not only offered many good suggestions but also lifted my spirits at times when it was most urgent. Thanks also go to my graduate assistants Jayna McIntire, Megan Pavlik, and Wendy Wasylovski for the hours they spent trying to track down references. This project all began with Allyn and Bacon's, specifically Steve Dragin's, encouragement. His continued support throughout the project has meant a lot. Also, thanks to Doris P. Bradley, University of Southern Mississippi; Michael W. Casby, Michigan State University; Julie Masterson, Southwest Missouri State University; and Leslie Plonsker, University of Wisconsin, Stevens Point, who reviewed earlier versions of this manuscript.

ARTICULATORY AND PHONOLOGICAL IMPAIRMENTS

CHAPTER 1

CLINICAL FRAMEWORK
BASIC TERMS AND CONCEPTS

CHAPTER OUTLINE

- Articulation and Articulation Disorders
- Phonetics and Its Relationship to Articulation Disorders
- Speech Sounds versus Phonemes: Clinical Application

- Phonology and Phonological Disorders
- Phonetics versus Phonology: Form and Function
- Articulation Disorders versus Phonological Disorders
- Summary

Basic terms and concepts are principal components of every discipline. They serve as building blocks for other important concepts within the field of study. As a discipline, communication disorders therefore has a core vocabulary. *Phonetics, phonology, speech sound, phoneme,* and *articulation,* for example, represent fundamental concepts that have been frequently defined and exemplified. Together with many other terms, they have been integrated into a conceptual framework that establishes a firm foundation for students and practitioners. However, the link between this knowledge base and clinical practice is often not clear. Questions arise, such as: How do these concepts relate to clinical practice? How does the understanding of these concepts guide my clinical decision making? This chapter attempts to bridge the gap between some fundamental terms and concepts of our discipline and clinical practice.

The goal of this beginning chapter is to define and demonstrate the applicability of certain terms that are fundamental to the assessment and treatment of articulatory and phonological disorders. Definitions as well as distinctions between concepts are presented. Naturally, new knowledge calls for new terminology. However, new terms often result in an ongoing discussion among professionals about their nature, exact delineation, and application to communication disorders. The terms *phonological disorder* and *articulation disorder* are examples of concepts that have generated differing clinical interpretations. The controversies surrounding the practical application of some of these concepts will be introduced as a means to a better understanding of the various ways they are used today in the assessment and remediation of communication disorders.

ARTICULATION AND ARTICULATION DISORDERS

Articulation and *articulate* are words that are often used to describe an individual's speech. They might appear in a referral statement or within a diagnostic report, for example:

Sandy was referred to the clinic because her parents were concerned about her articulation *skills.*

Bob could articulate *the sound correctly in isolation, but not in word contexts.*

Joe's articulation disorder *affected his speech intelligibility.*

For the purpose at hand, **articulation** refers to the totality of motor processes involved in the planning and execution of sequences of overlapping gestures that result in speech (Fey, 1992). According to Fey (1992), this definition implies that, first, the learning of articulatory skills is an acquisitional process involving the gradual development of the ability to move the articulators in a precise and rapid manner. Thus, *learning to articulate is a specific kind of motor learning.* Just as children become more adept at certain motor skills as they grow older, their articulation skills develop as well. We cannot and do not expect the same level of articulatory abilities from a 2-year-old child as from a 6-year-old. Second, the definition implies that errors in articulation must be seen as relatively peripheral disturbances of articulatory processes. Therefore, *peripheral motor processes, not central linguistic abilities, are impaired.* In summary, articulation is a specific, gradually developing motor skill that involves mainly peripheral motor processes. Articulation errors must be

examined in light of the child's stage within this developmental articulatory process. This is typically referenced by the child's age. Thus, certain articulation errors will be considered normal given the age of the child while others might not be considered age-appropriate.

If an individual's articulation deviates significantly from the norm, it may be diagnosed as an articulation disorder. An **articulation disorder** refers to difficulties with the motor production aspects of speech, or an inability to produce certain speech sounds (Elbert and Gierut, 1986). Articulation disorders represent deficiencies in the relatively peripheral motor processes that result in speech. This leads us to a discussion of phonetics.

PHONETICS AND ITS RELATIONSHIP TO ARTICULATION DISORDERS

Generally stated, phonetics is the science of speech (Grunwell, 1987). However, the domain of what is considered "speech" seems to vary somewhat from author to author. Some define phonetics in a broad, encompassing way by including speech sound production, transmission, and perception (Crystal, 1987; Halle and Stevens, 1979; Kantner and West, 1960; Waengler, 1983). Others state that phonetics entails only the study of the production and perception of speech sounds (Shriberg and Kent, 1995; Wise, 1958). And there are some authors who equate phonetics with just the study of speech sound production (Creaghead and Newman, 1989; Heffner, 1975). Why are these definitions so different? Perhaps Crystal (1987) offers a valid explanation:

Articulation is rooted in the Latin word *articulatio,* which stood for the "joining of separate entities." In anatomy, zoology, and biology, this basic definition is preserved, as in "The thyroid cartilage articulates with the cricoid cartilage." Musicians, too, use the word to refer to the joining of separate entities, for example, tone groupings, as in, "She played the sonata with feeling and superb articulation." When used by dentists, *articulation* alludes to the joining of teeth, as in "The articulation of the new dentures was better than that of the patient's set of natural teeth." Within communication disorders, the original *articulatio* is exemplified by the joining of the many separate movements needed to establish speech, as in "The child's articulation was characterized by multiple sound errors."

The description and classification of speech sounds is the main aim of phonetic science, or phonetics. Sounds may be identified with reference to their production (or "articulation") in the vocal tract, their acoustic transmission, or their auditory reception. The most widely used descriptions are articulatory, because the vocal tract provides a convenient and well-understood reference point.... (p. 152)

Thus, differences in the definitions of phonetics may reflect common usage or the special importance delegated to the different descriptors of speech. For the discussion at hand, a broader definition, such as Crystal's, is more suitable. It delineates speech in its entirety and effectively indicates the various subdivisions of phonetics. **Phonetics** is the study of speech emphasizing the description and classification of speech sounds according to their production, transmission, and perceptual features. See Table 1.1.

One branch of phonetics, **articulatory phonetics**, deals with the production features of speech sounds and their categorization and classification according to specific parameters of their production. How sounds are actually *articulated*, their objective similarities, and their differences are central aspects of this branch of phonetics. The transmission properties of speech are dealt with in **acoustic phonetics.** Here, the frequency, intensity, and duration of speech sounds, for example, are described and categorized. Within **auditory phonetics**, investigators focus on how we perceive sounds. Our ears are not objective receivers of acoustic data. Rather, many factors influence our perception. Such factors are examined in the area of auditory phonetics.

In the context of this discussion, we are primarily interested in articulatory phonetics. This specialty area deals with the actualities of how speech sounds are formed. Directly related to this area of phonetics is, of course, articulation. Although articulation represents all motor processes resulting in speech in its entirety, in articulatory phonetics, only specific motor processes responsible for the production of speech sounds are described and classified.

The description and classification of speech sounds is an integral portion of both

TABLE 1.1 Articulation, Articulation Disorder, Phonetics, and Articulatory Phonetics

TERM	DEFINITION	EXAMPLES
Articulation	The totality of motor processes involved in the planning and execution of speech.	Describes the speech sound production of individuals, e.g., "He mis*articulated* the [s] sound." Describes tests that examine speech sound production ability, e.g., "He administered an *articulation* test."
Articulation disorder	Difficulties with the motor production aspects of speech, or an inability to produce certain speech sounds.	A diagnostic category that indicates that an individual's speech sound productions vary widely from the norm, e.g., "He was diagnosed as having an *articulation disorder.*"
Phonetics	The study of speech emphasizing the description and classification of speech sounds according to their production, transmission, and perceptual features.	Used in a narrow sense to refer to the production of speech sounds, e.g., "Clinicians use *phonetic* transcription." Indicates branches of study that are related to speech sound production, transmission, or perception, e.g., acoustic *phonetics* and auditory *phonetics.*
Articulatory phonetics	Categorization and classification of speech sounds according to specific production parameters.	How individual sounds are formed, e.g., their place, manner, and voicing characteristics.

the assessment and the treatment of articulation disorders. Knowledge of the production features of speech sounds will guide clinicians when they are evaluating the various misarticulations noted in a clinical evaluation. One important step involves gathering phonetic information on the exact way an individual misarticulates sounds. This type of phonetic clinical work is indispensable in the assessment and treatment of our clients with articulation disorders.

SPEECH SOUNDS VERSUS PHONEMES: CLINICAL APPLICATION

Speech sounds and phonemes are central units in any discussion of disordered articulation and phonology. Although the human vocal tract is capable of producing a wide array of sounds, including coughing and burping, speech sounds are special sounds because they are associated with speech. **Speech sounds** represent physical sound realities; they are end products of articulatory motor processes. When talking about a child's s-production in the context of an articulation test, for example, we refer to the *speech sound* production of [s].

Speech sounds, then, are real, physical sound entities used in speech. But in addition to their articulatory form, they also have a linguistic function. The smallest linguistic unit that is able, when combined with other such units, to establish word meanings and distinguish between them is referred to as a **phoneme.** Words that differ in only one phoneme value among their sound constituents are called **minimal pairs.** Examples are *dog* versus *log* and *dog* versus *dot.*

> The conceptual nature of the phoneme is more fully developed in Chapter 4.

The term *phoneme* designates a linguistic concept, not a physical actuality. If one wants to refer to the physical reality, to the actual production, the term *speech sound* is used. See Table 1.2. From early to contemporary publications, such phoneme realizations have also been labelled **allophonic variations** (e.g., Trubetzkoy, 1939; Shriberg and Kent, 1995) or **phonetic variations** (Grunwell, 1987). As far as notation is concerned, real sound productions are always placed within brackets in phonetic transcription whereas phoneme values are symbolized by slanted lines, or virgules. For example, [s] indicates that it was a sound someone actually pronounced in a specific manner. On the other hand, /s/ signifies the phoneme "s." Speech sounds or phonetic variations can be examined, and usually are, without reference

TABLE 1.2 Phoneme versus Speech Sound

PHONEME	SPEECH SOUND
The smallest unit within a language that is able, when combined with other units, to establish word meanings and distinguish among them	Actual realizations of phonemes; referred to as allophonic variations or phonetic variations
Linguistic unit	Concrete, produced, transmitted, and perceived
Used in reference to a particular language system	Can be examined without referring to a specific language system
Basic unit within phonology	Basic unit within phonetics
Notation is within virgules / /, e.g., "the /s/ phoneme"	Notation is within brackets, e.g., "the [f] speech sound"

to a given language system. This is not the case with phonemes. Using the term *phoneme,* we refer exclusively to the function of the sound in question, to its ability to signify differences in word meaning within a specific language.

How do these terms relate to our clinical decision making? Speech sounds as end products of articulatory motor processes are the units we are describing when we use phonetic transcription to capture an individual's actual productions on an articulation test or spontaneous speech sample. Speech sounds and speech sound errors relate to articulation abilities. However, what if we notice that a child's productions of *swing, sing, ring,* and *wing* all sound the same, for example, that they all sound like *wing*? The child is not using the necessary sound units to signal differences between these words. Both listener and speaker will probably not be able to differentiate between these words because they sound the same. Now we are analyzing the child's phoneme system, the child's ability to use phonemes to establish and distinguish between word meanings. If this occurs consistently throughout the child's speech, we could conclude that the child's phoneme system is limited, that is, restricted when compared to the norm. Phonemes and difficulties in using phonemes contrastively to distinguish meanings relate to *linguistic* abilities, to the individual's language system.

PHONOLOGY AND PHONOLOGICAL DISORDERS

The term *phonology* is basic to the understanding of phonological disorders. **Phonology,** a branch of linguistics, pertains to the description of the systems and patterns of phonemes that occur in a language. It involves determining the language-specific distinctive phonemes and the rules that describe the changes

Some phoneme combinations do not occur in General American English words. An example would be /ʃ/ + /v/. General American English does have other /ʃ/ combinations, such as /ʃ/ + /r/ (e.g., *shrink*) or /ʃ/ + /t/ (e.g., *wished*). The /ʃ/ + /v/ combination does, however, occur in the phonological system of German. Words such as *Schwester* (/ʃvɛstəʀ/) document this as a *phonotactic* possibility in German.

Other consonant clusters that do occur in General American English are restricted in use to certain positions. For example, the clusters "sk" and "ks" cannot occur in the same places. Words or syllables can begin or end with "sk" (e.g., *skate, risk*). This, though, is not the case with "ks." This cluster can occur only at the end of a syllable or word (e.g., *kicks*). This is a *phonotactic* characteristic of the phonological system of General American English.

that result when these phonemes occur in different relationships with other phonemes (Ladefoged, 1993). Phonology includes the inventory of phonemes of the language in question. For example, a list of all the vowels and consonants that function in American English to differentiate meaning would give us this inventory. However, phonology also focuses on how these phonemes are *organized* to convey meaning within a language system. Such a description would include how the phonemes can and cannot be arranged to form meaningful words. The term **phonotactics** refers to the description of the allowed combinations of phonemes in a particular language.

Phonological disorder refers to an impaired system of phonemes and phoneme patterns within the context of spoken language. The term represents an individual's impairment of the representation and organization of phonemes within the language system. Therefore, it is hypothesized that a phonological disorder reflects a more central deficiency, specifically a neurolinguistic dysfunction at the phonological level (Grunwell, 1987).

Assessment of a child with a phonological disorder would include gathering information about all the phonemes that the child uses to distinguish meaning—the phonemic inventory. When compared to the phonemic inventory of General American English, we might find that certain phonemes are not present in the child's speech, that is, that the child's phonemic inventory is restricted. In addition, we might analyze the child's phonotactics by examining the position in the word where these phonemes occur, that is, at the beginning, middle, or end of the word. Children who have difficulties with the organization of their phoneme system might not realize the phonotactics that are typical for American English. Their speech may demonstrate *phonotactic constraints,* in other words, that the phonemes are not used in all possible word positions.

CLINICAL APPLICATION

Inventory and Phonotactics

Jeff was referred to the school speech-language pathologist by his kindergarten teacher, who was worried about the lack of intelligibility of his speech. The clinician noted that Jeff's phonemic inventory was very restricted. The following phonemes were present in Jeff's speech: /p, b, t, d, k, g, m, n, ŋ, f, v, h, w/. Jeff's phonemic inventory did not include the following phonemes: /s, z, ʃ, ʒ, θ, ð, j, l, r, ʧ, ʤ/. In addition, certain phonotactic constraints were noted. At the beginning of a word, Jeff always realized all noted speech sounds. However, at the end of a word or syllable, only voiced sounds were used. Jeff's phonotactics did not employ voiceless sounds to terminate a word or syllable. Not only was Jeff's phonemic inventory limited, but also phonotactic constraints were discovered.

Phonology is closely related to other constituents of the language system, such as morphology, syntax, semantics, and pragmatics. A child's phonological system, therefore, can never be regarded as functionally separate from other aspects of the child's language growth. Several recent studies (e.g., Paul and Jennings, 1992; Ratner, 1994; Rescorla and Ratner, 1996; Scarborough and Dobrich, 1990; Stoel-Gammon, 1989) have documented that delayed phonological development occurs concurrently with delayed lexical and grammatical development. Although the direct relationship between phonological and grammatical acquisition remains unclear, interdependencies certainly exist between these areas.

PHONETICS VERSUS PHONOLOGY: FORM AND FUNCTION

The speech sounds which are investigated within the area of phonetics have a great many acoustic and articulatory properties which are all important for the phonetician…. However, for the phonologist most of them are totally irrelevant as long as they do not function as distinguishing marks between words. Therefore, the speech sound of the phonetician does not coincide with the sound segment of the phonologist. The phonologist considers the sound segment only insofar as it fulfills a certain linguistic function. (Translated from Trubetzkoy, 1939, p. 14)

Any understanding of phonology presupposes its distinction from phonetics. The difference between *form* and *function* has often been used to characterize this distinction. While phonetics emphasizes the form of speech sounds, that is, their concrete actualities, phonology stresses their function as phonemes within the language system (see Table 1.3).

How do we practically differentiate between the form and the function of a specific sound segment in question? When analyzing the speech sound form, a clinician examines all the distinct properties that are associated with its production. It might be noted that [ʃ]

TABLE 1.3 Phonetics versus Phonology

TERM	MAJOR EMPHASIS	EXAMPLES
Phonetics	The actualities of speech production	Describes how individual speech sounds are produced, their form
Phonology	The function and organization of phonemes within a given language system	Includes inventory of phonemes within a specific language that functions to differentiate meaning in that language
		Examines how phonemes can and cannot be arranged to establish meaningful words, i.e., phonotactics

is produced without the normal lip rounding or that [s] is produced with the tongue too far forward, giving it a dull rather than its characteristic sharp s-quality. The **phonetic inventory** is the repertoire of speech sounds for a particular client, including all his or her characteristic production features.

On the other hand, if the phoneme function is the goal of the assessment, the clinician would examine the child's phoneme system to determine whether a child employs specific phonemes contrastively, that is, for the purpose of differentiating between word meanings. A phonemic analysis ignores all the production characteristics of the sound segment except those that distinguish between word meanings in that language. In a phonemic analysis, if a child produces [ʃ] without lip rounding but the sound segment is still perceived as /ʃ/, then the lack of lip rounding would not be relevant. However, if the child's production of [ʃ] is so far off that it is perceived as /s/, this would be important. Its importance lies in the fact that /ʃ/ and /s/ are two separate phonemes in American English; they can be used contrastively to differentiate word meanings, as in *ship* versus *sip*. The **phonemic inventory** is the repertoire of phonemes used contrastively by an individual. A phonemic analysis would also examine the phonotactics of a particular client to determine if all sound segments are used in all possible positions.

ARTICULATION DISORDERS VERSUS PHONOLOGICAL DISORDERS

Although the term *phonology* has been a conceptual entity for linguists at least since the beginning of the twentieth century, it is only within the last few decades that it has gained wide usage by speech-language pathologists. For example, describing *phonological processes* when analyzing a child's speech error patterns or diagnosing a child as having a *phonological disorder* both have their theoretical basis in phonology. In addition, a gradual shift has occurred in the 1970s and 1980s away from use of the term *articulation disorder* to use of the term *phonological disorder*. For some, this change was considered necessary as "phonological notions provided a much richer framework for describing normal and disordered speech development" (Kamhi, 1992, p. 262). However, for many, this change in terminology created confusion. One reason for this confusion was the various ways in which the term *phonological disorder* was defined. Another confusing issue concerned how these new theoretical concepts were to be applied to the assessment and management of children with speech sound/phoneme difficulties. Based on the conceptual framework discussed earlier, articulation disorders were defined as disturbances in the relatively peripheral speech motor processes. They result in sounds that are notably different from norm productions. When comparing these characteristics to the previously given definitions, it becomes clear that *articulation disorders are phonetic in nature.*

On the other hand, phonological disorders represent impairments of the representation and organization of phonemes within a language system. They result in an inadequate phoneme system or in phoneme patterns that are different from those normally noted within a particular language. Phonological disorders are seen as deficiences in *phoneme function.* Thus the child may demonstrate the ability to realize the sound in question but also the inability to use it appropriately within the phoneme system. *Phonological disorders are phonemic in nature.* See Table 1.4.

TABLE 1.4 Articulation Disorders versus Phonological Disorders

ARTICULATION DISORDER	PHONOLOGICAL DISORDER
Phonetic errors	Phonemic errors
Problems in speech sound production	Problems in the language-specific function of phonemes
Difficulties with speech sound forms	Difficulties with phoneme function
Disturbances in relatively peripheral motor processes that result in speech	Disturbances are more central in nature, concerning the phonological level of the organization of the language system
Speech sound production difficulties do not typically impact other areas of language development such as morphology, syntax, or semantics	Phoneme difficulties may impact other language areas such as morphology, syntax, or semantics

While it does not seem difficult to separate an articulation disorder from a phonological disorder definitionally, opinions vary as to the relationship and interdependencies between the two. Is it important for the assessment and remediation process to distinguish between the terms? Or should professionals choose one term to represent both?

For certain speech sound problems, many believe that the term *phonological disorder* is a better label. First, it places speech sound disorders into the broader framework of language. Within this broader framework, attention is focused on the whole system rather than on only one part of the system (Elbert, 1992). This viewpoint also seems more in line with findings that suggest that phonological performance is influenced by pragmatic, morphosyntactic, and semantic levels of organization (e.g., Hoffman, 1990; Panagos and Prelock, 1982; Panagos, Quine, and Klich, 1979; Paul and Shriberg, 1982; Shriberg and Kwiatkowski, 1994). Phonological development is seen as directly linked to the child's developing cognitive and language systems. In addition, it seems clear that some of the sound errors made by children cannot be due to faulty control of the articulators, that is, they cannot be viewed as articulation disorders

Historically, the term *articulation disorder* has been used as a label for all clients who evidenced speech sound production difficulties. Observed errors were thought to be caused by faulty control of the peripheral articulators. Remediation consisted of increasing precision, speed, and/or mobility of these articulators within the context of speech production. This viewpoint did not emphasize the decisively important fact that speech sounds function within the language system as phonemes. This limited understanding of disordered articulation probably set the stage for embracing a new, more encompassing concept.

(Edwards, 1992; Fey, 1992). Although these children may demonstrate adequate production of speech sounds, their rule-governed use in specific contexts or word positions is impaired. For these children, then, the speech sound form is adequate; speech sound function, however, is not.

In an attempt to resolve this labelling issue, Shriberg and Kwiatkowski (1982a) suggested that the term *phonological disorder* be used as a cover term for any problem that involves the speech production process. Thus, both groups of children, those with faulty control of the articulators *and* those with faulty phonemic system organization, would be considered to have a phonological disorder.

Using the term *phonological disorder* in such a broad manner creates several theoretical and practical problems. Definitionally, a phonological disorder represents difficulties with the organization and function of the phoneme system. Does this mean that all children who have speech impairments, even those with so-called simple problems—for example, a distorted [s] or an [r] that is not quite correct—now have problems with the organization and function of their phoneme system? Certainly not. And what about those disorders that have historically been considered articulation disorders, such as the dysarthrias or cerebral palsy? Should these now be considered phonological disorders, too? By labelling all children with speech production problems as "phonologically disordered," more confusion than coherence is gained.

The distinction between articulation and phonological disorders remains decisively important. It keeps definitions clear and is practically applicable to diagnostic and intervention procedures. For the purpose at hand, therefore, a distinction will be made between *phonetic errors,* those in which the peripheral motor processes are disturbed, and *phonemic errors,* those in which the organization and function of the phoneme system is impaired. While this description of phonetic versus phonemic sound errors is not without problems, the distinction between the two will be applied throughout this text: Phonetic errors result in articulation disorders, while phonemic errors represent phonological disorders.

Delineating phonetic and phonemic errors is clinically not an either/or proposition. Often, a child will display characteristics of both phonetic and phonemic errors. Although this division between phonetic and phonemic errors may remain at times unclear, a systematic attempt to distinguish between them is one important aspect of clinical decision making.

There is no doubt that the application of phonological principles has added considerably to our understanding of speech errors in children. However, zealously embracing these newer concepts, many professionals have started to ignore phonetics due to its alignment with traditional motor-based approaches. The conceptual framework offered by phonetics continues to be a central portion of the assessment and treatment process. "Clearly one cannot employ phonological concepts and techniques without phonetic knowledge, and that knowledge informs clinical assessment and treatment" (Grunwell, 1997, pp. 63–64). Accordingly, after analyzing various treatment perspectives, Shelton (1993) concluded that "both articulatory and phonological concepts contribute to the understanding of children's speech-sound system and related language disorders, but neither is sufficient by itself as a framework for clinical work" (p. 175). For decades, phonetic principles have been the core of assessment and treatment of speech disorders in children and adults. Although phonological principles add to our understanding, they do not replace the valuable knowledge phonetics has to offer.

CLINICAL APPLICATION

Phonetic Disorder

Sandy is a 6-year-old child who was seen in a diagnostic session at the speech and hearing clinic. Her parents were concerned about her inability to produce an "s" sound. Based on an analysis of a spontaneous speech sample and an articulation test, it was found that Sandy misarticulated "s" and "z" in all transcribed situations. The child was also able to differentiate her mispronunciations from norm productions of [s] and [z]. No other speech sounds were in error, and language skills were found to be within normal limits. Sandy used her distorted realizations in every position where [s] and [z] should occur. Thus, she seemed to understand the organization of /s/ and /z/ within the language system. The clinician hypothesized that this child was having difficulties with the actual production level only, with the speech sounds [s] and [z], whereas the understanding of their phoneme function was intact.

CLINICAL APPLICATION

Phonemic Disorder

Travis was a 6-year-old first-grader who was referred by his classroom teacher to the speech-language pathologist. The teacher said that although Travis's speech was fairly intelligible, she was concerned about speech and language problems she had noticed in class. Her second concern was that these difficulties might be impacting his emerging literacy skills. According to the teacher, Travis was having difficulty distinguishing between certain sounds and words as the class progressed with elementary reading tasks.

An articulation test and a spontaneous speech sample were analyzed with the following results: Travis had difficulties with s-productions. At the end of a word or syllable, [s] was always deleted. At the beginning of a word or syllable, [s] was produced as [ʃ]. Interestingly enough, when the clinician analyzed

other words, she found that Travis could produce [s], but not in its proper context. Thus, several words that contained [f] were articulated with a normal sounding [s] realization. Testing of minimal pairs containing /s/ and /ʃ/ revealed that Travis was having difficulty distinguishing between the phonemic value of the two sounds.

On language tests and in spontaneous conversation, Travis deleted the plural -s and the third person singular -s (e.g., "He, she, it walk"). Comprehension of these grammatical forms was also often in error.

The clinician hypothesized that Travis had a phonological disorder—that he had difficulties with the phoneme function and the phonotactics of /s/. This problem was impacting his morphological development. Due to the noted problems in discrimination, this could also have an effect on his beginning reading skills.

SUMMARY

This chapter refamiliarized students and clinicians with several terms that are fundamental to the assessment and treatment of articulatory and phonological disorders. Definitions and clinical applications were provided for *articulation, phonetics, speech sound, phonology,* and the *phoneme* as a foundation for this understanding. Form versus function was used to distinguish between phonetics, with its basic unit the speech sound, and phonology, with its basic unit the phoneme. Phonetics emphasizes the form of speech sounds, while phonology stresses the function of phonemes within a language system. Based on these definitions, a differentiation between articulation disorders and phonological disorders was presented. The problems of such a division were discussed in light of the diversity of viewpoints on the subject as well as of the clinical consequences of such a separation.

CHAPTER 2

ARTICULATORY PHONETICS
SPEECH SOUND FORM

CHAPTER OUTLINE

- Vowels versus Consonants
- Sounds in Context: Coarticulation and Assimilation

- Syllable Structure
- Summary

Articulatory phonetics deals with the categorization and classification of the production features of speech sounds. A thorough knowledge of how vowels and consonants are generated remains essential for successful assessment and remediation of articulatory and phonological disorders. Although contemporary phonological theories have provided new ways of viewing assessment and treatment of these disorders, only knowledge of the speech sounds' production features secure a firm basis for utilizing such procedures. Without this knowledge, phonological process analysis, for example, is impossible.

This chapter discusses articulatory-phonetic aspects of the speech sounds of General American English. The specific goals are

1. to provide a review of the form of vowels and consonants, that is, to examine their production features;
2. to introduce the concepts of coarticulation and assimilation as a means of describing how sounds change within a given articulatory context; and
3. to examine the structure of syllables and their clinical applicability in the assessment and treatment of impaired articulation and phonology.

The production of vowels and consonants, as well as their language-specific arrangements into syllables and words, depends entirely on articulatory motor processes. If these processes are disordered, speech sound production will be impaired. Articulatory motor processes depend in turn on many anatomical-physiological prerequisites, which can be classified as respiratory, phonatory, or resonatory. For example, the problems that render the speech of children with cerebral palsy difficult to understand often originate in abnormal respiratory, resonatory, and/or phonatory prerequisites for articulation. The proper function of such prerequisites, therefore, must first be secured before any articulatory improvement can be expected. Articulatory motor ability is embedded in many different anatomical-physiological prerequisites of fundamental importance to speech-language pathologists.

Basic knowledge in these areas is typically gained from courses and textbooks covering anatomy and physiology of the speech and hearing mechanisms

> For more information about the respiratory, phonatory, resonatory, and articulatory characteristics of cerebral palsy, see Chapter 10.

rather than from those covering impaired articulation and phonology. This is because the clinical significance of anatomical-physiological knowledge and its application to articulatory and phonological disorders is not always recognized. The anatomical-physiological aspects of such disorders are not within the scope of this chapter, but Box 2.1 offers references as an incentive for the reader to rediscover the wealth of anatomical-physiological information essential to the clinical assessment and remediation of articulatory and phonological impairments.

VOWELS VERSUS CONSONANTS

Speech sounds are commonly divided into two groups: *vowels* and *consonants*. The distinction between the vowels and the consonants relates both to their form and to their function (see Table 2.1). Productionally, vowels are articulated with a relatively open vocal tract whereas consonants are not. A **vowel** is a speech sound that is formed without significant constriction of the oral (and pharyngeal) cavities. This

TABLE 2.1 Vowels and Consonants: Form and Function Differences

FORM DIFFERENCES	
Vowels	*Consonants*
No significant constriction of the vocal tract	Significant constriction of the vocal tract
Sagittal midline of vocal tract remains open	Constriction occurs along sagittal midline of vocal tract
Open sounds	Constricted sounds
Voiced	Voiced or unvoiced

FUNCTION DIFFERENCES	
Vowels	*Consonants*
Typically serve as syllable nuclei	Only specific consonants can serve as syllable nuclei
More intensity than other elements of the syllable	Less intensity than vowels as syllable constituents
Carry prosodic features such as intonation and stress	Do not typically carry prosodic features

Box 2.1_____

Selected Readings in Anatomy and Physiology of the Speech and Hearing Mechanisms

Culbertson, W. R., & Tanner, D. C. (1997). *Introductory speech and hearing anatomy and physiology workbook.* Boston: Allyn & Bacon.

Kahane, J. C., & Folkins, J. F. (1984). *Atlas of speech and hearing anatomy.* Columbus, OH: Charles E. Merrill.

Kent, R. D. (1997). *The speech sciences.* San Diego: Singular.

Seikel, J. A., King, D. W., & Drumright, D. G. (1997). *Anatomy and physiology for speech and language.* San Diego: Singular.

Zemlin, W. R. (1988). *Speech and hearing science: Anatomy and physiology* (3rd ed.). Englewood Cliffs, NJ: Prentice-Hall.

means that there are no major obstructions along the passage from the vocal folds to the mouth opening (Kent, 1997). In spite of different positionings of the articulators for the vowels [i] and [u], for example, the expiratory airstream can always pass freely; the sagittal midline of the vocal tract remains open.

In contrast, **consonants** are speech sounds with a significant constriction within the vocal tract, mainly in the oral and pharyngeal cavities, foremost along the sagittal midline of the oral cavity. Whether we articulate [p] or [v], for example, there is al-

The *sagittal midline of the vocal tract* refers to the median plane that divides the vocal tract into right and left halves.

ways a partial or complete obstruction in the way of the expiratory airstream. In the case of [p], the lips form this barrier, whereas for the generation of [v], the contact of the lower lip with the upper teeth impedes the voiced airstream. The transcription of the various vowels and consonants together with examples of words in which these sounds can be heard are contained in Table 2.2.

There are other production features that distinguish vowels from consonants. Although vowels, under normal speech conditions, are produced with vocal fold vibration (i.e., they are voiced), consonants may be generated with or without vibration of the vocal folds (i.e., they can be voiced or voiceless). Voicing features constitute the main linguistically relevant differences that separate consonants such as [s] from [z] or [f] from [v].

Although vowels have been labelled "open" sounds and consonants "constricted" sounds, these working definitions remain relative. The obstruction of the expiratory airstream characterizing consonants is not always present. If we say [m] or [j], for example, the expiratory airstream is actually not impeded. For [m], although the lips are closed, the expiratory airstream flows freely through the nasal cavity. Indeed, this nasal airflow is characteristic of [m]. Also, only minimal differences are found in the constriction of the expiratory airstream if we contrast [j] to the [i] vowel, for example. Certain consonants have less obstruction of the airstream during their production, while others have more. Those consonants that have less obstruction are labelled sonorants. **Sonorant consonants** (or **semivowels**) are produced with a relatively open expiratory passageway. The sonorants include the nasals [m], [n], and [ŋ]; the liquids [l] and [r]; and the glides [w] and [j]. The sonorants are distinguished from the **obstruents**, which are characterized by a complete or narrow constriction between the articulators hindering the expiratory airstream. The obstruents include the stops [p], [b], [t], [d], [k], [g]; the fricatives [f], [v], [s], [z], [ʃ], [ʒ], [θ], [ð]; and the affricates [tʃ] and [dʒ].

There are also functional differences between vowels and consonants. In this context, *functional* indicates linguistic function. Vowels and consonants fulfill different tasks within the language system, that is, they play different linguistic roles. This has often been referred to as the "phonological difference"

TABLE 2.2 IPA Symbols (Wise, 1958)

CONSONANTS		VOWELS	
Symbol	Commonly Realized in	Symbol	Commonly Realized in
[p]	pay	[i]	eat
[b]	boy	[ɪ]	in
[t]	toy	[eɪ]	ape
[d]	doll	[ɛ]	egg
[k]	coat	[æ]	at
[g]	goat	[a]	father*
[m]	moon	[u]	moon
[n]	not	[ʊ]	wood
[ŋ]	sing	[oʊ]	boat
[θ]	think	[ɔ]	father*
[ð]	those	[ɑ]	hop
[f]	far	[aɪ]	tie
[v]	vase	[aʊ]	mouse
[s]	sun	[ɔɪ]	boy
[z]	zoo	[ɜ]	girl*
[ʃ]	shop	[ɝ]	bird*
[ʒ]	beige	[ɚ]	winner
[tʃ]	chop	[ʌ]	cut
[dʒ]	job	[ə]	above
[j]	yes		
[w]	win		
[ʍ]	who		
[l]	leep		
[r]	red		
[h]	hop		

*May be regional or individual pronunciations.

between vowels and consonants (Crystal, 1987; Hyman, 1975). The term *consonant* indicates this: *con* meaning "together with" and *-sonant* reflecting the tonal qualities that characterize vowels. Accordingly, consonants are those sounds that function linguistically only *together with* vowels, suggesting a certain functional priority of vowels over consonants.

In agreement with such a position, vowels serve as the center of syllables, as *syllable nuclei*. Vowels can constitute syllables all by themselves, as in the words *a-bove* or *a-way*,

> The notation *C* refers to a consonant, *V* to a vowel. Examples: CV structure—*go, no;* VC structure—*up, on;* CVC structure—*hot, ball;* CVCC structure—*milk, want.*

or together with one or more consonants, as in *win-dow* or *bridge*. Although there are many types of syllables—such as CV, VC, CVC, or CVCC—the vowel is always the center of the syllable, its nucleus. Vowels as "open" sounds also have more acoustic intensity than do other elements of the syllable. Therefore, they typically carry the prosodic features of a syllable or word. Hence, intonation and stress are common characteristics of vowels and not of consonants.

There are exceptions to this rule. A small group of conso-

> When transcribing, syllabic consonants need a special notation. This is discussed in Chapter 3.

nants can serve as the nuclei of syllables. A consonant that functions as a syllable nucleus is referred to as a syllabic.

American English Vowels

Vowels are commonly described according to certain parameters (Abercrombie, 1967; Crystal, 1987; Heffner, 1975; Kantner and West, 1960; Kent, 1998; Shriberg and Kent, 1995):

1. The *part* of the tongue that is raised. Example: *front* versus *back* vowels.
2. The *extent* to which the tongue is raised in the direction of the palate. Example: *high* versus *low* vowels.
3. The *kind* of opening made at the level of the lips. Example: *rounded* versus *unrounded* vowels.

The vowel quadrilateral of General American English describes vowels according to a horizontal and a vertical dimension. Divisions along a horizontal plane yield front, central, and back vowels, while points along a vertical plane give high, mid, and low vowels (see Figure 2.1).

The terms *tense/lax* and *open/close* are also used to describe vowels. *Tense* and *lax* refer to the degree of muscular activity involved in the articulation and to the length of the vowels in question (Shriberg and Kent, 1995). Therefore, tense vowels are considered to

	FRONT	CENTRAL	BACK
High	[i]		[u]
	[ɪ]		[ʊ]
	[e]		[o]
Mid		[ɜ] [ɝ]	
	[ɛ]	[ə] [ɚ]	
		[ʌ]	[ɔ]
	[æ]		
Low		[a]	[ɑ]

FIGURE 2.1 Vowel Quadrilateral of General American English Vowels

have relatively more muscle activity and are longer in duration than lax vowels. The vowel [i] is considered to be a tense vowel, while [ɪ] is lax. When contrasting tense versus lax, one has to keep in mind that these oppositions refer to paired productions of similar vowels only, that is, to vowel cognates. For example, [i] and [ɪ] are considered to be "ee" type vowels and [u] and [ʊ] are "oo" type vowels.

The terms *close* and *open* refer to the relative closeness of the tongue to the roof of the mouth (Abercrombie, 1967). Again, only similar vowels are usually characterized with these terms. Using the previous examples, [i] is more close and [ɪ] more open, [u] close and [ʊ] open.

There are two types of vowels: monophthongs and diphthongs. **Monophthongs** remain qualitatively the same throughout their entire production. They are pure vowels (Abercrombie, 1967; Shriberg and Kent, 1995). **Diphthongs** are vowels in which there is a change

> "It should be noted that although monophthongs are often referred to as "pure" vowels, no special virtue attaches to them" (Abercrombie, 1967, p. 60).

in quality during their duration (Ladefoged, 1993). The initial segment, the beginning portion of such a diphthong, is phonetically referred to as the **onglide,** its end portion as the **offglide.** Using this notation system, the following descriptions for the most common vowels of General American English are offered.

Front Vowels

[i]   a high-front vowel, unrounded, close and tense.

[ɪ]   a high-front vowel, unrounded, open and lax.

[e]   a mid-front vowel, unrounded, close and tense. In General American English, this vowel is typically produced as a diphthong, especially in stressed syllables or when articulated slowly.

[ɛ]   a mid-front vowel, unrounded, open and lax.

[æ]   a low-front vowel, unrounded, open and lax.

[a]   a low-front vowel, unrounded, close and tense. In General American English, the use of this vowel depends on the particular regional dialect of the speaker. In the New England dialect of the Northeast, one might often hear it.

All front vowels show various degrees of unrounding (lip spreading), with the high-front vowels showing the most. The lip spreading becomes less as one moves from the high-front vowels to the mid-front vowels, finally becoming practically nonexistent in the low-front vowels.

Back Vowels

[u]   a high-back vowel, rounded, close and tense.

[ʊ]   a high-back vowel, rounded, open and lax.

[o]   a mid-back vowel, rounded, close and tense. Again, this vowel is typically produced as a diphthong, especially in stressed syllables or when articulated slowly.

[ɔ]   a low mid-back vowel, rounded, open and lax (Heffner, 1975). The use of this vowel depends on regional pronunciation.

[ɑ]   a low-back vowel, unrounded, open and lax (Kantner and West, 1960). There seems to be some confusion in transcribing [ɔ] and [ɑ], although acoustic differences certainly exist. One distinguishing feature: the [ɔ] shows some degree of lip rounding, whereas [ɑ] does not.

Back vowels display different degrees of lip rounding in General American English. The high-back vowels [u] and [ʊ] often show a

There are differences of opinion as to whether certain vowels (specifically [ɔ] and [ɑ]) are tense or lax. This is based partially on definitional differences. Heffner (1975) and Kantner and West (1960) define tense and lax according to the degree of muscular activity. Shriberg and Kent (1995) point out that this has not been verified by experimental studies (e.g., Neary, 1978; Raphael and Bell-Berti, 1975), and they add the dimension of length: tense vowels are longer in duration than lax ones. Ladefoged (1993) defines tense and lax according to the type of syllable in which the vowel can occur. Only tense vowels can occur in open syllables, that is, in those without a consonant following the vowel (as in the words *bee* or *do*); all other vowels must be considered lax.

fairly high degree of lip rounding, whereas the low-back vowel [ɑ] is commonly articulated as an unrounded vowel.

Central Vowels

[ɝ]   a central vowel, rounded, tense with r-coloring. Rounding may vary, however, from speaker to speaker. [ɝ] occurs usually in stressed syllables of words.

[ɚ]   a central vowel, rounded, lax with r-coloring. Again, lip rounding may vary from speaker to speaker. This lax vowel is heard primarily in unstressed syllables.

[ɜ]   a central vowel, rounded, tense. [ɜ] is very similar in pronunciation to [ɝ], but it lacks any r-coloring. This vowel is heard in certain dialects. [ɜ] might be found in a Southern dialect pronunciation of *bird* or *worth*, for example. Also, it could be heard in the speech of children having difficulties producing the "r" sound.

[ʌ]   a lax, unrounded central vowel. In General American English, it is pronounced in stressed syllables of words.

[ə]   a lax, unrounded central vowel. It is typically used in unstressed syllables.

CLINICAL APPLICATION

Do Children Have Difficulties Producing Vowels?

Vowel errors in children developing phonological skills in a normal manner are relatively uncommon. However, children with phonological disorders may show deviant vowel patterns. Several studies (e.g., Pollock and Keiser, 1990; Reynolds, 1990; Stoel-Gammon and Herrington, 1990) have documented the presence of specific vowel problems in phonologically disordered children. Although certain vowel substitutions seem to be articulatory simplifications that could also occur in normal development, other errors appear to be idiosyncratic. Assessment of vowel qualities should be a portion of every diagnostic protocol. This can be easily achieved with any formal articulation test by transcribing the entire word rather than just the sound being tested.

Diphthongs.   As previously defined, a diphthong is a vowel sound that demonstrates articulatory movement during its production. Its initial portion, the onglide, is acoustically more prominent and usually longer than the offglide. Typically, only *rising* diphthongs are articulated in the standard pronunciation of General American English (Heffner, 1975). This means that in producing these diphthongs, essential portions of the tongue move from a lower onglide to a higher offglide position; thus, the tongue moves in a rising motion. This can be demonstrated on the vowel quadrilateral as well (see Figure 2.2).

There are several different ways to characterize diphthongs as single phonemic units in contrast to two separate vowels. Some transcribers use a bar or bow either above or below the two vowel symbols—[e͞ɪ], [e͜ɪ], or [eɪ], for example. The author has chosen to use the transcription that elevates the offglide portion of the diphthong to indicate its typically lesser intensity and length.

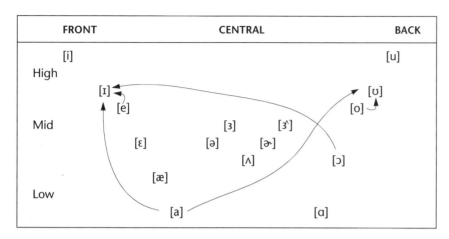

FIGURE 2.2 Vowel Quadrilateral with Rising Diphthongs

Discrepancies may be noted between the transcriptions of diphthongs offered in this text and the ones in other books. Because phonetic transcription is purely *de*scriptive, never *pre*scriptive, any transcription will, of course, vary according to the actual pronunciation. See Shriberg and Kent (1995) for a thorough discussion of the various ways diphthongs have been transcribed.

[eᴵ] a **nonphonemic diphthong**

It is nonphonemic in the sense that the meaning would *not* change if in a particular word the vowel was to be pronounced as a monophthong [e] or as a diphthong [eᴵ]. Words pronounced [beᴵk] or [bek], for example, would be recognized as the same word.

[oᵁ] a nonphonemic diphthong.

[aᴵ] a **phonemic diphthong**

It is phonemic in the sense that the meaning *would* change if in a particular word the vowel was produced as a monophthong or as a diphthong. A realization of [a] instead of [aᴵ] will change the meaning in General American English as the words *sod* [sad] versus *sighed* [saᴵd] demonstrate.

[ɔᴵ] a phonemic diphthong

The opposition [dʒɔ], *jaw*, versus [dʒɔᴵ], *joy*, exemplifies its phonemic value as a meaning-differentiating sound feature of English.

[aᵁ] a phonemic diphthong

Oppositions such as [mas], *moss*, versus [maᵁs], *mouse*, exemplify its phonemic value.

CLINICAL APPLICATION

Analyzing the Vowel System of a Child

Occasionally, the vowel system of a client may be restricted or show deviant patterns. In this case, a more in-depth analysis of the vowels produced may be necessary. Vowel systems can be analyzed using the vowel quadrilateral and knowledge of the diphthongs as guiding principles. Front, back, and central vowels as well as diphthongs can be checked in relationship to their accuracy and their occurrence in the appropriate contexts. George, age 5;3, is an example of a child with a deviant vowel system.

George was being seen in the clinic for his phonological disorder. He was a gregarious child who loved to talk and would try to engage anyone who would listen in conversation. The only problem was that George was almost unintelligible. This made dialogue difficult, possibly more so for those who would patiently and diligently try to understand his continuing attempts to interact.

In addition to his many consonant problems, the following vowel deviations were noted:

VOWEL ERRORS

Norm Production	→	Actual Production	Word Examples	Transcriptions
[eɪ]	→	[ɛ]	grapes	[greɪps] → [dɛ]
			table	[teɪbl] → [tɛboʊ]
[i]	→	[ɪ]	feet	[fit] → [fɪ]
			teeth	[tiθ] → [tɪ]
			three	[θri] → [dɪ]
[ɛ]	→	[æ]	bed	[bɛd] → [bæt]
			feather	[fɛðɚ] → [fævə]
[u]	→	[u]	shoe	[ʃu] → [tu]
			spoon	[spun] → [mun]
[ʊ]	→	[ʊ]	book	[bʊk] → [bʊ]
[oʊ]	→	[oʊ]	stove	[stoʊv] → [doʊ]
			nose	[noʊz] → [noʊ]
[ɑ]	→	[ɑ]	car	[kɑɚ] → [dɑ]
			blocks	[blɑks] → [bɑ]

George's productions of the back vowels [u], [ʊ], [oʊ], and [ɑ] are on target. The front vowels do show a deviant pattern, however. Not only is the diphthong [eɪ] produced as a monophthong, but also the articulatory position of the vowel substitution is realized lower than [e], as [ɛ]. This tendency to lower vowels is also noted in the other productions with front vowels, where [i] becomes [ɪ] and [ɛ] becomes [æ].

American English Consonants

Four phonetic categories are used to transcribe consonants: (1) organ of articulation, (2) place of articulation, (3) manner of articulation, and (4) voicing features. Most textbooks state that only place, manner, and voicing are used to characterize individual consonants (Edwards, 1997; Lowe, 1994; Shriberg and Kent, 1995). However, they nevertheless often include the organ of articulation. For example, the general term *lingual* as in *lingua-dental* or *lingua-palatal*, is used to designate a consonant in which the tongue is the active organ of articulation. When contrasting the lingua-dental sounds [θ] and [ð] with the lingua-palatal sounds [ʃ] and [ʒ], it becomes clear that different portions of the tongue are actively involved in the articulation. The term *lingual* does not specify these differences. This text emphasizes the detailed knowledge of production features for specific therapy goals. By adding a category specifically designating the active articulator, the organ of articulation, valuable clarification of consonant articulation is achieved.

TABLE 2.3 Phonetic Description: Organ of Articulation

ORGAN OF ARTICULATION	PHONETIC DESCRIPTOR	EXAMPLES
lower lip	labial	[p], [b], [m], [f], [v], [w], [ʍ]
tip of tongue	apical	[s], [z], [θ], [ð], [ɾ],[1] [l]
lateral rims of tongue[2]	coronal	[t], [d], [n], [ʃ], [ʒ]
surface of tongue	dorsum	
anterior portion	predorsal	[s], [z]
central portion	mediodorsal	[j], [r]
posterior portion	postdorsal	[k], [g], [ŋ]

1. The phonetic transcription [ɾ] denotes the retroflexed r-sound, while the [r] represents the bunched r-production.

2. The term *coronal* designates the apex and the lateral rims of the tongue. While the term *blade* of the tongue also includes its apex, it characterizes an extension into predorsal areas as well. In order to delineate the action of the organ of articulation as closely as possible, the terms *coronal* and *predorsal* will be used instead of *blade*.

Organ of Articulation. Consonants are sounds characterized by a partial or total obstruction by articulators impeding the expiratory airstream. There are active and passive articulators. Active articulators, the so-called **organs of articulation**, are the parts within the vocal tract that actually move to achieve the articulatory result (Crystal, 1987). In describing the consonants of General American English, we are referring specifically to the movements of the lower lip and portions of the tongue. The structures actively involved in the articulation of the consonants of General American English and the resulting phonetic descriptors are contained in Table 2.3. Figure 2.3 displays the divisions of the tongue.

Place of Articulation. The **place of articulation** denotes the area within the vocal tract that remains motionless during consonant articulation, that is, the passive articulator; it is the part that the organ of articulation, or active articulator, approaches or contacts directly (Crystal, 1987). The upper lip and teeth, the palate, and the velum are the main places of articulation when describing the

consonants of General American English. The passive structures of articulation and their resulting phonetic descriptors are contained in Table 2.4. Figure 2.4 displays the structures of the oral cavity as organs and places of articulation.

Manner of Articulation. The **manner of articulation** refers to the type of constriction

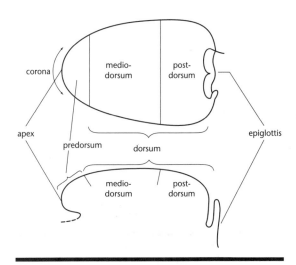

FIGURE 2.3 Divisions of the Tongue

TABLE 2.4 Phonetic Description: Place of Articulation

PLACE OF ARTICULATION	PHONETIC DESCRIPTOR	EXAMPLES
upper lip	labial	[p], [b], [m], [w], [ʍ]
upper teeth	dental	[f], [v], [θ], [ð]
alveolar ridge	alveolar	[t], [d], [n], [s], [z], [l]
surface of hard palate	palatal	
anterior portion	prepalatal	[ʃ], [ʒ],[1] [ɾ]
central portion	mediopalatal	[j], [r]
posterior portion	postpalatal	(does not normally occur in General American English)
soft palate	velar	[k], [g], [ŋ]

1. [ʃ] and [ʒ] are also referred to as postalveolar sounds, indicating a place of articulation just posterior to the highest point of the alveolar ridge. This text will include both of these places of articulation to describe [ʃ] and [ʒ].

the organ and place of articulation produce for the realization of a particular consonant. There are various manners of articulation, ranging from complete closure for the production of stop-plosives to a very limited constriction of the vocal tract for the production of glides. The following manners of articulation are used to account phonetically for the consonants of General American English.

Stop-Plosives. During the production of stop-plosives, complete occlusion is secured at specific points in the vocal tract. Simultaneously, the velum is raised so that no air can escape through the nose. The expiratory air pressure builds up naturally behind this closure (stop); compression results, which is then suddenly released (plosive). Examples of stop-plosives are [p] and [b].

Fricatives. Fricatives result when organ and place of articulation approximate each other so closely that the escaping expiratory airstream causes an audible friction. As with the stops, the velum is raised for all fricative sounds. Two examples of fricatives are [f] and [v]. Some fricatives, referred to as **sibilants,** have a sharper sound than others due to the presence of high-frequency components. In General American English [s], [z], [ʃ], and [ʒ] belong to the fricative subclass of sibilants.

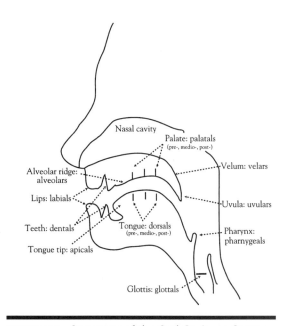

FIGURE 2.4 Structures of the Oral Cavity as Organs and Places of Articulation

Stop-plosives are sometimes referred to as stops and sometimes as plosives, depending on the phase of production one wants to draw attention to. Such a division appears at first glance rather academic. There are situations, however, when this distinction becomes important. For example, a client has difficulties realizing a complete occlusion of the lips. This can occur in cases of paralysis of the facial nerve, such as in myasthenia gravis (Thiele, 1980). Such a client has trouble with the stop portion of the production. Other clients, for example children with developmental verbal dyspraxia, have difficulties with rapid movement patterns of speech. These children can realize the static articulatory postures of the occlusion, but they cannot necessarily release it suddenly enough (Velleman and Strand, 1994). They therefore have problems with the plosive phase of the realization and need to be treated quite differently.

Nasals. These consonants are produced with the velum lowered so that the air can pass freely through the nasal cavity. However, there is complete occlusion within the oral cavity between organ and place of articulation. Because of this closure and the ensuing lack of any air passage through the oral cavity, these sounds have sometimes been called oral stops (Heffner, 1975). [m], [n], and [ŋ] are the nasal speech sounds of General American English.

Affricates. In affricates, a complete closure is formed between organ and place of articulation while, at the same time, the velum is raised. As a consequence of these articulatory conditions, expiratory air pressure builds up behind the blockage formed by the organ and place of articulation which is then slowly (in comparison to the plosives) released orally, resulting in the friction portion of the speech sound. Affricates should not be viewed as a stop plus fricative combination similar to con-

sonant blends or clusters, such as [ks], in which the stop portion is formed by a different organ and at a different place of articulation than the fricative portion. Rather, affricates are single uniform speech sounds characterized by a slow release of a stopping phase into a homorganic (*hom* = same) friction element. The two most prominent affricates of General American English are [tʃ] and [dʒ].

Glides. For the realization of glides, the constriction between organ and place of articulation is not as narrow as for fricatives. In addition to this relatively wide articulatory posture, glides are also characterized by a gliding movement of the articulators from a relatively constricted into a more open position. The sounds [w] and [j] are considered glides.

Laterals. These sounds are established by a midline closure but lateral openings within the oral cavity. Consequently, the expiratory airstream can pass only around one or both sides of the tongue. [l] is the only lateral consonant of General American English. The laterals together with the rhotics are collectively referred to as liquids.

Rhotics. The rhotics' phonetic characteristics are especially difficult to describe. First, there

According to the symbols used by the International Phonetic Association (IPA), the two types of rhotics, bunched versus retroflexed, are transcribed in a different manner. The bunched "r" is officially transcribed as [ɹ], an upside down r, while the retroflexed is characterized by [ɻ], an r with a retroflexed diacritic. The [r] symbol is reserved for the dental trilled "r" sound. Because trilled "r" sounds do not exist in General American English, and in order not to complicate matters unnecessarily, it is customary to use the [r] symbol for both the bunched and the retroflexed "r" sounds.

are at least two types of rhotic productions: *retroflexed* and *bunched* (Shriberg and Kent, 1995). Second, the actual forming of rhotics is highly context dependent. Thus, the production easily changes depending on the features of the surrounding sounds (Kantner and West, 1960). In addition, the positioning of the tongue is for individual speakers highly variable (Shriberg and Kent, 1995). Generally, the *retroflexed* rhotics are produced with the tongue tip in a retroflexed position (*retro* = back, *flex* = turn). The bunched rhotics, on the other hand, show an elevation of the whole corpus of the tongue toward the palate. Table 2.5 contains the various manners of articulation with examples of the consonants of General American English.

Voicing.   **Voicing** is the term used to denote the presence or absence of simultaneous vibra-

tion of the vocal cords resulting in voiced or voiceless consonants. The voiced and voiceless consonants of General American English are summarized in Table 2.6.

Far more precision may often be necessary to describe how specific consonants are produced. However, this framework of organ of articulation, place of articulation, manner of articulation and voicing provides a fairly accurate description of General American English consonants.

CLINICAL APPLICATION

When Organ, Place, Manner, and Voicing Are Not Enough

In analyzing the articulatory requisites for the realization of [ʃ], we find that it can be described—according to articulatory organ, place, manner, and voicing—as

TABLE 2.5   Phonetic Description: Manner of Articulation

MANNER OF ARTICULATION	PHONETIC DESCRIPTOR	EXAMPLES
Complete blockage	Stop-plosive	[p], [b], [t], [d], [k], [g]
Partial blockage	Fricative	[f], [v], [s], [z], [ʃ], [ʒ], [θ], [ð]
Nasal emission	Nasal	[m], [n], [ŋ]
Release of stop portion to a homorganic fricative portion	Affricate	[tʃ], [dʒ]
Gliding motion from a more closed to a more open position	Glide	[w], [ʍ], [j]
Lateral airflow	Lateral	[l]
Retroflex blade or bunched dorsum	Rhotic	[r], [ɻ]

TABLE 2.6   Phonetic Description: Voicing

VOICING	PHONETIC DESCRIPTOR	EXAMPLES
With vocal fold vibration	Voiced	[b], [d], [g], [m], [n], [ŋ], [v], [z], [ʒ], [ð], [w], [j], [l], [r], [ɻ]
Without vocal fold vibration	Voiceless	[p], [t], [k], [f], [s], [ʃ], [θ], [ʍ], [h]

a coronal-prepalatal fricative that is voiceless. Although that is a generally satisfactory phonetic description, another production characteristic is lip rounding. Describing such an additional feature becomes necessary because some children with "sh" problems do not realize the rounding. In fact, the resulting aberrant production may be due entirely to the absence of this lip-rounding feature.

The following phonetic descriptions classify the consonants of General American English according to the parameters of voicing, organ, place, and manner.[1]

[p] voiceless bilabial stop-plosive
(Because both organ and place of articulation are the lower and upper lips, respectively, one should actually say labio-labial. However, the term *bilabial* is usually preferred.)

[b] voiced bilabial stop-plosive

[t] voiceless coronal-alveolar stop-plosive

[d] voiced coronal-alveolar stop-plosive

[k] voiceless postdorsal-velar stop-plosive

[g] voiced postdorsal-velar stop-plosive

[f] voiceless labio-dental fricative

[v] voiced labio-dental fricative

[s] voiceless apico-alveolar or predorsal-alveolar fricative
[s] (and [z]) can be produced in one of two ways: with the tongue tip up (i.e., as apico-alveolar fricative [sibilant]) or with the tongue tip resting behind the lower incisors (i.e., predorsal-alveolar fricative [sibilant]).

[z] voiced apico-alveolar or predorsal-alveolar fricative

[ʃ] voiceless coronal-prepalatal or coronal-postalveolar fricative with lip rounding

[ʒ] voiced coronal-prepalatal or coronal-postalveolar fricative with lip rounding

[θ] voiceless apico-dental or interdental fricative
The [θ] and [ð] are typically produced with either the tongue tip resting behind the upper incisors (i.e., apico-dental) or with the tongue tip between the upper and lower incisors (i.e., interdental).

[ð] voiced apico-dental or interdental fricative

[m] voiced bilabial nasal

[n] voiced coronal-alveolar nasal

[ŋ] voiced postdorsal-velar nasal

[w] voiced bilabial glide with high-back tongue position

[ʍ] voiceless bilabial glide with high-back tongue position

[j] voiced mediodorsal-mediopalatal glide

[l] voiced apico-alveolar lateral

[r] voiced mediodorsal-mediopalatal rhotic (bunched)

[ɹ] voiced apico-prepalatal rhotic (retroflexed)
Here, the term *apico* refers to the underside of the apex of the tongue.

[h] voiceless unlocalized open consonant that is, an aspirate
Although this sound is sometimes classified as a laryngeal fricative, in General American English, there is normally no constriction at the laryngeal, pharyngeal, or oral levels. See Heffner (1975) for a discussion of the [h] production in General American English.

[tʃ] voiceless coronal-alveolar affricate

[dʒ] voiced coronal-alveolar affricate

---

1. The organ, place, manner, and voicing features are based on the phonetic descriptions provided by Bronstein (1960) and Kantner and West (1960). These features are seen as descriptive and may, therefore, vary somewhat from speaker to speaker.

CLINICAL APPLICATION

Rhotic Errors versus Central Vowels
with R-Coloring

Children with "r" problems, thus, rhotic consonant difficulties, often produce the central vowels with r-coloring ([ɝ] and [ɚ]) in error as well. However, that is not always the case. Note the following patterns seen in Latoria's speech from the Word Articulation Subtest of the Test of Language Development, Primary, Second edition. (Newcomer and Hammill, 1988).

Norm Production	→	Actual Production	Word Example	Transcriptions
Rhotics				
[tr]	→	[tw]	tree	[tri] → [twi]
[br]	→	[bw]	bridge	[brɪʤ] → [bwɪʒ]
[r]	→	[w]	ring	[rɪŋ] → [wɪŋ]
[br]	→	[bw]	zebra	[zibrə] → [zibwə]
[r]	→	[w]	garage	[gəraʒ] → [ʤəwa]
[θr]	→	[θw]	thread	[θrɛd] → [θwɛd]
[tr]	→	[tw]	treasure	[trɛʒɚ] → [twɛʒɚ]
Central Vowels with R-Coloring				
[ɚ]	→	[ɚ]	feather	[fɛðɚ] → [fɛdɚ]
[ɚ]	→	[ɚ]	soldier	[soʊldʒɚ] → [soʊʒɚ]
[ɚz]	→	[ɚz]	scissors	[sɪzɚz] → [sɪzɚz]
[ɝ]	→	[ɝ]	birthday	[bɝθdeɪ] → [bɝdeɪ]

On the one hand, Latoria has a [w] for [r] substitution ([r] → [w]) for the rhotic consonant [r]. On the other, she can produce the central vowels with r-coloring accurately.

SOUNDS IN CONTEXT: COARTICULATION AND ASSIMILATION

Up until now, this textbook has discussed articulatory characteristics of General American English speech sounds as discrete units. The articulators do not move from sound to sound in a series of separate steps, however. Speech consists of highly variable and overlapping motor movements. Sounds within a given phonetic context influence one another. For example, if the [s] production in *see* is contrasted to the one in *Sue*, it can be seen that [s] in *see* is produced with some spreading of the lips, whereas there is lip rounding in *Sue*. This difference is due to the influence of the following vowel articulations: [i], a vowel with lip spreading, facilitates this feature in the [s] production in *see*, whereas the lip rounding of [u] influences the production of [s] in *Sue*. These types of modifications are grouped together under the term *coarticulation*. **Coarticulation** describes the concept that the articulators are continually moving into position for other segments over a stretch of speech (Fletcher, 1992). The result of coarticulation is referred to as assimilation. The term **assimilation** refers to adaptive articulatory changes by which one speech sound becomes similar, sometimes identical, to a neighboring sound segment. Such a change may affect one, several, or all of a sound's phonetic constituents, that is, a sound may change its organ, place, manner, and/or voicing properties under the articulatory influence of another sound. Assimilation processes are perfectly natural consequences of normal speech production and by no means are restricted to developing speech in young children. Because the two segments become more alike, assimilatory processes are also referred to as *harmony processes*.

There are different *types* and *degrees* of assimilatory processes. In regard to the different types of assimilatory processes, the following should be noted:

1. Assimilatory processes modifying directly adjacent sounds are called *contact* (or *contiguous*) *assimilations*. If at least one other segment separates the sounds in question, especially when the two sounds are in two different syllables, one speaks of *remote* (or *noncontiguous*) *assimilation* (Heffner, 1975).

The following assimilation processes were noted in the results of children's articulation tests:

Contact

"jumping" [ʤʌmpɪn] → [ʤʌmbɪn]

The voiced [m] impacts the normally voiceless [p].

"skunk" [skʌŋk] → [stʌŋk]

The organ and place of articulation for [s] influences the stop-plosive, changing it from a postdorsal-velar to a coronal-alveolar.

Remote

"yellow" [jɛloᵘ] → [lɛloᵘ]

Organ, place, and manner of articulation are impacted when the [j] at the beginning of the word becomes identical to the following [l].

"telephone" [tɛləfoᵘn] → [tɛdəfoᵘn]

Manner of articulation is impacted when the [l] is changed from a lateral to a stop-plosive, similar to the [t] at the beginning of the word.

2. Assimilations can be either *progressive* or *regressive*. In progressive assimilation, a sound segment influences a following sound. This is also referred to as *perseverative assimilation* (Crystal, 1987; Ladefoged, 1993). The previously noted contact assimilations for *jumping* and *skunk* and the remote assimilation for *telephone* are examples of progressive assimilation. A previously articulated sound influenced a following sound.

In regressive assimilation, a sound segment influences a preceding sound. If "is she" [ɪz ʃi] is pronounced [ɪʒ ʃi], changing [s] into [ʒ], regressive assimilation was at work. Regressive assimilations are also known as *anticipatory* assimilations (Crystal, 1987; Ladefoged, 1993).

The following are examples of progressive and regressive assimilation processes:

Progressive

"ice cream" [aɪskrim] → [aɪstrim]

Organ and place of articulation for [s] influence the following stop-plosive, changing it from a postdorsal-velar to a coronal-alveolar stop-plosive production: This is progressive contact assimilation.

"television" [tɛləvɪʒən] → [tɛdəvɪʒən]

Manner of articulation is impacted when the stop-plosive [t] impacts the following [l], changing it from a lateral to a stop-plosive: this is progressive remote assimilation.

Regressive

"pumpkin" [pʌmkɪn] → [pʌŋkɪn]

Organ and place of articulation of [k] influence [m], which is changed from the bilabial to the postdorsal-velar nasal [ŋ]: this is regressive contact assimilation.

"bathtub" [bæ<u>θ</u>tʌb] → [<u>θ</u>æ<u>θ</u>tʌb]

Organ, place, and manner of articulation are impacted as [θ] influences the previous segment [b]: this is regressive remote assimilation.

In regard to the different degrees of assimilatory influence, one distinguishes between *total* (or *complete*) and *partial assimilatory processes* (Heffner, 1975). If a sound is forced by another sound to change all of its phonetic properties (organ, place, and manner) into the sound category of the influencing sound, this is referred to as *total* or *complete assimilation*. Total assimilation is also termed *coalescence* when the features from two adjacent sounds are combined so that one sound replaces two other sounds (Bankson and Bernthal, 1998). If, on the other hand, only parts of the phonetic characteristics become modified, resulting in a higher degree of similarity between the respective sounds, we refer to *partial assimilation*. An example of partial (re-

gressive) assimilation would be the realization of *sandwich* [sænwɪtʃ] as [sæmwɪtʃ]. The bilabial organ and place of articulation for [w] have regressively impacted the organ and place of articulation of the original coronal-alveolar nasal, which now becomes a bilabial nasal [m].

The following are examples of total and partial assimilation processes:

Total   "window"   [wɪndoʊ] → [wɪnoʊ]
         "Pontiac"   [pɑntiæk] → [pɑniæk]
Partial "Christmas" [krɪsməs] → [krɪsnəs]

Children at different stages of their speech-language development tend to utilize assimilation processes in systematic ways.

> Typical assimilation processes and the ages at which these processes occur in children are discussed in Chapter 5.

This is of obvious interest to clinicians whose task it is to separate normal from impaired phonological development.

CLINICAL APPLICATION

Assimilation Processes and Articulation Testing

Assimilatory or harmony processes often occur during an articulation test. It is important to recognize these processes so that the test scoring will not be negatively impacted. The following assimilation processes have been frequently observed by the author:

Word	Expected Response	Child's Response	Impact on Scoring
Santa	[sæntə]	[sænə] total assimilation	Could be scored as an omission of [t]
sandwich	[sænwɪtʃ]	[sæmɪtʃ] total assimilation (coalescence)	Could be scored as an omission of [w] and an [m]/[n] substitution
window	[wɪndoʊ]	[wɪnoʊ] total assimilation	Could be scored as an omission of [d]

A less common example was observed for Danny, age 4;3:

Word	Expected Response	Child's Response	Impact on Scoring
bath	[bæθ]	[θæθ]	[θ]/[b] substitution
bathtub	[bæθtʌb]	[θæθtʌb]	[θ]/[b] substitution

However, Danny could produce [b] correctly in all other contexts. Note the correct production of [b] at the end of *bathtub*. This was an example of a regressive remote assimilation.

SYLLABLE STRUCTURE

If we are asked to break words down into component parts, syllables seem to be more natural than sounds. For example, speakers of unwritten languages will characteristically use syllable, not sound, divisions. They may even resist the notion that any further breakdown is possible (Ladefoged, 1993). Also, preschool children use syllabification if they try to analyze a word. It is only after children are exposed to letters and writing that they begin to understand the possibility of dividing words into sounds. Thus, syllables appear to be easily recognizable units.

Counting the number of syllables in a word is a relatively simple task. Probably all will agree on the number of syllables in the words *away* or *articulation*, for example. What we might disagree on are the beginning and end points of the syllables in question. To arrive at a consensus, it is first necessary to differentiate between written and spoken syllables.

If one consults a dictionary, written syllabification rules are found. We learn that the word *cutting* is to be divided between the two *t*s. However, differences may, and often do, exist between written and spoken syllables. The written syllabification rules for *cutting* do not reflect the way we would syllabify the words when speaking. The divisions [kʌ tɪŋ] would be more probable during normal speech. An awareness of existing differences between spoken and written syllable boundaries is important for speech-language specialists.

This is especially critical because a dictionary of rules for the boundaries of *spoken* syllables does not exist. Thus, two competent speakers of a given language may syllabify the same word in different ways. Words such as *hammer* and *window* would probably not cause problems. However, how should one syllabify *telephone,* as [tɛ lə foʊn] or as [tɛl ə foʊn]? That is, does [l] belong to the second or to the first syllable? Variations in the syllabification of spoken words do indeed exist between speakers.

Structurally, the syllable can be divided into three parts: *peak, onset,* and *coda* (Sloat, Taylor, and Hoard, 1978). The **peak** is the most prominent, acoustically most intense part of the syllable. A peak may stand alone, as in the first syllable of the word *a-way,* or it can be surrounded by other sounds, as in *tan* or *bring.* Although vowels are clearly more prevalent as syllable peaks, consonants are not strictly excluded. Consonants that serve as the syllable peak are referred to as *syllabics.*

The **onset** of a syllable consists of all the segments prior to the peak, while the **coda** comprises all the sound segments of a syllable following its peak. The segments that compose the onset are also termed *syllable releasing* sounds, while those that compose the coda are termed *syllable arresting* sounds. Thus, the onset of *meet* [mit] is [m], that is, [m] is the syllable releasing sound. The coda, or syllable arresting sound, of *meet* is [t]. This applies also to consonant blends within one syllable. The onset of *scratched* is [skr], its peak is [æ], and the coda [tʃt]. Not all syllables have onsets or codas. Both syllables of *today* [tu deɪ] lack a coda, while *off* [ɑf] does not have an onset. The number of segments that an onset or a coda may contain is regulated by rules of the language in question. General American English syllables can have one to three segments in an onset (ray, stay, stray) and one to four segments in a coda (sit, sits, searched, sixths).

Syllables that do not contain codas are called **open** or **unchecked syllables.** Examples of open, unchecked syllables are *do* [du], *glee* [gli], or the first syllable of *rebound* [ri baʊnd]. Syllables that do have codas are called **closed** or **checked syllables,** such as in "stop" [stɑp] or the first syllable in "window" [wɪn].

The use of specific syllable structures is often neglected when analyzing the speech characteristics of children. However, they do seem to play an important developmental role. A child's first words consist typically of open or unchecked syllables, such as [bɑ] for *ball* or [mɪ] for *milk*. If children start to produce closed syllables, they usually contain only single-segment codas. Similarly, two-syllable words at this stage of development consist usually of open syllables (e.g., Ingram, 1976; Menn, 1971; Velten, 1943; Vihman, Ferguson, and Elbert, 1986). Productions such as [beˈbi] for *baby* or [ti pɑ] for *teapot* are examples.

Syllable Structure: Clinical Implications

The syllable is also an important unit when assessing and treating children with articulatory or phonological disorders. Sometimes, the syllable unit can give us a more accurate picture of the child's articulatory capabilities than can individual sound productions. The ease of syllable production can be affected by at least three circumstances: (1) the *number of syllables* an utterance contains, (2) the *type of syllable* (open versus closed), and (3) the *degree of syllable stress* (stressed or unstressed) (Fleming, 1971; Kent, 1982). Generally, fewer syllables, open syllables, and stressed syllables usually facilitate accurate productions of specific target sounds.

The designs of most articulation tests document a striking lack of attention to these variables. Most assessment instruments focus on the beginning-initial, the middle-medial, and the end-final sound positions within words. At first glance, it may seem as if initial could be related to the syllable onset, medial to syllable peak, and final to syllable coda. This may work somewhat adequately as long as only one-syllable words are considered. However, as soon as the test items become multisyllabic, as is often the case, difficulties arise with this procedure. What is the medial

sound position within a word? Assume that the word *window* is used in an articulation test to assess the production of the word-medial [d] sound. The same test uses the word *bathtub* to test the word-medial [θ] and [t] sounds. [m], again labelled medial, is tested by the elicitation of the words *Christmas tree*. From these examples, it appears that *medial* indicates anything between the beginning and the end of an utterance.

Is there any comparability between these "medial" positions? Let's examine the syllable structures of these three words:

"window" [wɪn-doᵘ]

1st syllable	stressed	onset-peak-coda
2nd syllable	unstressed	onset-peak

"bathtub" [bæθ-tʌb]

1st syllable	stressed	onset-peak-coda
2nd syllable	unstressed	onset-peak-coda

"Christmas tree" [krɪs-məs-tri]

1st syllable	stressed	onset-peak-coda
2nd syllable	unstressed	onset-peak-coda
3rd syllable	unstressed	onset-peak

As one can see, the "medial" sound [d] in *window* is actually the onset of an unstressed, open syllable. The preceding syllable ends with a coda, thus, two consonants (i.e., [n] + [d]) must be produced in immediate succession. The "medial" [θ] tested in *bathtub* poses a different problem. It represents the coda of a stressed syllable. Again, there is the complication of two consonants in sequence, [θ] and [t]. The word-medial [t] now appears as a syllable onset in a closed syllable, which varies from the *window* example, in which the medial sound occurred in an open syllable. The third example of "medial" [m] in *Christmas tree* exemplifies a quite different articulatory situation again. Here, a three-syllable phrase is elicited in which the "medial" [m] is actually an onset of an unstressed closed syllable. Oddly enough, this same test instrument evaluates the consonant blend [tr] in *Christmas tree* as an "initial" production. According to the original definition of *medial*, indicating all segments between the beginning and end of an utterance, this [tr] should also be classified as medial. In order for [tr] to be classified as initial, the child would have to pause between *Christmas* and *tree*, a highly unlikely occurrence.

An analysis of such an articulation test according to the syllable structure rather than the word unit would eliminate these problems. If onset, peak, and coda for each syllable are examined, the results also become more accurate and, therefore, clinically more valid. Accuracy of any assessment process is the key to successful treatment. The information attained from examining sound articulation with the syllable as a basic structural unit complement the word-based results and give additional insight into the child's true articulatory abilities.

SUMMARY

This chapter presented an overview of the form and function of vowels and consonants of General American English. Both vowels and consonants were classified according to their articulatory production features and their linguistic functions. Phonetic descriptors were given to provide the clinician with a detailed account of articulatory action during norm production of vowels and consonants. These features can later be contrasted to those noted in the impaired sound realizations of children and adults with articulatory-phonological impairments.

In the second portion of this chapter, coarticulation, assimilation processes, and syllable structure were defined and examined. Coarticulation and resulting assimilatory processes were described as normal articulatory consequences that regularly occur in the speech of individuals. Assimilatory processes were defined according to the type and degree of sound modification. Examples were given of assimilatory processes in children as well as of the possible impact these processes could have on articulation test results. The last section, on syllable structure, defined the parts of the syllable. Variations in syllable structure do not seem to be accounted for when testing individual sounds within most articulation tests. However, this may be a factor that could affect the articulatory proficiency of children and adults with impaired speech. An analysis of syllable structures would provide the clinician with additional knowledge when evaluating individuals with articulatory-phonological disorders.

CHAPTER 3

PHONETIC TRANSCRIPTION
AND DIACRITICS

CHAPTER OUTLINE

- Phonetic Transcription as a Notational System
- Why Use Phonetic Transcription?

- Diacritics
- Clinical Implications
- Summary

Virtually every book on articulatory-phonological disorders contains a brief discussion of phonetic transcription. In such a section, the symbols and diacritics of the International Phonetic Alphabet are listed together with a comment on the importance of accurate transcription for the assessment procedure. This underplays its importance, however; accurate transcription forms *the* basis for the diagnosis of articulatory-phonological impairments. If clinicians cannot correctly identify and transcribe the productions of their clients, their therapy will not be as goal directed as it should be.

Nevertheless, in training and in clinical practice, phonetic transcription seems to be one of the most neglected areas of study. Although transcription skills are as indispensable as they are difficult to master, the chance to learn them is often limited to one undergraduate course. This meager knowledge base is seldom systematically expanded or revisited in other courses or in most clinical experiences. Many practicing clinicians simply do not feel comfortable with phonetic transcription and therefore, unfortunately, use it as infrequently as possible.

Phonetic transcription involves not just transposing perceived sounds into "strange" symbols, it is above all a process of fine-tuning the auditory perception for the purpose of successful clinical intervention. Perceptual skills improve with methodical efforts to listen carefully to, and to differentiate accurately between, subtle changes in sound quality. Although this is not a workbook on phonetic transcription (this section does not offer nearly enough information for such a course), phonetic transcription will be emphasized and treated in considerably more detail than is usually the case in textbooks on articulatory-phonological disorders.

The first goal of this chapter is to introduce the International Phonetic Alphabet as the notational system used to document norm productions of vowels and consonants of General American English. However, the transcription of disordered speech requires more than that. It needs additional signs, diacritical marks, which can be added to basic transcription symbols to indicate aberrant sound values. They provide a means of documenting irregular articulatory events. Therefore, this chapter's second goal is to present and discuss some of the most common diacritical markers. This presentation includes clinical comments exemplifying the use of these diacritics. The third goal of this chapter is to consider the clinical implications of phonetic transcription, including the use of diacritics. Examples are provided to demonstrate how phonetic transcription can be used in the assessment process. Familiarity with, and the proper use of, phonetic transcription is seen as an invaluable tool for the diagnosis and treatment of articulatory-phonological impairments.

PHONETIC TRANSCRIPTION AS A NOTATIONAL SYSTEM

Speech is a fleeting event, existing for only the shortest period of time. So short, in fact, that if we don't employ artificial means to preserve speech, we couldn't prove that it had ever existed, even immediately after the event. Historically, all writing systems were invented to make speech events last longer, to preserve them.

Traditional writing systems do a great job in preserving *what* has been said, but they fall grossly short in indicating *how* it has been said, even though this can be just as important. Take a linguist, for example, who wants to describe and preserve for others how the San people produce some speech sounds totally unfamiliar to us, say, klicks. Which letters or letter combinations of our traditional writing system should the linguist use to make the reader understand the phonetic nature of such sounds? There are none available to do the job. Or, take a speech pathologist who needs to document the details of a child's aberrant sound realization. There are no letters in our alphabet for lateral s-sounds, for instance. In both cases, the professionals clearly need more information about *how* a specific speech event has been executed than

about *what* has been said. In fact, what has been said doesn't help their tasks at all. For these special purposes, all traditional writing systems are useless. Special ones had to be invented to serve these needs. *Phonetic transcription* systems were devised in order to document real actualizations of speech events.

Over a period of several hundred years, countless transcription systems have been created for different purposes. They can be divided into two groups: *alphabetical* and *analphabetical* systems (Abercrombie, 1967). Alphabetical transcription systems are, as a rule, monotypic, that is, there exists a one-to-one relationship between a speech sound produced and a transcription symbol indicating it. That makes them relatively user-friendly, but they seldom reach a very high level of accuracy in the representation of sound components. That can be handled much better by analphabetical systems. Analphabetical notation systems provide descriptive labels for a segment in abbreviated form. They are like chemical formulas signifying all elements of the actual sound production with various types of letters and numbers. Such a description might take a dozen or more different markers to characterize the realization of just a single sound. Analphabetic transcription systems are polytypic, that is, one phoneme realization can have several symbols. They can thus be very exact in representing actual speech. But they are bothersome to use. For this reason, alphabetical transcription systems are favored for clinical purposes.

There have been and still are numerous alphabetical transcription systems in use. These include Wilkins (1668), Bell (1867), Sweet (1890), Copenhagen Conference (1925), Jakobson, Fant, and Halle (1951), Chomsky and Halle (1968) and, of course, the International Phonetic Alphabet (IPA), to name just a few. The IPA originated with Paul Passy, a French language teacher, in 1886.

One analphabetic system was devised by Jespersen (1889). The following was the notation for the vowel that is typically produced in *all.*

$$α7^bβgγ7_kδ0εl$$

Each Greek letter referred to an active organ of articulation, while the numbers and letters following the Greek letters indicated the posture and activity of the articulators during the production.

Pike (1943) worked out an even more complex analphabetical system when attempting to describe sounds based on the mechanics of their production. In his system, a vowel was described using a string of more than eighty characters, while a consonant required many more.

Today, the frequently revised IPA is probably the most widely accepted transcription system in the world. In a way, the IPA system is a compromise between alphabetic and analphabetic systems. There is a one-to-one correspondence between phoneme realizations and sound symbols; however, at the same time, many additional signs can be used to identify modifications in the original production. Generally, the IPA serves the professional interests of speech-language pathologists well. Its symbols capture much of what we are interested in. Occasionally, one may be forced to add to the inventory of available symbols in order to characterize an aberrant production. That, though, is to be expected, because phonetic transcription systems are typically designed to transfer standard (but highly impermanent) speech events adequately into (more durable) readable signs. In *aberrant* speech, just about anything can happen, and this may well necessitate additional characters for unusual articulatory events. If such an additional characterization becomes necessary, the specific phonetic value of any added sign must, of course, be described precisely and in detail. If other professionals cannot reliably "read" the transcribed materials, they cannot accurately retransform the symbols into the original phonetic events, that is, they still won't know what the child produced, how the sound was actualized. Under such circumstances, any phonetic transcription becomes pointless.

CLINICAL APPLICATION

The Necessity of Using Phonetic Transcription

Ben had just moved to town and his parents were anxious to begin speech therapy. According to his parents, Ben had just been given an articulation test by a clinician in the town where they had previously lived. The parents presented me with a copy of this articulation test. I noticed that certain words from the test had a large X through them while others were marked with a D. There was no key on the test indicating what these markers might mean. The parents did not really understand why I thought it was necessary to repeat the same articulation test—after all, I did have the results in my hand. I tried to explain in a relatively calm manner that I had no idea what the symbols that the clinician had used meant. The situation was awkward: Ben's father asked why, if we "professionals" used the same test, we didn't speak the same language. The parents finally agreed that I should repeat the test; however, it was not a good beginning. Ben's father was right, professionals should be able to interpret each other's test results. I later concluded from my test results that the X was used to describe final consonant deletions while the D characterized distortions of varying kinds and degrees. Such a system does not represent phonetic transcription.

Any phonetic transcription is a purely *descriptive* enterprise. It is nothing but the "spelling out" of an actual speech event by means of special symbols invented to represent the sounds of the utterance in question. This statement is of fundamental importance for our understanding of what phonetic transcription really is and how it can serve our task.

Occasionally, beginning transcription materials consist of lists of orthographically presented words (*book, table, snail,* and so on) that students then have to transfer into phonetic symbols. Such a practice is misleading. It supports the mistaken notion that there is a *prescriptive* part to phonetic transcription, that it provides some guiding principle about how words are supposed to be pronounced. This is also suggested by dictionaries: Each entry tells the reader how to spell a word correctly, and the following transcription indicates how the word "should be" pronounced. There is, of course, nothing wrong with spelling out how words are commonly pronounced, but any jump from how they *are* pronounced to how they *should be* pronounced has nothing to do with the idea behind, and practice of, phonetic transcription.

There is not a prescribed way to pronounce and transcribe a word that is comparable to the rules of how to spell a word in an orthographically "correct" way. Phonetic transcription is used solely *to indicate the articulatory makeup of real utterances by means of written symbols.* In other words, for a valid phonetic transcription, one always needs a spoken event, preferably realized by a person "right here and now."

In addition, a thorough phonetic transcription offers a long-lasting, verifiable document, which also provides accountability. Assessment and therapeutic accountability are without question fast-growing issues. To secure both we need, of course, to select a widely used transcription system—the IPA system, for instance.

WHY USE PHONETIC TRANSCRIPTION?

Accurate phonetic transcription is an indispensable clinical tool for speech-language pathologists. That is why it has to be taken so seriously, especially when dealing with the assessment and remediation of impaired articulation and phonology. Without a reliable record of how a child or adult realized a particular speech sound, we simply do not have enough information for goal-directed intervention. Phonetic transcription provides a reasonably accurate written record of what was said and what it sounded like.

But, one might argue, why not make a high-quality audio-recording? That should create an acceptable likeness of not only what was said but also how it sounded. Such a recording is also repeatable as well as relatively durable. Audio- (and video-) recordings are important aids in our field; however, they can never replace a reliable phonetic transcription. The main reason: Clinicians are interested in how a specific segment was *produced*—its production properties are inferred from the way the segment sounded.

There is typically a direct relationship between how a sound was generated and its audible result. If, for example, during an apical [s] production, the tip of the tongue is too near the front teeth, [s] will sound "dull." This is a direct result of the fronted tongue position. On the other hand, one cannot deduct from any "dull" [s] that it came into existence by way of a tongue tip that was placed too far forward. Other phonetic events can create quite similar acoustic effects. In the case of our "dull" [s], abnormal air pressure conditions, for example, even in the presence of perfectly "proper" tongue positioning, can cause the same kind of auditory impression. Phonetic transcription provides an initial impression of how a sound is produced (this must, however, always be verified).

In addition, certain recording conditions can create the impression of abnormal articulation. Acoustic properties of the recording room, the distance of the microphone from the speaker's mouth, and the effects of too high an input level, for example, can easily cause such impressions. Some people with considerable recording and listening experience might be able to distinguish between the audible effects of certain recording conditions and a speaker's abnormal sound realization. However, absolute certainty cannot be achieved even by these experts. Therefore, to base an assessment of an articulatory or phonological disorder only on phonetic transcriptions of taped materials is unacceptable. Taped transcriptions should only complement those formerly obtained through direct contact with the speaker. By using phonetic transcription in such a manner, we secure a reliable record of the status quo, prerequisite not only for systematic treatment but also for the purpose of documenting professional services.

Admittedly, phonetic transcription is somewhat troublesome and time-consuming. In addition, it certainly has its own problems. Some rules have to be strictly observed in order to overcome these problems. The first thing any aspiring transcriber has to understand is that the human ear is not a microphone. We are unable to *re*ceive only; we must always *per*ceive, that is, people automatically judge incoming acoustic signals based on their experience with those signals. In respect to spoken language, this means that when listening to the incoming acoustic signal, the listener unwillingly "distorts" it in the direction of former experiences, including how the listener would have produced it. This "built-in" tendency is the greatest danger to any serious transcription effort. Any higher degree of accuracy achieved while listening to, and then describing the *how* of, spoken language is very difficult to attain if perceptual biases rule transcription efforts. To overcome the tendency to "interpret" what was heard requires considerable goodwill, patience, and special training.

There are several other problems that must be considered when using phonetic transcription. For example, many circumstances can affect our transcription, such as the age of the client or an unusual vocal quality. Other factors may produce large variations in the inter- and intrajudge reliability of transcriptions, including the intelligibility of the client (Shriberg and Lof, 1991), the position of the sound in the word (Philips and Bzoch, 1969; Shriberg and Lof, 1991), and whether narrow or broad transcription is used (Shriberg and Lof, 1991). Shriberg and Kent (1995) provide an excellent overview of the sources of variation and the factors that affect the reliability of phonetic transcription. These problems are very real, and caution must be exercised when using phonetic transcription. On the other hand, we cannot simply disregard transcription because of its inherent problems or use a private system of noting sound realizations. Instead, the importance of developing good, reliable transcription skills should be stressed. They will prove to be an invaluable resource in the assessment and treatment of articulatory-phonological disorders.

> Interjudge reliability denotes the percentage of agreement between two or more people's transcriptions. Intrajudge reliability is how well a person agrees with his or her own former transcription.

DIACRITICS

Diacritics are marks added to sound transcription symbols in order to give them a particular phonetic value. The set of basic phonetic transcription symbols represents language-specific norm productions. Because speech-language pathologists deal mostly with aberrant articulatory events, it follows that diacritical markers are of special importance to the characterization of the speech of their clients. Diacritics are needed to note the clients' deviant sound qualities.

There are numerous diacritics in use today. Most of them are part of the IPA notation system. Others will have to be modified to meet our clinical needs. Still others may have to be invented to represent a special articulatory situation. The following is a list of diacritics used often. Unless otherwise noted, these diacritics are those proposed by the latest modification of the International Phonetic Alphabet (IPA, 1996). The diacritic markers and additional symbols presented in this chapter are summarized in Table 3.1, found on page 45.

Diacritics Used with Consonants

Changes in Place of Articulation for Consonants. These symbols describe deviations from normal tongue placement for consonants.

Dentalization. *Dentalization* refers to an articulatory variation in which the tongue approaches the upper incisors. It is marked by [̪] placed under the IPA symbol. For example, the symbol [d] stands for a coronal-alveolar voiced stop. A dentalized realization results when a child places the tip of the tongue not against the alveolar ridge, as the IPA symbol indicates, but against the inside of the upper incisors. A dentalized realization is transcribed as

[d̪] = dentalized [d].

[d̪] occurs quite often as the result of coarticulation. Compare [d]-productions in the words *widow* and *width*. The articulatory influence of the following [θ], an addental or even interdental sound, will probably "dentalize" normally alveolar [d] realizations. Dentalized s-sounds, [s̪] and [z̪], frequently occur in the speech of children (Van Riper, 1978; Weiss, Gordon, and Lillywhite, 1987).

Palatalization. Another modification of consonant articulation is *palatalization*. Only sounds for which the palate is not the place of articulation can be palatalized. Therefore, pal-

atalization can occur with sounds that have a place of articulation anterior or posterior to the hard palate region. If the place of articulation is the alveolar ridge or the upper incisors, palatalization occurs if the anterior portions of the tongue approach anterior parts of the palate, that is, when organ and place of the production are articulated somewhat posteriorly. For velar consonants, palatalization indicates the movement of the place and organ of articulation in the direction of the palate, to a more anterior articulation. Palatalization causes a typical change in the quality of the sound(s) in question. The diacritical mark for palatalization is a tail-like appendix added to the basic IPA symbol:

[s̡] = palatalized [s]

[t̡] = palatalized [t]

Velarization. *Velarization* refers to the posterior movement of the tongue placement (in the direction of the velum) for palatal sounds. The auditory impression of this change in place of articulation can be exemplified by the so-called dark [l], which in General American English is usually heard in word-final positions (also as a syllabic), preceding a consonant, and following back vowels (Bronstein, 1960; Carrell and Tiffany, 1960). The velarization in these cases is often so prominent that even main phonetic characteristics of [l], the articulation of the tongue tip against the alveolar ridge, are sometimes no longer present. In such a case, the velarization actually replaces the typical apicoalveolar l-articulation. The velarized production is an allophonic variation of [l]. Velarized [l]-productions are transcribed [ɫ]:

> The so-called dark and light l-sounds are discussed in more detail in Chapter 8.

[fuɫ] = velarized [l]-sound

Lateralization. [l] is the only lateral in General American English. It cannot be lateralized because it is a lateral already; only nonlateral speech sounds can be lateralized. If during any consonant production other than [l] air is released laterally, we speak of *lateralization*. Not too seldom, [s] becomes lateralized. Articulations of [s] and [z] require a highly accurate placement of frontal parts of the tongue (apical or predorsal) *approximating* the alveolar ridge. This precarious position must be maintained throughout the entire sound duration, a motorically difficult task, especially for young children. To make things motorically easier, children sometimes establish direct contact between the organ and place of articulation. Under these circumstances, the airstream cannot, of course, escape centrally any longer. In an attempt to maintain the fricative effect of [s], the child now releases the air laterally into the cheeks. The result is a conspicuous [s] variation, a lateral lisp. Lateralization is noted by the following diacritic marker from Shriberg and Kent (1995):

$$[slip] \rightarrow [\underset{\sim}{s}lip]$$

CLINICAL COMMENTS

Dentalized, palatalized, and lateralized [s] realizations are frequent distortions noted in children. In some children, the dentalized [s̪] may co-occur with a "th" for "s" substitution ([s] → [θ]), as in the following production:

"Santa Claus" [θæn tə klɑs̪] for [sæn tə klaz]

   The too-fronted tongue position of the child's [s]-productions may fluctuate slightly, so that it is perceived at times as [s̪], at other times as [θ]. It is interesting to note, however, that certain children may also use this dichotomy systematically: [θ] may be realized initiating words or syllables, while [s̪] is produced terminating words or syllables, for example. Such a possibility should be considered in our assessment.

   Differentiating between dentalized, palatalized, and lateralized [s]-productions may seem difficult at first. However, there are clear perceptual qualities that distinguish the three forms of [s] actualization. Dentalized [s]-sounds, [s̪], have a "dull" quality; they lack the sharp, high-frequency characteristic of norm [s]-productions. On the other hand, lateralized [s]-sounds, [ɬ], have a distinct noise component to them that is typically as disagreeable as it is conspicuous. Palatalized [s] variations, [s̠], approach perceptually a [ʃ] characteristic. Palatalization that is marked by the anterior portions of the tongue approaching parts of the palate results in a somewhat posterior placement of the organ and place of articulation. Comparing the production features of [s] to [ʃ], one notes that [ʃ] realizations require a more posteriorly placed organ and place of articulation (apico-alveolar [s] versus coronal-prepalatal [ʃ]).

Voice Symbols

Devoicing of Voiced Consonants.   Under normal circumstances, vowels and more than half of our consonants are voiced. If these sounds become devoiced in a speech sample, it needs to be marked. In cases of total devoicing, the IPA symbol for the voiceless counterpart of the voiced sound, its unvoiced cognate, is usually indicated:

[ʃus] for "shoes"
[brɛt] for "bread"

Partial Devoicing.   Often, however, the sound in question is only partially devoiced. The diacritic for partial devoicing is a small circle placed under the sound symbol:

[suz̥]
[brɛd̥]

If that placement interferes with the clarity of the basic symbol, it is acceptable to put the circle above the sound symbol:

[dɑg̊] instead of [dɑg]

Voicing of Voiceless Consonants.   Voiceless consonants may also be voiced, especially if they occur between two vowels. A casual pronunciation of the name Betty might serve as an example. If voiceless consonants become totally voiced, the segment is transcribed with the respective symbol:

[bɛti] → [bɛdi]

Partial Voicing. If voiceless consonants become partially voiced, the diacritical mark is a lowercase *v* under the respective sound symbol:

[bɛt̬i] for "Betty"

CLINICAL COMMENTS

Partial voicing and devoicing are difficult to discern and to transcribe correctly. The first impression of transcribers is often some minor qualitative variance—the sound is somehow "off." Such a first impression is usually a good reason to focus subsequently on the voicing–devoicing opposition. This two-step procedure makes it easier to arrive at the difficult judgment: partially voiced or partially devoiced.

Also, in General American English, there is a tendency to devoice (or partially devoice) final consonants. The following are examples from Daniel, age 4;7.

"stove"	[stoᵁv]	→	[stoᵁf]	total devoicing
"slide"	[slaɪd]	→	[slaɪd̥]	partial devoicing
"flag"	[flæg]	→	[flæg̊]	partial devoicing
"nose"	[noᵁz]	→	[noᵁs]	total devoicing

The general devoicing tendency in final positions suggests that realizations like these should probably not be considered aberrant productions.

Aspiration and Nonaspiration of Stop-Plosives.

Stop-plosives (as well as other consonants) are often described according to two parameters: fortis and lenis. **Fortis** refers to relatively more articulatory effort, whereas **lenis** refers to comparatively less. Most voiceless sounds are realized as fortis consonants, while voiced sounds are usually articulated as lenis productions. (One can note the increased articula-

tory effort on the level of air pressure by contrasting [t] and [d] with a hand in front of the mouth.) The sudden release of the articulatory effort in fortis stop-plosives leads typically to aspiration. This aspiration is noted by using a small elevated *h* following the voiceless stop-plosive sound:

"table" [tʰeɪbəl]

Stop-plosives, which are normally aspirated, are not marked unless the aspiration is excessive.

Voiceless stop-plosives that are typically aspirated may be produced without this fortis aspiration. In this case, the diacritic for unaspirated stops, [˭], could be added.

"pie" [p˭aɪ]

This example indicates that a normally aspirated [p] has occurred without aspiration.

CLINICAL COMMENTS

Voiceless stop-plosives are usually aspirated at the beginning of words; however, they are not aspirated in consonant clusters. Word-final aspiration is variable (Edwards, 1997).

Unreleased Stop-Plosives. Stop-plosives can be modified in yet another manner. Unreleased consonants result when the articulatory closure is maintained and not—as usual—released. Although voiceless unreleased stops are more obvious because of their loss of aspiration, voiced stops can be unreleased as well. Unreleased stops can occur at the end of an utterance or in one-word responses. To indicate an unreleased articulation, the diacritical mark [˺] is added:

Boy, was it hot.

[bɔɪ wʌz ɪt hat˺]

CLINICAL COMMENTS

Unreleased consonants should be noted *during* the simultaneous transcription of a client's speech. Just listening to and transcribing from tape recordings can be misleading because, when taped, unreleased consonants can sound similar to consonant omissions. While children and adults do not often realize many unreleased consonants, confusing this production variation with a final consonant deletion could lead to an inaccurate diagnosis. During live transcriptions, we can hear and at least partially see the actual articulation. This provides a much better basis for our judgment: unreleased consonant production or consonant deletion.

The following transcriptions come from an articulation test of Billy, age 4;3:

"cup"	[kʌp]	→	[tʌp˺]
"music"	[mjuzɪk]	→	[mudɪk˺]
"book"	[bʊk]	→	[bʊk˺]
"feet"	[fit]	→	[fit˺]
"watch"	[wɑtʃ]	→	[wɑt˺]
"sandwich"	[sænwɪtʃ]	→	[gæmɪt˺]

Unreleased consonants seldom warrant therapeutic intervention. Billy's case was different. Coming in addition to his many articulation errors, they contributed substantially to a decrease in his intelligibility.

Syllabic Consonants. Unstressed syllables easily become *reduced syllables*. This means that their vowel nucleus practically disappears. If the vowel nucleus is reduced, the following consonant becomes a syllabic, that is, it becomes the peak of that syllable. This is especially the case in unstressed final syllables when a nasal or the lateral [l] follow the preceding vowel (Heffner, 1975). The proper diacritic mark for such an occurrence is a straight line directly under the syllabic consonant:

fɪʃɪŋ → fɪʃən → fɪʃn̩

CLINICAL COMMENTS

In spontaneous speech, adults often reduce the unstressed final syllable, as in the following example:

Yesterday, we went swimming.

[jɛstə˞deɪ wi wɛnt swɪmn̩]

In spontaneous speech, and often during an articulation test, children will also demonstrate the use of syllabics. For example:

"chicken" [tʃɪ kn̩]

"scratching" [skræ tʃn̩]

The boy is fishing; he has a fishing pole.

[ðə ˌbɔɪ ɪzˈfɪʃn̩ hi hæz əˈfɪʃn̩ poʊl]

While such syllabics, obviously, need to be noted and transcribed, they are considered norm realizations.

Labialization/Nonlabialization of Consonants. Consonants, with the exception of [ʃ], are typically unrounded. Lip rounding is a production feature of [ʃ]. If a normally unrounded consonant is produced with lip rounding, this is referred to as labializing the sound in question. When the [ʃ] is produced without lip rounding, this is a nonlabialized production. The diacritics for labialized or nonlabialized consonants are a right-side-up or upside-down lowercase version of the Greek letter omega, [ω] or [ɯ], placed under the sound symbol in question. Labialized consonants can be the result of assimilation processes, as in the following example:

"soup" [s̫up] = labialized [s]

The labialized [s] could be a regressive assimilation due to the lip rounding of the following [u]. Labialization of normally unrounded consonants due to assimilation is noted, but it is not considered a speech sound problem. On the other hand, [ʃ] is usually produced with at least some degree of lip rounding. The following example indicates [ʃ] without lip rounding:

"ship" [ʃ̫ɪp] = nonlabialized [ʃ]

Unrounded [ʃ] realizations can also be due to assimilation; however, there are children who unround [ʃ] in all contexts. This should be noted and is considered an aberrant production.

CLINICAL COMMENTS

Rounded [s]- and unrounded [ʃ]-sounds are frequent sibilant realizations of children. These may be aberrant productions or context-based assimilation processes. The following is an excerpt from a transcription of Matt, age 4;6:

The boy is swinging really high.

[ðə bɔɪ ɪz s̹wɪŋən rili haɪ]

My mommy made vegetable soup.

[maɪ mɑmi meɪd vɛdʒəbļ s̹up]

In addition to Matt's unorthodox pronunciation of *vegetable,* we note that his [s]-sounds are rounded. In the given context, they may be just assimilation processes regressively influenced by the rounding of the following [w] or [u].

This does not seem to be the case in Chris's transcription, based on an articulation test and a spontaneous speech sample.

"fish"	[fɪʃ]	→	[fɪʃ̹]
"watch"	[wɑtʃ]	→	[wɑʃ̹]
"chicken"	[tʃɪkən]	→	[ʃ̹ɪkən]
"shovel"	[ʃʌvəl]	→	[ʃ̹ʌvəl]

At lunch I ate a peanut butter sandwich.

[æt lʌntʃ̹ aɪ eɪt ə pinət bʌtɚ ʃ̹ænɪtʃ]

I wish I had some new tennis shoes, like Michael Jordan.

[aɪ wɪʃ aɪ hæd sʌm nu tɛnəʃuz laɪk maɪkļ tʃ̹ordən]

Chris, in contrast to Matt, *un*rounds his "sh"-sounds even when they precede a rounded vowel, as in the word *shoes.* He also occasionally uses [ʃ] for [s]- and [tʃ]-sounds.

Derhotacization. Derhotacization is the loss of r-coloring for the consonant [r] and the central vowels with r-coloring, [ɝ] and [ɚ].

Derhotacized central vowels are transcribed as [ɜ] and [ə]. However, [r] often becomes derhotacized as well. The symbol used for a derhotacized [r] is [ɹ̠].

CLINICAL COMMENTS

Children often have difficulty with [r]-sounds. One common substitution is [w]. However, when listening to these r-productions, one should try to differentiate between the w/r substitution and a derhotacized [r]. Shriberg and Kent (1995) suggest that most [r] problems labelled as w/r substitutions are in fact derhotacized [r]-productions. If [r] is in error and is not a "true" [w] but also "not quite" an [r], it may be a derhotacized realization and should be transcribed as [ɹ̠].

Diacritics Used with Vowels

Rounding/Unrounding of Vowels. There are vowels that are normally rounded and others that are normally unrounded—[u] versus [i], for example. The rounding or unrounding of the lips is an important feature of vowel realizations. However, for several reasons, some clients may delete or inappropriately add these characteristics. This results in a distortion of the respective sound quality. IPA offers four diacritics grouped as two pairs to indicate rounding and unrounding of vowels. The signs are placed directly under the vowel symbol in question and consist of a small *c*-type notation, which indicates unrounding (or less rounding than is considered normal) when open to the right. When this *c* is inverted, creating an opening to the left, it denotes rounding (or more rounding than is normally the case):

[u̹] = unrounded [u]
[ɛ̹] = rounded [ɛ]

Changes in Tongue Placement for Vowels. Deviations in tongue positioning affect vowel as well as consonant articulations. Different vowel qualities are established essentially by different sizes and forms of the vocal tract. Two main factors determining these sizes and forms pertain to the location of the raised portion of the tongue (front and back dimensions) and to the extent to which the tongue is raised in the direction of the hard or soft palate (high and low dimensions).

Raised/Lowered Tongue Position. The IPA system offers a set of diacritics that signal the direction of tongue heights on the vertical plane leading to deviations from norm vowel productions. There are tongue symbols for too raised or too lowered a "hump" location for the norm production of the vowel in question. The diacritic [˕] under the vowel symbol marks a lower elevation, while the diacritic [˔] under the vowel marks a higher elevation of the tongue than is normally the case for the production of the vowel in question. For example,

[s ɪ̞ t]

would state that the high-front elevation of the tongue for standard [ɪ] articulation has not been reached in this realization; that is, the tongue articulation was lower than normal, resulting in a perceptible off-quality for [ɪ]. Trying to describe our auditory impression of this sound, we would say that it shifted in the direction of (but not reaching) the sound quality of [e].

Similarly, the transcription

[b ɪ̝ t]

would indicate a higher-than-normal elevation of the tongue for [ɪ], resulting in a quality that approaches [i] characteristics.

The same principle applies to all vowels. A question that logically follows is whether it makes a difference which symbol we use if the vowel is somewhere in between two qualities. In other words, do a raised [e] ([e̝]), and a lowered [ɪ] ([ɪ̞]) signify the same vowel quality? The answer is no. Therefore, in our previ-

ous example, one has to make a decision as to whether this vowel realization sounded more like an [e]- or an [ɪ]-type vowel. Based on the transcriber's auditory perception, the basic vowel quality must first be chosen, and then the modifying diacritic mark must be added to it.

Advanced/Retracted Tongue Position. There are also diacritics signalling tongue variations on the horizontal plane that lead to deviations from norm productions. They indicate a "hump" location too far forward or too far back for a norm production of the vowel in question. The diacritic for vowels produced with a tongue elevation more advanced than usual is [˖]. More retracted protrusions are marked by the diacritic [˗]. Both are placed under the vowel symbol: [ɛ̠], for example.

CLINICAL COMMENTS

Changes in the position of the tongue for vowel realizations are often perceptually difficult to target. Although transcribers are aware that the vowel quality is "off," they may not be sure in which direction. If the tongue has been lowered or raised, the vowel quality will sound somehow similar to the neighboring vowel on the vertical plane of the vowel quadrilateral. Thus, a lowered [ɛ] will have a certain [æ] quality, or a raised [ʊ] will approach a [u]. The best reference source in these cases is the vowel quadrilateral. However, this is

Think of the symbol as a pointer with its base the top of the *T*-type notation. If the pointer projects down [˕], the tongue has been lowered; if it points up [˔], the tongue has been raised. This also works for a tongue position too far forward or too far back. If it points to the left, toward the front of the vowel quadrilateral ([˖]), this indicates an advanced tongue placement. If it points to the right, toward the back of the vowel quadrilateral ([˗]), this would signify a retracted tongue position, one that is too far back.

not as simple if the tongue movements pertain to the horizontal plane, that is, to a tongue position too advanced or retracted. One point of reference is that front vowels that demonstrate a retracted tongue position and back vowels that demonstrate too forward a tongue position sound somewhat "centralized," that is, their distinct qualities appear reduced. Therefore, although the vowel can still be identified as the respective front or back vowel, it approaches a [ʌ]-type quality.

Nasality Symbols. During the production of most General American English speech sounds, the velum is elevated to block the expiratory air's escape through the nasal cavity. There is only one exception to this rule: the nasals. This is what—quite correctly—the textbooks tell us. However, in reality, the conditions are not always so clear-cut. If a nasal follows a vowel, for example, nasality often seeps into the vowel segment; the preceding vowel becomes nasalized:

$$[tæn] \rightarrow [t\tilde{æ}n]$$

As long as the nasality doesn't overstep the boundary line of natural assimilatory processes, this nasality remains unmarked. Speakers and listeners perceive these variations as normal. However, if the nasality is perceived as being excessive, or hypernasal, we need to place the "tilde" (which you may have encountered in Spanish language classes) over the respective sound(s). As speech-language specialists, we encounter hypernasality prominently in the speech of clients with dysarthria and cleft palates.

Denasality is also encountered in the speech of our clients. The symbol for denasality is the tilde with a slash through it, placed above the nasal consonant:

$$ni \rightarrow \tilde{n}i$$

This symbol refers to a reduction of nasal quality caused by velar elevation or blockage within the nasal cavity. Only nasal consonants can be denasalized. If nasal consonants are perceived as having a total lack of nasal quality (having a completely oral quality), then the symbol for the resulting homorganic voiced stop is used:

$$ni \rightarrow di$$

CLINICAL COMMENTS

One of the characteristics of African American dialect is the total regressive assimilation of postvocalic nasals (e.g., Haynes and Moran, 1989; Wolfram, 1986). The assimilation process is regressive in that the nasal following the vowel changes the characteristic of the preceding vowel into a nasalized vowel. In other words, the central feature of a following sound, nasality, impacts the previous vowel. It is considered a *total* assimilation process because the postvocalic nasal consonant is totally replaced. The following examples demonstrate this process:

| "pen" | [pɛn] | → | [pɛ̃n] | → | [pɛ̃] |
| "thumb" | [θʌm] | → | [θʌ̃m] | → | [θʌ̃] |

These pronunciations were noted on an articulation test from a child, age 4;3, speaking African American dialect:

"broom"	[brum]	→	[brũ]
"airplane"	[ɛɚ pleɪn]	→	[ɛɚ pleɪ̃]
"sandwich"	[sæn wɪtʃ]	→	[sæ̃ wɪtʃ]
"clown"	[klaʊn]	→	[klæ̃õ]

Since these variations are dialectal in nature, they would not be considered aberrant pronunciations. In African American dialect, they represent a regular pronunciation possibility.

Diacritics for the Suprasegmentals: Stress, Duration, and Juncture

Stress Markers. Every multisyllabic word has its own stress pattern, which may or may not be realized in a regular manner by our clients. The main purpose for all stress realizations is to emphasize certain syllables over others, thus creating a hierarchy of prominence among them.

Primary Stress.   The order of prominence is actualized by differences in loudness, pitch, and duration, the loudness differences being the most striking of the three. Generally, three different loudness levels are observed. The loudest syllable is said to have the *primary* stress. It is marked by a superscript short straight line in front of the respective syllable.

"syllable"	[ˈsɪ lə bəl]
"railway"	[ˈreɪl weɪ]
"superior"	[sə ˈpɪr iɚ]

Secondary Stress.   The next loudest syllable bears the *secondary stress.* It is indicated by a subscript short straight line in front of the syllable in question.

"supermarket"	[ˈsu pɚ ˌmɑr kət]
"signify"	[ˈsɪg nə ˌfaɪ]
"phonetic"	[fə ˈnɛ tɪk]

Some people find it difficult to distinguish between subtle loudness differences. For them, it may be of help to know that in General American English, different loudness levels characterizing stress go usually (but not

---

Stress patterns that extend beyond primary and secondary stresses include a feature known as *tertiary stress.* Tertiary stresses commonly display very small loudness differences from unstressed syllables. Therefore, they usually remain unmarked. Occasionally, though, it is necessary to distinguish a syllable with tertiary stress from an unstressed syllable within the same utterance. This may be important if a client shows a very peculiar stress pattern. If this is the case, one can number the syllables. Numerals (1 for primary stress, 2 for secondary stress, 3 for tertiary stress, etc.) are placed above the vowel nucleus of the corresponding syllable:

$$\overset{2\quad 1\ 4\ 3\ 5}{[dɪs\ ɑn\ ə\ rə\ bəl]}$$

---

always) hand in hand with changes in pitch. Thus, the louder the syllable, the higher the pitch. To pay attention to pitch differences first, then, may aid in discriminating between differing levels of loudness in stressing. It is also helpful to know that many (but again not all) words in General American English have their primary (or secondary) stress emphasis on the first syllable. A third possibility for those with difficulty in distinguishing stress differences is to vary systematically the loudness in each of the syllables of the word in question, [ˈdʒɛ ˌloʊ] versus [ˌdʒɛ ˈloʊ], for example. Typically, one version of that particular word will sound clearly more acceptable than the other. By a process of elimination, then, one can often ascertain the appropriate stressing pattern.

CLINICAL COMMENTS

Clients with dysarthrias have typical difficulties with stressing. The following transcription exemplifies such a possible displacement of stress.

	"birthday"
Norm speaker:	[ˈbɝθ ˌdeɪ]
Dysarthric speaker:	[ˌbɝθ ˈdeɪ]

	"umbrella"
Norm speaker:	[ˌəm ˈbrɛ lə]
Dysarthric speaker:	[ˈʌm ˌbrɛ lə]

Duration Symbols.   Sounds take up different amounts of time in continuous speech. We are so used to these measurable differences in sound duration that we register differences in usual lengths automatically as "too short" or "too long." If that is our perceptual impression, we have to indicate it by means of diacritic markers. Normal (i.e., inconspicuous) sound duration remains unmarked.

Lengthening. Longer than normal duration is signalled by either one or two dots following the sound symbol in question. The more dots, the longer the sound.

[fit]   standard vowel duration
[fi·t]   slightly longer than normal vowel duration
[fi:t]   clearly longer than normal vowel duration

The notation for lengthening from the 1925 Copenhagen Conference's revision of the IPA included up to four dots to signify lengthening. These could be used in special situations:

[fi:t] distinctly longer than normal vowel duration
[fi::t] exceedingly long vowel duration, as we might hear in dysarthric speakers

Shortening. Shorter than normal speech sound productions also occur. Different degrees of shortening are, as a rule, not indicated. The diacritic mark for any shortened sounds is [ˇ] placed above the respective sound symbol.

Shortening of sounds can lead to cutting off a portion of their phonetic properties. Young children with still unstable [s]-sounds sometimes shorten the (normally fairly long) segments to something that may sound like the release portion of [t]. If onset and holding portions of [t] are also identifiable, the obvious transcription would be [t]. However, if that is not the case, that is, if we indeed had an [s]-impression, we would transcribe this as [š].

> The phonetic symbol and diacritic [š] indicating shortening of [s] should not be confused with the same symbol [š], which is sometimes used in texts to indicate [ʃ].

Juncture Symbols. During continuous speech, all sounds seem to connect seamlessly. Occasionally, however, short gaps separating some of them are necessary to avoid misunderstandings. Consider the realizations of the following sentences:

He's a nice man.
He's an ice man.

In cases like this, the placement of the gaps, or *open junctures,* becomes the most important distinguishing element between the two different meanings. Yet, some of our clients may make open junctures where they do not belong, thus endangering the conveyance of their intended meaning.

In phonetic transcription, open junctures can be marked with the diacritic sign + between the symbols of slightly separated sounds. The sample sentences would then be transcribed as follows:

[hiz ə + naɪs mæn]
[hiz ən + aɪs mæn]

A *closed juncture,* on the other hand, is a normal state of affairs during speaking. It remains unmarked in phonetic transcription.

Terminal junctures mark the end of an utterance. In General American English, they are typically characterized by falling pitch for statements and *wh-* questions and by rising pitch for yes–no questions. The diacritic sign is an arrow pointing in the respective directions:

Never!   [ˈnɛ v ɚ↘]
Where are you going? [wɛɚ ɑɚ ju ˈgoʊɪŋ↘]
Really?   [ˈriə li↗]

If a speaker intends to continue talking after a pause, or if he wants to invite a response from another person, the *checked* or *held juncture* is normally used. To indicate this, an arrow is placed horizontally, signalling the speaker's suspended intonation:

tə ˈdeɪ →
ˈsu zi →

CLINICAL COMMENTS

Dysarthric speakers often have difficulty with sound durations and juncture. The following transcription is from Peter, age 22, with acquired spastic quadriplegia following an automobile accident.

I used to work as a mechanic, in a big shop.

[aɪ nus + tu wɝ::k æs ə 'mʊ:: + kɛni + nɪnə bɪk sɑp]

I could fix motorcycles, too.

[aɪ kʊt fɪs mʊ::to saɪ + soᵘš + tu]

I like motorcycles. I used to have one.

[aɪ nɑk mʊtə saɪtəs aɪ nu + tu hæ:: + fən]

Additional Symbols. The following symbols are not diacritics but are often used when transcribing aberrant speech.

Glottal Stop. The glottal stop ([ʔ]) is produced when a closed glottis is suddenly released after a build-up of subglottal air pressure. The release of air pressure creates a popping noise. The glottal stop is considered an allophonic variation of some stop-plosive productions and can serve to release vowels in stressed syllables (Edwards, 1997) or separate successive vowels between words (Wise, 1958):

| "oh" | [ʔoᵘ] | releasing a vowel |
| "Anna asks" | [æ nə ʔæsks] | separating successive vowels |

Some children with articulatory or phonological impairments use the glottal stop as a sound substitution (Stoel-Gammon and Dunn, 1985).

> The bilabial fricatives are phonemes in several languages. For example, [ɸ] is a phoneme of Japanese, while [β] has phonemic value in Spanish.

Bilabial Fricatives. The voiceless ([ɸ]) and voiced ([β]) bilabial fricatives are not phonemes of General American English but can also be used as sound substitutions in aberrant speech. Both sounds are produced by bringing the lips together so that a horizontally long but vertically narrow passageway is left between them for the voiceless or voiced breath stream to pass (Heffner, 1975).

Flap, Tap, or One-Tap Trill. The flap, tap, or what is also known as the one-tap trill [ɾ], is a frequent allophonic variation of [t] and [d]. This variation often occurs when stop-plosives are preceded and followed by vowels, as in *city* or *butter.* A single tap of the tongue tip against the alveolar ridge or with a gesture of the tongue tip in that direction characterizes these sounds (Wise, 1958).

CLINICAL IMPLICATIONS

Phonetic transcription and, especially, its diacritic marks appear at first glance complicated to handle and difficult to remember. Is this an exercise in pointless detail that has no practical application to the real clinical situation, a purely academic exercise? The obvious question arises as to how these diacritics could be helpful in our assessment and therapeutic process. The answer is threefold.

First, accurate phonetic transcription involves ear training, a sharpening of our auditory discrimination abilities. These skills are indispensable for clinical expertise, something that can never be emphasized enough. Second, phonetic transcription, and especially the use of diacritic markers, provides a generally agreed upon, professional way to note certain deviations from norm productions. This system allows clinicians to communicate freely with other professionals within the field of communication sciences and disorders. Transcription symbols can be translated back into actual speech events in the same way that musicians can read notes and translate them back into tunes. Third, by being aware of the many variations that can occur, accurate phonetic transcriptions open up diagnostic possibilities that we might not have considered without this knowledge. If we don't know

TABLE 3.1   Summary of Diacritic Markers and Additional Symbols

DIACRITICS USED WITH CONSONANTS	SUPRASEGMENTAL DIACRITICS
Changes in place of articulation	*Stress*
Dentalization [s̪]	Primary ['] as in ['æ pəl]
Palatalization [s̠]	Secondary [ˌ] as in [fʌ 'nɛ tɪk]
Velarization [ɫ]	*Duration*
Lateralization [s̩]	Lengthening [ˑ], [ː], [ːˑ], [ːː]
Voice symbols	Shortening [s̆]
Partial devoicing [z̥]	*Juncture*
Partial voicing [s̬]	Open juncture [+]
Aspiration of stop-plosives [ʰ]	Terminal junctures
Nonaspiration of stop-plosives [⁼]	Falling [↘]
Unreleased stop-plosive [̚]	Rising [↗]
Syllabic consonants [n̩]	Checked/held [→]
Labialization [s̫]	
Nonlabialization [ʃ̫]	
Derhotacization [ɹ̴]	

DIACRITICS USED WITH VOWELS	OTHER USEFUL SYMBOLS
Rounding [æ̹]	Glottal stop [ʔ]
Unrounding [ʊ̜]	Voiceless bilabial fricative [ɸ]
Changes in tongue placement	Voiced bilabial fricative [β]
Raised [ɛ̝]	Flap, tap, or one-tap trill [ɾ]
Lowered [ɛ̞]	
Advanced [ɛ̟]	
Retracted [ɛ̠]	
Nasality [ɑ̃]	
Denasality [ñ]	

what to listen for—unreleased stops or partial devoicing, for example—we might not identify some of the abnormal variations.

[s]-sound realizations illustrate well how the use of diacritics can have valuable practical consequences for assessment and intervention. Knowing what to listen for, we find that what once sounded like simply a distorted [s] can now be specified as the actual aberrant form presented: a palatal versus a lateral versus a dentalized [s] distortion, for example. All these variations can be noted using the respective diacritic markers. In addition, aside from the clarification the notation system provides, detailed knowledge about actual realizations is indispensable for the assessment and successful remediation of [s] errors. By establishing that the [s] appears distorted, we are saying only that its typical production is "off." We have addressed the *acceptability* issue of the sound realization, but not its aberrant *production* features, the most important information for clinical purposes. However, by comparing the child's actual articulatory features with the known features for regular [s]-productions, we will know precisely which placement characteristics need to be changed therapeutically.

By identifying an [s]-distortion as a palatal [s̪], for example, detailed information that can be used when planning therapy is given. A palatal [s̪] is produced with the tongue tip too far back in the direction of the palatal area. Due to this tongue position, the palatal [s̪] has a [ʃ]-like quality. All other production features are usually in accordance with norm [s]-articulations; the lateral edges of the tongue are raised, and the sagittal grooving necessary for the [s] is present as well. It may be possible, therefore, that the child needs only to move the tongue tip to a more anterior position to produce a regular [s]. Applying this knowledge, therapy becomes not only more goal directed but also much simpler—with the consequence of saving time and possible frustration.

The advantage of knowing how the child actually produces the distorted speech sound becomes even more obvious if we compare two distorted sound productions, one palatal [s̪], ([ş]), one dentalized [s], ([s̪]), for example. The [s̪] is characterized by a tongue placement too far forward. In this case, the child needs to move the tongue back, posteriorly, to obtain a regular [s]. This would be in direct contrast to the procedure necessary for the [ş], in which fronting of organ and place of articulation becomes necessary. Detailed knowledge of the client's production features, then, proves to be an important asset leading to expedient and thorough therapeutic intervention.

Theoretically and practically, the importance of the preceding discussion seems rather obvious. Its essential ingredient is our ability to note and differentiate between changes in sound quality as the basis for our remedial task. By fine-tuning transcription skills, not only are the transcriber's discrimination and notational recording capabilities increased, but also the effectiveness of the whole intervention process improves.

CLINICAL APPLICATION

Using Diacritics in the Assessment Process

Andy, age 6;2, was referred to the speech-language specialist by his classroom teacher. According to the teacher, his main problem seemed to be his "speech," which she described as being somewhat difficult to understand and containing many sound errors. After a thorough appraisal, the speech-language specialist was concerned that Andy might have a phonological disorder. When first listening to Andy's spontaneous speech, in addition to his w/r substitutions, she thought that he used [θ] realizations for th-, s-, and sh-sounds. The clinician was worried that Andy was not able to differentiate between these phonemes. She had to admit, though, that there had been some qualitative differences between the productions which she could not quite describe. She decided to continue with her assessment, paying special attention to these sounds. She also used some pictures that pinpointed the th-, s-, and sh-sounds in an elicited speech sample. After carefully listening to Andy's actual productions and later to the recording, the clinician arrived at the following results:

One-Word Articulation Test Results

Norm Production	→	Actual Production	Word Examples	Transcription
[s]	→	[s̪]	sun	[sʌn] → [s̪ʌn]
			bus	[bʌs] → [bʌs̪]
			zoo	[zu] → [z̪u]
			all consonant clusters with [s]	[s] + consonant → [s̪] + consonant

One-Word Articulation Test Results (continued)

Norm Production	→	Actual Production	Word Examples	Transcription
[ʃ]	→	[ʂ]	shoe	[ʃu] → [ʂu]
			fish	[fɪʃ] → [fɪʂ]
			dishes	[dɪʃəz] → [dɪʂəʐ]
[θ]	→	[θ]	thumb	[θʌm] → [θʌm]
[ð]	→	[ð]	feather	[fɛðɚ] → [fɛðə]

Selected Spontaneous Speech Sample:

I have a red toothbrush. My mommy tells me every night to brush my teeth.
[aɪ hæv ə wɛd tuθbwəʐ maɪ mɑmi tɛlʐ mi ɛvri naɪt tu bwʌʂ maɪ tiθ]

Today in school we made an art picture.
[tudeɪ ɪn ʂkul wi meɪd ən at pɪkʂəl]

We cut out all sorts of things with scissors and pasted them on this sheet of paper.
[wi kʌt aʊt al ʂowəts ʌv θɪŋz wɪθ ʂɪʐəʐ ænd peɪʂtəd ðɛm ɑn ðɪʂ ʂit ʌv peɪpə]

Andy did actually differentiate between the th-, s-, and sh-sounds with a dentalized production—[s̪, z̪] for /s/ and /z/, a palatalized [ʂ] for /ʃ/, and correct "th" re- alizations. In this case, careful transcription made a large difference in the outcome of this assessment.

SUMMARY

Assessment procedures and results should be accurate, professional, and accomplished in an accountable manner. This chapter introduced the International Phonetic Alphabet (IPA) as a widely used system that can provide these requisites for the assessment of articulatory and phonological disorders. The IPA system was developed to document actual phonetic realizations of speech events. It is a means of transferring highly impermanent speech events into more durable graphic representations. Such a system offers the speech-language specialist a way to substantiate assessment results as well as to communicate effectively with other professionals. Transcription should never be considered just an option; accurate transcription is a necessity for professional evaluations.

To increase the effectiveness of the IPA system, certain diacritic markers are used to add production details to the meaning of the basic symbol. These markers are indispensable to the documentation of many of the unusual realizations of our clients. Such diacritics were itemized, explained, and exemplified in the second section of the chapter. This section also offered clinical comments on many of the diacritics as well as actual phonetic transcriptions utilizing these marks.

The last section of this chapter demonstrated how phonetic transcription and the detailed knowledge acquired through its use in assessment procedures also benefits the intervention process. First, the accuracy needed for the transcription task promotes the fine-tuning of perceptual skills, a clinical proficiency that will, by its very nature, enhance the likelihood of successful intervention. Second, the specificity gained through phonetic transcription, including diacritics, translates into a far more goal-directed treatment approach, which increases clinical efficacy.

THEORETICAL CONSIDERATIONS

Many students and clinicians are skeptical about theories. They are viewed as unnecessarily difficult to understand, impractical, and not really relevant to diagnostic and therapeutic issues. Some theories may indeed be somewhat difficult to understand because they are attempts to explain highly complex behaviors. For example, Schwartz (1992a) states that a theoretical framework that addresses any aspect of language acquisition requires

1. a theory of abstract knowledge and representation,
2. theories that address the processing of input, how it is represented, and how it is produced, and
3. a theory of developmental change.

It is easy to see why a theoretical framework that attempts to consider all these aspects might be complex.

The second objection to theories is that they are impractical. Actually, theories can be very practical. Theories are based on confirmed observations or systematic experiments. As such, they try to abstract from many practical experiences, allowing the realization of order and rules amidst seemingly entangled details. Theories can also serve as blueprints for practical tasks. For example, phonological theories attempt to explain the structure and function of phonological systems. The structure and function outlined by a specific theory can in turn be used to analyze a particular phonological system. This analysis procedure can then be applied to both the normal and the disordered phonological systems of our clients. Various theories, such as distinctive feature theory or generative phonology, have resulted in analysis procedures that are used daily to evaluate the phonological systems of children.

The third objection to theories is that they are not relevant to the diagnosis and treatment of individual clients. On the contrary, because theories guide and direct clinical work, they are fundamentally important and relevant to the diagnostic and therapeutic process. For example, many students and clinicians are currently using phonological processes to describe patterns of errors and to determine therapeutic goals. The concept of phonological processes evolved from a theory of natural phonology (Donegan and Stampe, 1979; Stampe, 1969, 1972, 1973). The theory of natural phonology applied certain principles of generative grammar, itself another theory that has revolutionized the way professionals view language. Both of these theories have resulted in major changes in diagnostic and therapeutic procedures. Different types of analyses are now employed diagnostically, and a major shift in therapy has occurred due to the impact of these theories. The relevance of theories to our profession cannot be overestimated.

Theories also offer a *variety* of clinical possibilities. Each theory provides a somewhat different perspective on the problem to be solved. Therefore, if one theory is used, assessment and treatment will vary from those suggested by a second theory. This gives clinicians several possible directions, and consequently approaches, from which to choose. Each theory and its application provide the clinician with unique problem-solving advantages. Without such problem-solving strategies, these features would go unnoticed; valuable diagnostic information would be lost. Thus, theories provide a means of maximizing diagnostic and therapeutic skills. They are significant to everything clinicians do professionally.

Chapters 2 and 3 dealt primarily with production features of articulation—with speech sound forms. The focus in Chapter 4 shifts to phonology—to speech sound function. This shift is a consequence of the fact that contemporary theories in our field are phonological theories; they clearly emphasize the function of the phoneme as a meaning differentiating unit.

The first goal of this chapter is to introduce the reader to some of the basic terminology and principles underlying many of the contemporary phonological theories. They are contained in the section on phonology. Care has been taken to keep the number of complex technical terms to a minimum. The second goal is to present several phonological theories that have been applied clinically within the

discipline. Each phonological theory will be discussed in relationship to its theoretical framework, how it developed, and how it functions. Finally, clinical implications will be suggested for each of the presented theories.

PHONOLOGY

What Is Phonology?

Phonology can be defined as the description of the systems and patterns of phonemes that occur in a language. It involves determining the language-specific distinctive phonemes and the rules that describe the set of changes that take place when these phonemes occur in different relationships with other phonemes (Ladefoged, 1993). Within this system, the smallest entity that can be distinguished by its contrasting function within words is called the *phoneme*. The phoneme is, thus, the central unit of phonology.

Many different theoretical frameworks for phonological investigations exist. Because phonology is a developing field of study striving to approach established goals in new ways, such differences seem only natural. However, these various approaches all have

Phonology as a concept and term has undergone considerable changes both in the name applied to the discipline concerned with the subject matter and in the basic understanding of what this discipline represents. The original French and German terms *phonologie* (Baudouin de Courtenay, 1872) and *Phonologie* (Trubetzkoy, 1931) were, under the influence of structuralism, replaced by *functional phonetics* (Jakobson, 1962; Martinet, 1960). The term *functional phonetics* emphasized the functional aspect of speech sounds. Phonology has also been called phonemics (Sapir, 1925), underlining the linguistic function of the phoneme. The term *phonology* is presently preferred and used by most professionals within the field of communication disorders.

one fundamentally important commonality, the differentiation between two levels of sound presentation:

1. the *phonetic level,* with sounds (phones, allophones) as central units
2. the *phonemic level,* represented by phonemes

How Does Phonology Work?

To understand the concept of phonology, it is important to differentiate clearly between speech sounds and phonemes. Speech sounds (phones, allophones) are physical *forms* that are the result of physiological processes and that have objectively verifiable acoustic properties. Phonemes, on the other hand, are defined in terms of their linguistic *function,* that is, in terms of their ability to establish meaningful units in a language.

How Did the Concept of the Phoneme Develop?

A definition of the phoneme and its relationship to phonology are found in Chapter 1.

The concept and term *phoneme* were born toward the end of the nineteenth century at a point when linguists and phoneticians found it necessary to expand the former single sound concept into a twofold sound concept:

1. speech sounds as production realities
2. speech sounds in their meaning-establishing and meaning-distinguishing function, as "phonemes"

In their works, the British phonetician Henry Sweet (1845–1912), the German Eduard Sievers (1850–1932), and the Swiss Jost Winteler (1846–1929) laid the foundation for the understanding of this duality. However, historically, Baudouin de Courtenay deserves the credit for introducing the concept of the phoneme in the year 1870. (The word *phoneme* existed prior to this time, but it was used as another label for speech sound.) N. H. Kruszewski (1881), a student of Baudouin de Courtenay's, further popularized the term in his dissertation. Baudouin de Courtenay interpreted the proposed sound duality as differences between a physiologically concrete sound realization and its mental image. Influenced by the thinking of his time, Baudouin de Courtenay interpreted phonemes as primarily *psychological* sound units, as "psychic equivalents of the sound" (Lepschy, 1970, p. 60), as the sound "intended" by the speaker and "understood" by listeners. This was in contrast to the actually articulated sound, which was seen as a physiological fact. Similarly, the Russian linguist L. V. Ščerba, who succeeded Baudouin de Courtenay, defined the phoneme as "the shortest general sound image of a given language which can be associated with meaning images, and can differentiate words" (Lepschy, 1970, p. 62).

Although still psychologically oriented, the British phonetician Daniel Jones presented a more language-based phoneme concept in the first half of the twentieth century (Jones, 1938, 1950). Jones defined the phoneme as a "family of sounds in a given language which are related in character and are used in such a way that no one member ever occurs in a word in the same phonetic context as any other member" (Jones, 1950, p. 10). According to Jones's definition, as long as speech sounds are understood as belonging to the same category, they constitute a phoneme of that language. For example, as long as [s] productions, with all their verifiable phonetic differences (different speakers, various circumstances), are evaluated by listeners as being the same, as belonging to the s-category, these allophonic variations represent the single phoneme /s/ in that language.

Today's prevalent phoneme concept is still more functionally oriented. The specific *use* of the phoneme in a language is the primary emphasis. This strictly functional phoneme concept was strongly influenced by Ferdinand de Saussure's (1916/1959) revolutionary new "structuralistic" ways to look at language and was introduced by Nikolai S. Trubetzkoy and Roman Jakobson. Trubetzkoy, cofounder of the Prague School of linguistics, wrote that "The phoneme can be defined satisfactorily neither on the basis of its psychological nature nor on the basis of its relation to the phonetic variants, but purely and solely on the basis of its function in the system of language" (Trubetzkoy, 1939/1969, p. 41).

When defining the phoneme, he added that it is "the sum total of the phonologically relevant properties of a sound" (p. 36). "References to psychology must be avoided in defining the phoneme, since the latter is a linguistic and not a psychological concept" (p. 38).

One important aspect of phonological systems of languages is each one's *phoneme inventory.* However, this is not the only variable used in characterizing different phonological systems. Edward Sapir (1921) pointed out that two languages having the same phoneme inventory can, nevertheless, have very different phonologies. Even though inventories may be identical, the way these sound segments can and cannot be arranged to form words may be quite different. Consequently, the *phonotactics,* or "permissible" sound arrangements within a language, is an important aspect of phonemes' "function" and is, therefore, an integral part of the phonology of a given language.

Speech Sound versus Phoneme: Clinical Implications

Every utterance has two facets: an audible sequence of speech sounds and their specific meaning conveyed through this sequence. For example, if someone says, "Hey Joe, over here," there is an audible sequence of sounds [heɪ dʒoʊ oʊvɚ hɪɚ] that conveys a specific meaning. Both the physical form of the

speech sound and its language-specific function need to be realized in order for the utterance to be meaningful. If only one aspect is realized, either speech sound form or function, a breakdown in the communicative process will occur.

Adequate form and function of all segments are basic requirements for meaningful utterances in any language. Form is established by the way the segment in question is produced, by articulatory events. Segment function presupposes the observance of the language-specific rules regarding the orderly arrangement of the speech sound segments. During an utterance, *form* and *function* become combined into meaning-conveying entities.

Segment form and function are also largely dependent on one another. Without acceptable production features, sound segments cannot fulfill their functional task. If, for example, the word *key* is realized as *tea,* a frequent error made by children with t/k substitutions, elements of sound production have interfered with sound function. In this case, the phonological opposition between /t/ and /k/ has been destroyed. Although a lateralized [s] production in General American English will not destroy any phonological oppositions, it will have an impact on the expected realization, thus influencing phoneme function as well. Segment function depends on normal segment form.

Also, segment form depends on proper segment function. Without observance of the phonotactic rules governing the language, an acceptable sound production will not transmit the intended message. If, for example, a child produces a correct [s] but does not realize the phonotactic rules that combine this [s] with other consonants in clusters, the meaning will be impaired. *Stop* might become *top,* or *hats* is realized as *hat.* For the purpose of effective verbal communication, regular segment form and function are indispensable.

Articulation and Phonological Theories and Therapies: Separation or Unity? In former times, "correct" single sound realizations were often the central focus of articulation work. The mastering of how sound segments can and cannot be joined together to establish and convey meaning within the respective language was largely neglected. The underlying assumption was that speakers with defective articulation either "know" these rules already or will "learn" them through the various exercises that incorporated the sound in various word positions and in consonant clusters, for example. Articulation therapies focused on the realization of acceptable speech sound forms.

Today, it is often the other way around. The main orientation is the mastering of the phonological rules that govern the language-specific utilization of the sound segments. Children with phonological disorders do not demonstrate difficulties primarily with the production of the sound segments but instead with their function, with the rule-governed arrangement of these segments. In these instances, mastery of the phonological rules, not the speech sound realization, will be the main goal. However, the mastery of phonological rules often becomes a central focus for children who demonstrate faulty segment production and for children with articulatory impairments. The underlying assumption is that mastery of the system-specific rules of speech sound use will generalize to the improvement of speech sound production. Phonological therapies focus on the realization of adequate segment function within a language system.

Both intervention approaches have contributed substantially to the treatment of impaired articulation and phonology. They represent outgrowths of different theoretical viewpoints. However, their high degree of mutual dependency implies that, for successful articulation work, these two approaches are clinically a matter not of "either or" but

of "as well as." Of course, based on the specific clinical characteristics of an individual client, one approach may take precedence. If, for example, emphasis on speech sound form was the chosen approach, functional aspects will, nevertheless, also have to be taken into consideration. On the other hand, if speech sound function needs to be emphasized, there may be a point in therapy when the clinician will need to consider aspects of speech sound form as well.

In summary, effective verbal communication always mirrors both aspects of speech sounds, acceptable form and function. Remediation must consider both sides of this duality, because they represent two sides of the same coin.

CLINICAL APPLICATION

Phonological and Articulation Therapies Working Together

Toby was 5;2 when he was seen by the new speech pathologist. Although he had previously received speech therapy, he was still considered very difficult to understand. A thorough assessment revealed that all fricative sounds were produced as stop-plosives. Thus, [f] and [v] were articulated as [p] and [b], and the voiceless and voiced [s] and [z], [ʃ] and [ʒ], as well as [θ] and [ð] were articulated as [t] and [d]. Toby's phonotactics for these sounds appeared intact. He did produce the noted substitutions consistently in all word positions. Toby often had difficulty discriminating words containing these phonemic oppositions. Thus, if the clinician asked the child to point to the picture of a "pin" versus a "fin" or of a "vase" versus a "base," Toby would often be in error. After completing the evaluation, the clinician decided that Toby had a phonological disorder: Toby did not understand the function of these phonemes in the language system.

The clinician began to work on differentiating and establishing these oppositions in meaningful contexts. Pictures and objects that contained these oppositions were used. The clinician noted that as Toby's discrimination abilities improved, he attempted to produce [f] and [v]; however, these realizations were consistently in error. As Toby struggled to correct the aberrant productions, the clinician realized that he was quickly becoming frustrated. The clinician used her knowledge of speech sound form to show Toby how to produce [f] and [v] in an acceptable manner. Toby was interested, responded quickly to this instruction, and soon could produce regular [f] and [v] sounds. He was very proud of his achievement and responded [naᵘ aɪ kæn teɪ ɪt waɪt].

DISTINCTIVE FEATURE THEORIES

To determine a single sound segment's linguistic role within the framework of meaningful communication, a means must be found of separating the phonetic differences that serve to signal meaning differences in a language from those that do not. The task is to determine which features are decisive for the identification of the various phonemes within a given language. Phonetic constituents that distinguish between phonemes are referred to as **distinctive features**.

What Are Distinctive Features?

How does one differentiate between apparent likenesses? For example, how do we distinguish between similar cars, houses, or streets? We look for discernible marks that might set the particular object apart from similar objects. A tree on the corner of a particular street, a brightly colored door on a house, for example, may serve as distinctive features that discriminate between streets or houses. "A distinctive feature is any property that separates a subset of elements from a group" Blache, 1978, p. 56).

Applying this broad definition of distinctive features to sound segments, it could be stated that any articulatory property that separates one sound segment from a group of similar sound segments is a distinctive feature. A sound component is said to be distinctive if it serves to distinguish one phoneme from another. These units, which are smaller than

sound segments, are considered to be "atomic" constituents of sound segments which cannot be broken down any further (Jakobson, 1949). An inventory of these properties would allow the analysis of the phonemes not only of General American English but also of all languages. Distinctive features allow the description of the oppositional function of phonemes, of their patterns, and of their systematic organization.

How Do Distinctive Features Work?

Distinctive features are the smallest indivisible sound properties that establish phonemes. An inventory of distinctive sound features would demonstrate similarities and dissimilarities between phonemes. These similarities and differences are marked by the presence of certain properties in some phonemes and the absence of these properties in others. The term *binary* is used in most distinctive feature analyses to indicate these similarities and differences. A **binary system** uses a plus (+) and minus (–) system to signal the presence (+) or absence (–) of certain features.

Many different distinctive features must be considered in order to arrive at those that distinguish between phonemes. For example, consonants must be distinguished from vowels, voiced consonants from voiceless

The *concept of binarity* goes back to Jakobson's influence on the evolution of distinctive feature theories. Jakobson, Fant, and Halle (1952) formulated that "any minimal distinction carried by the message confronts the listener with a two-choice situation" (paragraph 1.1). It follows that distinctive features are two-valued and require a yes/no decision concerning their presence or absence within sound segments. The concept of binarity has essentially been accepted by later distinctive feature systems. The Ladefoged (1971) system is the clear exception. Its nonbinary set of "Prime Features" uses multivalued features in its description.

consonants, nasals from nonnasals, to mention just a few. If /k/ and /g/ are considered, the following binary oppositions could be established:

/k/	/g/
is a consonant =	is a consonant =
+ consonantal	+ consonantal
is not a vowel = − vocalic	is not a vowel = − vocalic
is not voiced = − voice	is voiced = + voice

In this representation of similarities and dissimilarities, voicing is the only feature that distinguishes /k/ from /g/. Two sound segments are considered distinct, and can, therefore, serve as phonemes *if at least one of their features is different.*

To expand slightly upon this feature system, consider the phonemes /k/, /g/, and /ŋ/. As previously noted, /k/ and /g/ are distinguished from one another by the feature of voicing. How could this feature system be expanded to include the distinctive features that distinguish between /k/, /g/, and /ŋ/?

/k/	/g/	/ŋ/
+ consonantal	+ consonantal	+ consonantal
− vocalic	− vocalic	− vocalic
− voice	+ voice	+ voice
− nasal	− nasal	+ nasal

Although voice distinguishes /k/ from /g/ and /ŋ/, nasality is the feature that differentiates /g/ and /ŋ/, because all their other features are the same. In this example, nasality is the distinctive feature that creates an opposition between the phonemes /g/ and /ŋ/.

Presence or absence of the sound segments' distinctive features can be displayed conveniently in a matrix form. Often, the Chomsky-Halle (1968) distinctive feature system is noted in textbooks for speech-language pathologists. However, this is not the only distinctive feature system. Over the years, many different distinctive feature systems have been developed (e.g., Jakobson, 1949; Jakobson, Fant, and Halle, 1952; Jakobson and Halle, 1956; Ladefoged 1971; Singh and Polen, 1972). Each of their authors had a somewhat different idea about which distinctive features were important when distinguishing between phonemes. Most of the feature systems were binary; however, Peter Ladefoged (1971, 1993) used multivalued features. In addition, most distinctive feature systems used articulatory dimensions to classify the phonemes, although acoustic parameters have been categorized as well (Jakobson, Fant, and Halle, 1952). One distinctive feature system is not necessarily superior to another. They were all developed to address somewhat different aspects of feature distinctions. In addition, many distinctive feature systems originated as a means of analyzing *universal* similarities and differences among the phoneme systems of many different languages. This goal would of necessity incorporate feature modalities that are not necessary when analyzing General American English speech sounds.

To summarize, distinctive feature systems are an attempt to document specific speech sound constituents that establish phonemes. Distinctive feature theories organize sound constituents according to some productional (or in some cases acoustic) properties that might be utilized in languages to establish

---

An example of multivalued features includes using 1, 2, 3, and 4 to distinguish between differences in vowel height. Thus, [æ] is considered [1 height], while [i] is [4 height] (Ladefoged, 1993).

The use of acoustic parameters to specify distinctive features resulted in features such as "compact" and "diffuse." Based on acoustic displays of vowels (+), compact was defined as a concentration of acoustic energy in the midfrequency region of the spectrum. Low vowels were considered (+) compact. The distinctive feature (+) diffuse was defined by a spread of acoustic energy over a wider frequency range. High vowels and labial, dental, and alveolar consonants were (+) diffuse (Jakobson and Halle, 1956).

meaning differences. The result is a system of contrastive, linguistically relevant sound elements. Many different feature systems exist. No one feature system has clear advantages over another. All distinctive feature systems reflect the authors' concept of those characteristics that most aptly define the phoneme.

How Did Distinctive Feature Theories Develop?

The original distinctive feature theories grew out of the phoneme concept, which was developed by the members of the Prague School in the 1930s. Very early in his work, Roman Jakobson, cofounder of the Prague School, hypothesized that the ultimate constituent of language was not the phoneme itself but its smaller components, its distinctive features. Jakobson stressed that these minimal differences serve the function of distinguishing between words that are different in meaning. It is these distinctive features that

are functioning to distinguish between *bat* and *pat,* for example.

The Jakobson, Fant, and Halle (1952) system used twelve *acoustic* features based on the sound segments' spectrographic display. Such descriptions soon proved unsatisfactory for linguistic use primarily because similar acoustic representations can be achieved by a number of different articulatory gestures. This led to a revision of the original system. In 1956, Jakobson and Halle published a new distinctive feature system which now included *articulatory* production features. Table 4.1 presents a brief explanation and examples of each of these distinctive features.

Many of the later distinctive feature systems (Chomsky and Halle, 1968; Halle, 1962; Ladefoged, 1971, 1993; Miller and Nicely, 1955; Singh, 1968; Singh and Black, 1966; Voiers, 1967; Wickelgren, 1966) were defined primarily according to articulatory features (or to a combination of articulatory and acoustic parameters).

CLINICAL APPLICATION

Distinctive Features versus Organ, Place, Voice, and Manner

Distinctive features are usually based on articulatory properties. At first glance, this might appear to be similar to the phonetic production features of speech sounds. However, these two analyses look very different in their results. Returning to Toby from the previous clinical application, we find:

[p] and [b] replace [f] and [v]
[t] and [d] replace [s], [z], [ʃ], [ʒ], [θ], and [ð]

If the misarticulations are analyzed according to phonetic production features, the following results:

[p] and [b]	voiceless and voiced bilabial stop-plosives replace	[f] and [v] voiceless and voiced labio-dental fricatives
[t] and [d]	voiceless and voiced coronal-alveolar stop-plosives replace	[s] and [z] voiceless and voiced coronal-alveolar apico-alveolar fricatives
		[ʃ] and [ʒ] voiceless and voiced coronal-prepalatal fricatives with lip rounding
		[θ] and [ð] voiceless and voiced apico-dental fricatives

Distinctive feature analysis would compare the (+) and (–) features for each of the phonemes. If only the features that are different are noted (e.g., in one category, a (+) for one sound and a (–) for the other sound), the following results:

[p] and [b]	(–) strident	[f] and [v]	(+) strident
	(–) continuant		(+) continuant
[t] and [d]	(–) strident	[s] and [z]	(+) strident
		[ʃ] and [ʒ]	(+) strident
	(–) continuant	[s] and [z]	(+) continuant
		[ʃ] and [ʒ]	(+) continuant
		[θ] and [ð]	(+) continuant
	(+) diffuse	[ʃ] and [ʒ]	(–) diffuse

Distinctive Feature Theories: Clinical Implications

Distinctive feature systems were developed as a means of analyzing phonemes and entire phoneme systems of languages. Each phoneme of the particular system was assessed to determine if the distinctive feature was present (+) or absent (–). Although originally devised to analyze the regular realization of phonemes within and across languages, its analysis potential for disordered speech could not be overlooked. When sound substitution features were compared to target sound features, similarities and differences could be noted.

Distinctive feature systems offered several advantages over the previous analysis systems of classifying errors according to substitutions, deletions, and distortions. First, they provide a more complete analysis. For example, sound substitutions can be broken down into several different feature components, which can then be compared and analyzed. Second, and perhaps more important, distinctive feature systems concentrate on the features that distinguish phonemes within a language. Previous analysis procedures had, at best, focused on phonetic production aspects of speech sounds. With the impact of phonol-

ogy on the field of communication disorders, this emphasis now shifted to the phoneme and its function within the language system.

The preceding clinical application with Toby exemplifies how the distinctive feature analysis works and which results could be drawn from such an analysis. Toby substitutes [p] and [b] for [f] and [v], and [t] and [d] for [s], [z], [ʃ], [ʒ], [θ], and [ð]. When only the distinctive features that differentiate between these phonemes are described, comparisons of the target and substitution distinctive features yield just three separating features: strident, continuant, and diffuse. First, this analysis shows that the error and target sounds have many features in common. From the list of eleven different distinctive features, only three are different. Second, a specific error pattern becomes obvious. Primarily, Toby substitutes nonstrident, noncontinuant phoneme realizations for strident, continuant phoneme realizations.

Therapeutic implications follow logically. If the child can differentiate between the presence and absence of the continuant, strident, and diffuse features, the aberrant sound productions should be easily remediated. However, can children really understand and differentiate between distinctive features? Jakobson's (1942/1968) hypothesis that chil-

TABLE 4.1   Features, Descriptions, and Examples of the Jakobson and Halle (1956) Distinctive Feature System

FEATURE	DESCRIPTION	EXAMPLES
+ consonantal	obstruction in vocal tract	consonants, excluding glides (/w/, /j/) and /h/
– consonantal	no vocal tract obstruction	vowels and glides +/h/
+ vocalic	glottal vibration with free passage of air through the vocal tract	vowels and liquids /l/ and /r/
– vocalic	no glottal vibration or free passage of air through the vocal tract	all other consonants
+ nasal	mouth resonator supplemented by the nasal cavity	nasals /m/, /n/, and /ŋ/
– nasal	mouth resonator excluding the nasal cavity	all nonnasal consonants, vowels
+ grave	peripheral articulation	labial and velar consonants, back vowels
– grave	medial articulation	dental and palatal consonants, front vowels
+ compact	forward-flanged, concentration of energy in the midfrequency region of spectrum	low vowels
– compact	lack of concentration of energy in the midfrequency region	high vowels
+ diffuse	backward-flanged, spread of energy over a wider frequency range	high vowels, labial, dental, and alveolar consonants
– diffuse	lack of spreading of energy over a wider frequency range	low vowels, palatal, velar, and back consonants
+ strident	more noisy sounds	fricatives (excluding /θ/ and /ð/), affricates
– strident	less noisy sounds	vowels, stops, glides, liquids, /θ/ and /ð/
+ flat	labialized, rounded, retroflexed, or velarized	/w/ and rounded vowels
– flat	"plain" vowels and consonants	all other consonants and vowels
+ voice	produced with vibration of the vocal folds	vowels, voiced consonants
– voice	produced without vibration of the vocal folds	voiceless consonants
+ continuant	noninterrupted	fricative, liquids, glides, and vowels
– continuant	interrupted, abrupt	stops, affricates
+ tense	produced with more tension, strain, or duration	voiceless stops, fricatives, and affricates, vowels with more muscular effort
– tense	produced with less tension, strain, or duration	voiced stops, fricatives, and affricates, vowels with less muscular effort

dren acquire features rather than sounds seems to support this assumption. If this is the case, their therapeutic utilization could facilitate this developmental process. In addition, if children acquire features rather than sounds, a certain amount of generalization must occur during the process. Consequently, children should be able to generalize features from sounds they can realize to others they cannot. This could be therapeutically utilized. A child who can produce, for example, a + stridency in one phonemic context should be able to generalize this + stridency to other phonemic contexts. Using the example from above, if Toby could produce the + and – stridency and + and – continuancy features that differentiate between /f/ and /p/ phonemes, this should generalize to other instances, such as /v/ versus /b/, /s/ and /θ/ versus /t/, and /z/ and /ð/ versus /d/. Therefore, treatment of one phonemic opposition with specific distinctive features should lead to the norm production of other phonemic oppositions with the same distinctive feature oppositions. This would be a means of treating more than one phoneme in a time-efficient manner.

Over time, several distinctive feature therapy programs were developed (Blache, 1989; Compton, 1970, 1975, 1976; McReynolds and Engmann, 1975; Weiner and Bankson, 1978). However, both the analysis procedures and the clinical applicability of distinctive features for speech-disordered children have been questioned by several authors (Carney, 1979; Foster, Riley, and Parker, 1985; Parker, 1976; Walsh, 1974). Some critical comments have focused on the fact that distinctive feature theory and distinctive features are abstract concepts: Distinctive features are theoretical concepts that were formulated to account for the sound patterns of languages. Carney (1979) further argued that a distinctive feature analysis, based on the phoneme concept, compels the clinician to ignore phonetic information. This phonetic information, exemplified by [s̪] or [ʃ], is not classifiable according to distinctive features and may lead to classifying errors inappropriately or not at all. For example, if the child produces a dentalized s-sound, [s̪], how is this classified? There is no distinctive feature for dentalized [s]. The clinician might ignore the distortion, declaring it a norm production, or could perhaps classify it as a [θ]. In both cases, valuable diagnostic and therapeutic information would be lost.

Naturalness and Markedness. One aspect of distinctive feature theory that seems to have more direct clinical applicability and can be found in later theoretical constructs is the concept of *naturalness* and *markedness*. Naturalness and markedness can be seen as two ends of a continuum. The term **naturalness** designates two sound aspects: (1) the relative simplicity of a sound production and (2) its high frequency of occurrence in languages. In other words, more natural sounds are those that are considered easier to produce and occur in many languages. **Markedness** on the other hand, refers to sounds that are relatively more difficult to produce and are found less frequently in languages (Hyman, 1975). For example, [p] is considered a natural sound. It is easy to produce and occurs in many languages around the world. The affricate [tʃ], though, is a marked sound: it is relatively more difficult to produce and is found infrequently in other languages.

The notion of markedness was first developed by the Prague School but has been elaborated on and applied to several different contexts. Markedness and naturalness theories also continue to play a central role in generative and natural phonologies. Therefore, they will be discussed in more detail in the section on generative phonology.

To summarize, specific analysis procedures and therapeutic approaches have been developed based on distinctive feature theory. The assessment results support contemporary attempts to examine the phoneme and its language-specific function as well as to detect patterns of errors in disordered speech. Although the theoretical construct appears solid, several authors have questioned its applicability to the assessment and treatment of phonological disorders.

GENERATIVE PHONOLOGY

What Is Generative Phonology?

Generative phonology represents a substantial departure from previous phonological theories. Pregenerative theories of phonology, that is, those occurring prior to generative phonology (e.g., Jakobson and Halle, 1956; Jakobson, Fant, and Halle, 1952), distinguished between phonetic and phonemic levels of realization. However, both the phonetic and phonemic levels of pregenerative theories were utilized by analyzing the actual productions, the concrete realizations, of speech—for example, by using tape recordings of different language samples to analyze the systems. Thus, pregenerative theories were developed around the *surface forms,* the actualities of speech production. Generative phonologies expanded this concept decisively to include what has been called the underlying form. The **underlying form** is a purely theoretical concept that is thought to represent a mental reality behind the way people use language (Crystal, 1987). Underlying forms exemplify the person's language competency as one aspect of his cognitive capacity. The underlying forms also serve as points of orientation to describe regularities of speech reality as they relate to other areas of language, notably morphology and syntax.

Generative phonology, then, assumes two levels of sound representation, an abstract underlying form called *phonological representation* and its modified surface form, the *phonetic representation.* Generative phonological theory is concerned with the various kinds of abstract, underlying representations that are necessary to explain the range and distribution of phonetic features establishing phoneme values in languages. **Phonological rules** are used to demonstrate the relationship between the underlying (phonological) and the surface (phonetic) forms.

How Does Generative Phonology Work?

Distinctive features are central to the concept of generative phonology. *Phonological rules* explain the differences between phonological and phonetic representations. These rules are usually stated in a formalized notation system. When compared to earlier theoretical constructs, both the distinctive features and phonological rules of generative phonology contain distinctions that are important to the understanding of this theory and its application.

Generative Distinctive Features. The first accounts of a generative distinctive feature theory were presented by Noam Chomsky (1957) and Chomsky and Morris Halle (1968). Chomsky and Halle's (1968) The Sound Pattern of English is often cited as the major work in this area. They developed a new set of distinctive features which were different from those proposed by Jakobson and Halle (1956). In The Sound Pattern of English, the authors describe five features which are able to establish and distinguish between phonemes: (1) major class features, (2) cavity features, (3) manner of articulation features, (4) source features, and (5) prosodic features.

The *major class features* characterize, and distinguish between, three sound production possibilities that result in different basic sound classes:

1. *Sonorant.* "Open" vocal tract configuration promoting voicing. American English vowels, glides, nasals, and liquids belong to this category.
2. *Consonantal.* Sounds produced with a high degree of oral obstruction, such as stops, fricatives, affricates, and nasals.
3. *Vocalic.* Sounds produced with a low degree of oral obstruction (not higher than required for the high vowels [i] and [u]), such as vowels and liquids.

Cavity features refer to organ and/or place of articulation:

1. *Coronal.* Sounds produced with the apical/predorsal portion of the tongue ("the

blade of the tongue raised from its neutral position," Chomsky/Halle, 1968, p. 304). This cavity feature marks [d], [t], [n], and [l], for example.

2. *Anterior.* Sounds produced in the frontal region of the oral cavity with the alveolar ridge being the posterior border, that is, labial, dental, and alveolar consonants. [m],[n], [b], [p], [d], and [t] are examples.

3. *Distributed.* Sounds with a relatively long oral-sagittal constriction, such as [ʃ], [s], and [z].

4. *Nasal.* Sounds produced with an open nasal passageway—exemplified by the nasals [m], [n], and [ŋ].

5. *Lateral.* Sounds produced with lowered lateral rim portions of the tongue (uni- or bilateral). The only American English example is [l].

6. *High.* Sounds produced with a high tongue position, vowels as well as consonants. Thus, [i], [u], [k], and [ŋ] would be [+ high].

7. *Low.* Vowels produced with a low tongue position—[ɑ], for example. The only consonants qualifying for this category are [h], [ʔ], and pharyngeal sounds. The latter are produced with the root of the tongue as organ of articulation.

8. *Back.* Vowels and consonants produced with a retracted body of the tongue, that is, back vowels and velar and pharyngeal consonants.

9. *Round.* Refers to the rounding of the lips for the production of vowels and consonants. [u] and [w] are [+ round].

Manner of articulation features specify the way organ and place of articulation cooperate to produce sound classes, signalling production differences between stops and fricatives, for example:

1. *Continuant.* "Incessant" sounds produced without hindering the airstream by any blockages within the oral cavity. Vowels, fricatives, glides, and liquids are [+ con-

tinuant]; stops, nasals, and affricates are [– continuant].

2. *Delayed release.* Refers to sounds produced with a slow release of a total obstruction within the oral cavity. Affricates such as [tʃ] and [dʒ] are examples.

3. *Tense.* Consonants and vowels produced with a relatively greater articulatory effort (muscle tension, expiratory air pressure). [p], [t], [k], [i], and [u], for example, are [+ tense]. [b], [d], [g], [ɪ], and [ʊ], by comparison, are [– tense].

Source features refer to subglottal air pressure, voicing, and stridency:

1. *Heightened subglottal pressure.* American English voiceless aspirated stops ([p], [t], [k]) are [+ HSP] because their production requires an added amount of expiratory airflow which, after freely passing the glottis, accumulates behind the occlusion within the oral cavity.

2. *Voiced.* Produced with simultaneous vocal fold vibration. All American English vowels, glides, liquids, nasals, and voiced stops, fricatives, and affricates are [+ voiced]. [p], [t], [k], [f], [s], and [ʃ], by contrast, are [– voiced].

3. *Strident.* The "strident" noise component of American English voiceless and voiced fricatives and affricates, for example, are [+ strident]. However, the interdental fricatives [θ] and [ð] are [– strident].

Prosodic features are named but not discussed in Chomsky and Halle (1968). To see how all these distinctive features apply to General American English vowels and consonants, see Tables 4.2 and 4.3.

Generative Phonological Rules. Generative phonology is an attempt to understand and explain the sound patterns of languages. Inherent in this theory is the idea that a phonological description is dependent on information from other linguistic levels. For

TABLE 4.2 General American English Consonant Matrix According to the Chomsky and Halle (1968) Distinctive Features

	p	b	t	d	k	g	θ	ð	f	v	s	z	ʃ	ʒ	tʃ	dʒ	m	n	ŋ	r	l	w	j	h
Sonorant	−	−	−	−	−	−	−	−	−	−	−	−	−	−	−	−	+	+	+	+	+	+	+	+
Consonantal	+	+	+	+	+	+	+	+	+	+	+	+	+	+	+	+	+	+	+	+	+	−	−	−
Vocalic	−	−	−	−	−	−	−	−	−	−	−	−	−	−	−	−	−	−	−	+	+	−	−	−
Coronal	−	−	+	+	−	−	+	+	−	−	+	+	+	+	+	+	−	+	−	+	+	−	−	−
Anterior	+	+	+	+	−	−	+	+	+	+	+	+	−	−	−	−	+	+	−	−	+	−	−	−
Nasal	−	−	−	−	−	−	−	−	−	−	−	−	−	−	−	−	+	+	+	−	−	−	−	−
Lateral	−	−	−	−	−	−	−	−	−	−	−	−	−	−	−	−	−	−	−	−	+	−	−	−
High	−	−	−	−	+	+	−	−	−	−	−	−	+	+	+	+	−	−	+	−	−	+	+	−
Low	−	−	−	−	−	−	−	−	−	−	−	−	−	−	−	−	−	−	−	−	−	−	−	+
Back	−	−	−	−	+	+	−	−	−	−	−	−	−	−	−	−	−	−	+	−	−	+	−	−
Round	−	−	−	−	−	−	−	−	−	−	−	−	−	−	−	−	−	−	−	−	−	+	−	−
Continuant	−	−	−	−	−	−	+	+	+	+	+	+	+	+	−	−	−	−	−	+	+	+	+	+
Del. Release	−	−	−	−	−	−	−	−	−	−	−	−	−	−	+	+	−	−	−	−	−	−	−	−
Voiced	−	+	−	+	−	+	−	+	−	+	−	+	−	+	−	+	+	+	+	+	+	+	+	−
Strident	−	−	−	−	−	−	−	−	+	+	+	+	+	+	+	+	−	−	−	−	−	−	−	−

example, morphological and syntactic levels influence phonological descriptions. Consider the following sound changes that occur when a derivational morpheme is added:

"noble" [noᵛbəl] "nobility" [noᵛbɪləti]
"mobil" [moᵛbəl] "mobility" [moᵛbɪləti]

In each case, a characteristic change occurs. The primary stress changes from the first to the second syllable and the schwa vowel [ə], which was originally the vowel nucleus of the second syllable, becomes [ɪ]. Other morphological changes cause alterations in both the vowels and the consonants of the original

TABLE 4.3 General American English Vowel Matrix According to the Chomsky and Halle (1968) Distinctive Features

	i	ɪ	e	ɛ	æ	ɑ	ɔ	o	ʊ	u	ʌ
Consonantal	−	−	−	−	−	−	−	−	−	−	−
Vocalic	+	+	+	+	+	+	+	+	+	+	+
Coronal	−	−	−	−	−	−	−	−	−	−	−
Anterior	−	−	−	−	−	−	−	−	−	−	−
High	+	+	−	−	−	−	−	−	+	+	−
Low	−	−	−	−	+	+	+	−	−	−	−
Back	−	−	−	−	−	+	+	+	+	+	+
Round	−	−	−	−	−	−	+	+	+	+	−
Tense	+	−	+	−	−	+	−	+	−	+	−

word. Examples include national → nationality, and rational → rationality or electric → electricity, and plastic → plasticity. The word root always undergoes specific changes in the presence of some suffixes. How is this related to the underlying phonological representations and the surface-level phonetic representation? Generative phonologists would hypothesize that there is an underlying phonological representation of the lexeme, or word root. Certain phonological rules operate on this underlying representation to establish the different surface-level phonetic representations when specific morphemes are used. Phonological rules describe the differences in sound patterns that occur between the underlying phonological representation of the lexeme and the surface-level phonetic reality. One phonological rule might state that if a morphological ending is added which changes the stress on that syllable, the vowel nucleus will change in quality. Phonological rules are attempts to establish certain relationships between underlying and surface-level sound representations.

Phonological rules are also used to describe pronunciation patterns that are not related to morphological changes. For example, phonological rules could be developed to describe the contexts in which voiceless stops are typically aspirated versus those in which they are not. Or, phonological rules could be generated to account for final consonant devoicing or the changes that might occur when /t/ is realized intervocalically (*Pete* [pit] versus *Peter* [piɾɚ]). Although not originally intended to serve such a purpose, phonological rules can also be used to describe the sound patterns of children with disordered phonological systems. In each case, an abstract underlying representation of distinctive features is assumed and certain phonological rules are then generated to account for the surface-level phonetic realization.

Phonological rules use the following notation:

A → B
This indicates that A becomes B; → indicates "becomes" or "changes to."

Using the previous example of *Pete* and *Peter*, this notation would be used:

[t] → [ɾ]
aspirated [t] becomes the flap [ɾ].

Next, the context or environment must be considered. The following notation system is used to indicate various contexts:

/
/ indicates "in the environment of" or "in the context of."

A → B/
A becomes or changes to B in the environment of...

[t] → [ɾ]/
[t] becomes or changes to [ɾ] in the environment of...

The specific context in which the change occurs is now described:

___
The blank ___ indicates the location of the changed segment.

#___
Changes that occur word-initially.

___#
Changes that occur word-finally.

V ___ V
Changes that occur intervocalically.

A → B/V ___ V
A becomes B in the environment of an intervocalic production.

[t] → [ɾ]/V ___ V
[t] becomes [ɾ] in the environment of an intervocalic production.

Many other notations are used. A few examples include:

ø
  Indicates the deletion of a segment.

[t] → ø/ ___#
  [t] is deleted word-finally.

C
  Indicates a consonant segment; may be represented by the symbol for the individual sound segment.

C → ø/ ___#
  Consonants become deleted word-finally.

CC(C)
  ( ) indicate that a segment may be optional.

CC(C) → C/#___
  Two- or three-member consonant clusters are reduced to one consonant word-initially.

When formulating phonological rules, distinctive features are often employed, allowing segments to be grouped into natural classes. **Natural classes** are phonemes that share one or more features and usually have similar patterns within a language system (Grunwell, 1987). The following distinctive feature notation could be used to describe the pattern that final voiced consonants have a tendency to be devoiced at the end of a word:

$$\begin{bmatrix} + \text{consonantal} \\ + \text{voice} \end{bmatrix} \rightarrow \begin{bmatrix} + \text{consonantal} \\ - \text{voice} \end{bmatrix} \Big/ \underline{\hspace{1em}} \#$$

Distinctive features are placed in a column and within brackets.

In summary, phonological rules describe changes that occur from the underlying phonological representation to the surface-level phonetic realization. Phonological rules are stated according to a specialized notation system. Distinctive features are a portion of this notation system. Distinctive features group phonemes according to natural classes which often function similarly in a particular language. Thus, distinctive features are helpful when attempting to describe patterns of sound changes.

Generative Markedness. The concept of markedness is another central aspect of generative phonology. As previously mentioned, unmarked sounds have two attributes: (1) they are acquired earlier in the speech of children, and (2) they are more universal, that is, they occur more frequently in languages around the world. Their early acquisition implies that more natural (= unmarked) sounds are "easier" to produce. For example, the nasal /n/ is a clearly natural segment. It is acquired early by children and appears in the inventory of most languages.

Marked and unmarked features are used when referring to cognate pairs, such as /t/ and /d/, and sound classes, such as nasals. Sloat, Taylor, and Hoard (1978) describe the following sounds and sound classes according to markedness parameters:

Voiceless obstruents are more natural (unmarked) than voiced obstruents.

Obstruents are more natural (unmarked) than sonorants.

> Obstruents include the stops, fricatives, and the affricates. See Chapter 2 for a more complete definition.

Stops are more natural (unmarked) than fricatives.

Fricatives are more natural (unmarked) than affricates.

Low front vowels appear to be the most natural (unmarked) vowels.

Close-tense vowels are more natural (unmarked) than open-lax vowels.

Anterior consonants are more natural (unmarked) than nonanterior consonants.

Consonants without secondary articulation are more natural (unmarked) than those with secondary articulation (such as simultaneous lip rounding).

Determining markedness in detail is a highly complex and difficult matter. This led Chomsky and Halle (1968) to develop a set of *marking conventions.* These marking conventions attempted to deal with the degree of markedness of consonants and vowels. Subsequent work in this area has been limited; however, newer models (Dinnsen, 1996; 1997; Dinnsen and Chin, 1993) postulate that markedness may be an important determinant in the acquisition process.

How Did Generative Phonology Develop?

Generative phonology represents the applications of principles of generative (or transformational) grammar to phonology. The concept of generative grammar was first introduced by Noam Chomsky in 1957 in a book titled *Syntactic Structures.* Generative grammar departed radically from structuralistic and behavioristic approaches to grammar, which dominated linguistic thought during the decades before Chomsky's work. Prior to the introduction of generative grammar, linguists had analyzed the surface forms of sentences into their constituent parts. This type of analysis was found to be inadequate in various respects. An often-used example illustrates this point:

> John is eager to please.
> John is easy to please.

If the two sentences are analyzed according to a structuralistic point of view, the results will indicate that both sentences have exactly the same structure. However, this analysis does not reveal that the two sentences have drastically different meanings. In the first sentence, John wants to please someone else—John is

the subject of pleasing. In the second sentence, someone else is involved in pleasing John—John is the object of pleasing.

One aim of generative grammar was to provide a way to analyze sentences that would account for such differences. To do this, a concept was developed that postulated not only a *surface* level of realization but also a *deep* level of representation. *Competence* and *performance* were also terms that distinguished between surface and deep levels of representation. Language competence was viewed as the individual's knowledge of the rules of a language, while performance was actual language use in real situations. Structuralists and behaviorists had focused on an individual's performance; generative grammar shifted this focus to include the concept of an individual's language competence. The formulation of rules governing the events between the deep-level competence and surface-level performance was an important goal for generative grammarians.

A description of these rules was not limited to a particular language. A grammar was sought that would be capable of evaluating not only individual languages but also of contributing to an understanding of the nature of human language as a whole. Such "linguistic universals" would in turn advance our understanding of the human mind.

Generative Phonology: Clinical Implications

Generative phonology was originally developed to analyze the phonological systems of languages. Its application to phonological development in children has its foundation in Smith's (1973) case study of his son Amahl. Other authors (e.g., Compton, 1975, 1976; Grunwell, 1975; Lorentz, 1976; Oller, 1973) extended these analysis principles to children with disordered phonological systems. Generative phonology, applied in this manner, compares the child's phonological system to the adult's. Phonological rules thus become formalized statements of the patterns of sound substitutions and deletions. For example, a child might demonstrate the following errors:

"coat"	[koʊ]	"window"	[wɪ doʊ]
"bed"	[bɛ]	"monkey"	[mʌ ki]
"house"	[haʊ]		

This child deletes consonants at the ends of words (*coat, bed, house*) and within words before another consonant (*window, monkey*). The following phonological rule states the *deletion* pattern for this context.

$$C \rightarrow \emptyset \,/ \begin{bmatrix} \underline{\quad} \,\# \\ \underline{\quad} + \text{cons} \\ - \text{voc} \end{bmatrix}$$

The top rule applies to the deletion of consonants word-finally, while the bottom rule depicts the deletion of consonants within a word before a consonant.

The following examples are given for sound substitutions:

"soap"	[toʊp]
"kiss"	[kɪt]
"zoo"	[du]
"nose"	[noʊd]

Chomsky's current grammatical theory (1982, 1988) is known as government and binding theory. Although it has its roots in generative transformational grammar, government and binding theory attempts to include descriptions of the constraints in language patterns. Thus, phrase structure rules and lexical insertion rules are formulated to account for the permissible structures of phrases and the placement restrictions of lexical items in phrases. Language learnability is also considered within this theory. One of the tasks of a language-learning child is to derive meaning from ambiguous surface-level structures. Government and binding theory attempts to explain how this can be achieved.

This child's speech is characterized by t/s (s → t) and d/z (z → d) substitutions. Using distinctive features, the following phonological rule for sound *substitutions* could be generated:

$$\begin{bmatrix} + \text{cons} \\ + \text{cor} \\ + \text{ant} \\ + \text{cont} \\ + \text{strid} \end{bmatrix} \rightarrow \begin{bmatrix} + \text{cons} \\ + \text{cor} \\ + \text{ant} \\ - \text{cont} \\ - \text{strid} \end{bmatrix} \Big/ \begin{matrix} \underline{\quad}\# \\ \#\underline{\quad} \end{matrix}$$

Often, only the specifications of the changed feature are used on the "output" side of the rule, implying that all other features are the same. Therefore, this rule could be presented in the following simplified manner:

$$\begin{bmatrix} + \text{cons} \\ + \text{cor} \\ + \text{ant} \\ + \text{cont} \\ + \text{strid} \end{bmatrix} \rightarrow \begin{bmatrix} - \text{cont} \\ - \text{strid} \end{bmatrix} \Big/ \begin{matrix} \underline{\quad}\# \\ \#\underline{\quad} \end{matrix}$$

Generative phonological rules are not widely used in clinical assessments to describe patterns of errors produced by children. This may have to do with the relatively complex notational system or with the fact that the whole concept of distinctive features has receded somewhat under the influence of phonological process analysis.

CLINICAL APPLICATION

Simplicity in Generative Phonological Rules

The following words were a portion of a sample from Ralph, age 5;9:

"spin"	→	[bɪn]	"snow"	→	[noʊ]
"star"	→	[dɑr]	"skate"	→	[geɪt]
"sled"	→	[wɛd]	"swing"	→	[swɪŋ]
"spoon"	→	[bun]	"skunk"	→	[gʌŋk]
"smoke"	→	[moʊk]	"slip"	→	[wɪp]
"sweet"	→	[swit]	"slide"	→	[waɪd]

These various consonant cluster substitutions and omissions can be summarized by the following generative phonological rules:

1. s + [+nasal]   → [+ nasal]   / #___

2. s + −continuant   → − continuant
   − nasal   − nasal   / #___
   − voice   + voice

3. s + + sonorant   + sonorant
   + continuant → + continuant   / #___
   + vocalic   − vocalic
   − consonantal

Rule 1 describes the deletion of [s] preceding nasals, as in *smoke* and *snow*. Rule 2 describes the deletion of [s] and the corresponding change from a voiceless to a voiced stop-plosive demonstrated in *skate* and *spoon*. Rule 3 describes the deletion of [s] and the change from a liquid to a glide production in *slide* and *sled*.

The concept of naturalness versus markedness became a relevant clinical issue when it was observed that children with phonological disorders have a tendency to substitute more unmarked, natural classes of segments for marked ones. For example, children substituted stops for fricatives and deleted the more marked member of a consonant cluster (Ingram, 1989b). Although the results of at least one investigation demonstrated contrary findings (McReynolds, Engmann, and Dimmitt, 1974), most investigations supported the notion that children and adults with speech disorders more frequently showed a change from marked segments to unmarked substitutions (Blumstein, 1973; Klich, Ireland, and Weidner, 1979; Marquardt, Reinhart, and Peterson, 1979; Toombs, Singh, and Hayden, 1981; Williams, Cairns, Cairns, and Blosser, 1970; Wolk, 1986).

Newer theoretical models (Dinnsen, 1997) suggest that markedness may be an important aspect in feature acquisition of children. However, some believe that this highly complex, theoretical construct may not be fully applicable to clinical reality. Grunwell (1987), for example, states that "The theory of markedness…is not fully developed, and this must be borne in mind in evaluating the findings" (p. 152). Further research into the applicability of markedness and naturalness theories to the speech disorders of children and adults will be necessary before any definitive conclusions can be drawn.

In summary, generative phonology, as an outgrowth of generative grammar, has had a major impact on the field of linguistics and the understanding of phonology. A central aspect of this construct pertains to phonological rules, which can also be used to describe the irregular productions of children. A theory of markedness offers insight into the acquisition of sound features and, possibly, the type of substitutions that may be seen in the speech of children with disordered phonological systems. This generative phonological model has laid the foundation for other phonological theories. The theory of natural phonology, for example, also has its basis in generative phonology.

NATURAL PHONOLOGY

What Is Natural Phonology?

"[Natural phonology] is a natural theory…in that it presents language as a natural reflection of the needs, capacities, and world of its users, rather than as a merely conventional institution" (Donegan and Stampe, 1979, p. 127). **Natural phonology** incorporates features of naturalness theories and was specifically designed to explain the development of the child's phonological system. The theory of natural phonology postulates that patterns of speech are governed by an innate, universal set of phonological processes. "A **phonological process** is a mental operation that applies in speech to substitute for a class of sounds or sound sequences presenting a common difficulty to the speech capacity of the individual" (Stampe, 1979, p. 1). Phonological processes are innate and universal; therefore, all children are born with the capacity to use the same system of processes. Phonological processes, as natural processes, are easier for the child to produce and are substituted for sounds, sound classes, or sound sequences when the child's motor capacities do not yet allow their norm realization. These innate, universal natural phonological processes are operating as all children attempt to use and organize their phonological systems. Therefore, all children begin with innate speech patterns but must progress to the language-specific system that characterizes their native language. Phonological processes are used to constantly revise existing differences between the innate patterns and the adult norm production. The theory points out prominent *developmental steps* children go through until the goal of adult phonology is reached in the child's adolescent years. Disordered phonology is seen as an inability to realize this "natural" process of goal-oriented adaptive change.

How Does Natural Phonology Work?

The theory of natural phonology assumes that the child's innate phonological system is continuously revised in the direction of the adult phonological system. Stampe (1969) proposed three mechanisms to account for these changes: (1) limitation, (2) ordering, and (3) suppression. These mechanisms reflect properties of the innate phonological system as well as the universal difficulties children display in the acquisition of the adult sound system.

Limitation occurs when differences between the child's and the adult's system become *limited* to only specific sounds, sound

classes, or sound sequences. It represents a step in the developmental process as children revise the innate system they are born with to accomodate the adult phonological system. Limitation can be exemplified by the following: A child might first use a more "natural" sound for a more marked one. For example, all fricatives might be replaced by homorganic stops (e.g., [f] → [p], [θ] → [t], [s] → [t]). Later, this global substitution of all fricatives by stops might become *limited* to sibilant fricatives only.

Ordering occurs when substitutions that appeared unordered and random become more organized. This mechanism represents another recognizable step in the gradual revision of the phonological system from its innate stage to the adult standard. Ordering can be exemplified by the following: A child's first revisions may appear unordered. To stay with the stop for sibilant example, a child might at first also devoice the voiced stops of the substitution ([s] → [t], [z] → [t]). Thus, *Sue* is pronounced as [tu], but *zoo* is also articulated as [tu]. Later, the child might begin to "order" the revisions by not devoicing initial voiced stops any longer while retaining the stop substitution. Now *Sue* is [tu] and *zoo* is [du].

The term **suppression** refers to the abolishment of one or more phonological processes as children move from the innate speech patterns to the adult norm production. *Suppression* can be exemplified by the following: Voiced obstruents are less "natural," more "marked" than voiceless obstruents. As one example, voiced stops are less natural than voiceless ones. Therefore, a child may substitute a voiceless, more natural stop for a voiced one: *hid* becomes [hɪt]; *pig* becomes [pɪk]. This phonological process is referred to as devoicing. As one stage in the development of the child's speech, the child begins to use the voiced stop; thus *hid* is now pronounced [hɪd] and *pig* [pɪg]: the phonological process of devoicing is suppressed, that is, not used any longer.

According to Stampe (1979), all children embark on the development of their phonological systems from the same beginnings. Stampe sees children as possessing a full understanding of the underlying representation of the adult phoneme system: that is, from the very beginning, the child's perceptual understanding of the phonemic system mirrors the adult's. Children just have difficulties with the peripheral, motor realization of the phonetic surface form. Many authors have questioned the validity of this idea (e.g., Fey, 1992; Oller, Jensen, and Lafayette, 1978; Stoel-Gammon and Dunn, 1985). In addition, Stampe's account of phonological development presents children as passively suppressing these phonological processes. Other contemporary authors, notably Kiparsky and Menn (1977), see children as being far more actively involved in the development of their phonological systems.

In spite of such shortcomings, Edwards (1992) states that "it is not necessary to totally discard the notion of phonological processes just because we may not agree with all aspects of Stampe's theory of Natural Phonology, such as his view that phonological processes are 'innate' and his assumption that children's underlying representations are basically equivalent to the broad adult surface forms" (p. 234). Phonological process analysis has found widespread clinical utilization, although it is used not so much to *explain* developmental speech events, as was the original intent of natural phonologists, as to *describe* the deviations noted in the speech of children.

Because phonological processes are so central to the workings of natural phonology, and to its clinical application, some of the more common processes are listed here with some explanatory remarks.

Phonological Processes

Although many different processes have been identified in the speech of normally developing children and of those with phonological disorders, only a few occur with any regularity. Those processes that are common in the speech development of children across languages are called **natural processes.**

Phonological processes are categorized as syllable structure processes, substitution processes, or assimilatory processes. **Syllable structure** processes describe those sound changes that affect the structure of the syllable. **Substitution processes** describe those sound changes in which one sound class is replaced by another. **Assimilatory processes** describe changes in which a sound becomes similar to, or is influenced by, a neighboring sound of an utterance.

Syllable Structure Processes

Cluster reduction. The articulatory simplification of consonant clusters into a single consonant, typically the more "natural" member of the cluster.

Example: [pun] for *spoon.*

Reduplication. This process is considered a syllable structure process because the syllable structure is "simplified," that is, the second syllable becomes merely a repetition of the first. Total reduplication refers to the exact reduplication of the first syllable. In partial reduplication, the vowel in the second syllable is varied (Ingram, 1976).

Example:

Total reduplication: [wɑwɑ] for *water.*
Partial reduplication: [babi] for *blanket.*

Weak syllable deletion. The omission of an unstressed syllable.

Example: [nænə] for *baˈnana.*

Final consonant deletion. The omission of a syllable-arresting consonant.

Example: [hɛ] for *head.*

Substitution Processes

Consonant cluster substitution. The replacement of one member of a cluster.

Example: [stwit] for *street.*

Note: This is additionally referred to as gliding to indicate the specific type of substitution.

Changes in Organ or Place of Articulation

Fronting. Sound substitutions in which the organ and/or place of articulation are more anteriorly located than the intended sound. Prominent types include *velar fronting* (t/k substitution) and *palatal fronting* (s/ʃ substitution).

Examples: [ti] for *key;* [su] for *shoe.*

Labialization. The replacement of a nonlabial sound by a labial one.

Example: [fʌm] for *thumb.*

Alveolarization. The change of nonalveolar sounds, mostly interdental and labio-dental sounds, into alveolar ones.

Example: [sʌm] for *thumb.*

Changes in Manner of Articulation

Stopping. The substitution of stops for fricatives or the omission of the fricative portion of affricates.

Examples: [tʌn] for *sun;* [dus] for *juice.*

Affrication. The replacement of fricatives by homorganic affricates.

Example: [tʃu] for *shoe.*

Deaffrication. The production of affricates as homorganic fricatives.

Example: [ʃiz] for *cheese.*

Denasalization. The replacement of nasals by homorganic stops.

Example: [dud] for *noon.*

Gliding of liquids/fricatives. The replacement of liquids or fricatives by glides.

Examples: [wɛd] for *red;* [ju] for *shoe.*

Vowelization (vocalization). The replacement of syllabic liquids and nasals, foremost [l], [ɚ], and [n], by vowels.

Examples: [teˈbo] for *table;* [lædʊ] for *ladder.*

Derhotacization. The loss of r-coloring in rhotics [r] and central vowels with r-coloring, [ɝ] and [ɚ].

Examples: [ɹɛd] for *red,* [lædə] for *ladder.*

Changes in Voicing

Voicing. The replacement of a voiced for a voiceless sound.

Example: [du] for *two.*

Devoicing. The replacement of a voiceless for a voiced sound.

Example: [pit] for *beet.*

Assimilatory Processes (Harmony Processes)

Labial assimilation. The change of a nonlabial into a labial sound under the influence of a neighboring labial sound.

Example: [fwɪŋ] for *swing.*

> Assimilation processes can also be classified according to the type and degree of the assimilatory changes. For definitions and examples, see Sounds in Context: Coarticulation and Assimilation in Chapter 2.

Velar assimilation. The change of a nonvelar into a velar sound under the influence of a neighboring velar sound.

Example: [gɑg] for *dog.*

Nasal assimilation. The influence of a nasal on a nonnasal sound.

Example: [mʌni] for *bunny.*

Note: The place of articulation is retained; only the manner is changed.

Liquid assimilation. The influence of a liquid on a nonliquid sound.

Example: [lɛloᵊ] for *yellow.*

According to natural phonology, phonological processes are recognizable steps in the gradual articulatory adjustment of children's speech to the adult norm. This implies a chronology of phonological processes, that is, specific ages at which the process could be operating and when the process should be suppressed (Grunwell, 1981, 1987; Vihman, 1984). As useful as a chronology of normative data might seem for clinical purposes, tables of established age norms can easily be misleading. Individual variation and contextual conditions may play a large role in the use and suppression of phonological processes.

> Ages of suppression of the various processes are discussed in Chapter 5.

To summarize, natural phonologists assume an innate phonological system which is progressively revised during childhood until it corresponds with the adult phonological output. Limitation, ordering, and suppression are the mechanisms for the revisions that manifest themselves in phonological processes. Phonological processes are developmentally conditioned simplifications in the realization of the phonological system in question. As these simplifications are gradually overcome the phonological processes become suppressed.

How Did Natural Phonology Develop?

David Stampe introduced natural phonology in 1969. However, several of its basic concepts had been established considerably earlier, most prominent among them being the concepts of naturalness (markedness) and underlying and surface forms, which are important aspects of generative phonology.

Jakobson (1942/1968) extended the concept of naturalness and markedness to *implied universals,* which could be found in different languages, children's acquisition of speech, and the deterioration of speech in aphasics. These universals were even used as a predictive device. Some examples include "fricatives imply stops" and "voiced stops imply voiceless stops." These examples would mean that if a language has fricatives, that language will have stops as well and if a language has voiced stops in its inventory, the language will also have voiceless stops. Applying these two examples to children's acquisition of speech, children will acquire stops before (homorganic) fricatives. Also, voiceless stops are acquired before their voiced cognates. In an aphasic condition, the breakdown of speech would be characterized by the loss of the later-acquired sounds before the earlier-acquired ones. Thus, aphasics would lose fricatives before (homorganic) stops and voiced stops before voiceless ones. Whether these universal "laws" are generally valid under all of the above-mentioned conditions has been repeatedly questioned. However, they clearly exemplify the concepts of naturalness and markedness as universal phenomena.

Markedness theory also plays a central role in generative phonology (see Chapter 9 of Chomsky and Halle, 1968). According to generative phonologists, markedness values are considered to be universal and innate. Thus, Jakobson, with his concept of universal naturalness, and Chomsky and Halle, with their understanding of universal and innate naturalness, set the stage for Stampe's natural phonology. Stampe incorporated the conceptual framework of naturalness, which was considered to be universal and innate, into his theory of natural phonology.

At the same time, the meaning and use of the term *underlying form* changed drastically as it was incorpotated into natural phonology. Within generative grammar, underlying forms, lexical as well as phonological, are highly abstract entities. They represent *assumed points of reference* that are necessary for the explanation of the many possible surface forms. In contrast, within the context of natural phonology, underlying forms as "models" for surface realizations suddenly gain some concrete reality. The underlying form is *the adult norm* that is the intended goal for children's production efforts.

Natural Phonology: Clinical Implications

The phonological processes concept at the center of natural phonology has impacted both the assessment and the treatment of disordered phonological systems. Assessment procedures using phonological processes consist of contrasting the target word to the child's production. Aberrant productions are identified and labelled according to the phonological process that most closely matches the sound change. Typically, the processes are listed and the frequency of occurrence of individual processes is noted. Frequency of occurrence and the relative age of suppression play a role in targeting a process or processes for therapy. Depending on the age of the child, more frequent processes that should have been suppressed are commonly targeted for therapy. Some authors (Hodson and Paden, 1991; McReynolds and Elbert, 1981) suggest that a process should occur a certain number of times in order for it to be considered a possibility for therapy.

Unlike other analysis procedures, phonological processes can account for changes in syllable or word structures and those due to assimilations. Although phonological processes are not commonly used to identify sound distortions, they could be. For example, [ʂ] could be labelled fronting and [ʂ] backing.

In addition to the phonological processes earlier identified and exemplified, many other phonological processes have been found in the speech of children with *phonological disorders.* The speech of children with disordered phonological systems often contains phonological processes different from those noted in the speech of normally developing children.

CLINICAL APPLICATION

Idiosyncratic Processes Found in the Speech of Children with Phonological Disorders

The following are a few examples of the relatively uncommon processes that have been found in the speech of children with phonological disorders:

Process	Example			
Initial consonant deletion	"duck"	[dʌk]	→	[ʌk]
Backing of stops	"tub"	[tʌb]	→	[kʌb]
Backing of fricatives	"sun"	[sʌn]	→	[ʃʌn]
Glottal replacement	"gun"	[gʌn]	→	[ʔʌn]
Denasalization	"knee"	[ni]	→	[di]

Process	Example		
Fricatives replacing stops	"toe"	[toʊ]	→	[soʊ]
Stops replacing glides	"yarn"	[jɑrn]	→	[dɑrn]
Metathesis (reversal of two sounds)	"nest"	[nɛst]	→	[nɛts]
Affrication (a nonaffricate becomes an affricate)	"top"	[tɑp]	→	[tʃɑp]
Migration (movement of a sound from one position in the word to another position)	"soap"	[soʊp]	→	[oʊps]
Unusual cluster reduction	"plane"	[pleɪn]	→	[leɪn]
Unusual substitution processes	"plane"	[pleɪn]	→	[reɪn]
Vowel processes, for example, centralization of vowels	"bed"	[bɛd]	→	[bʌd]

Source: Bauman-Waengler and Waengler (1988, 1990), Dodd and Iacano (1989), Leonard and McGregor (1991), Roberts, Burchinal, and Footo (1990), Stoel-Gammon and Dunn (1985), Waengler and Bauman-Waengler (1989).

Children with phonological disorders use these processes in their speech somewhat differently than do normally developing children. Grunwell (1987) provides five different classifications to account for these differences: (1) persisting normal processes, (2) chronological mismatch, (3) systematic sound preference, (4) unusual/ idiosyncratic processes, and (5) variable use of processes.

Persisting normal processes are exemplified by the child who makes active use of commonly noted phonological processes but beyond the age at which they are typically seen. Thus, a 4-year-old child demonstrating very early processes, such as reduplication or final consonant deletion, might be considered within this category.

Chronological mismatch is evidenced by a child who demonstrates the persistence of early simplifying processes together with patterns that are characteristic of later stages of phonological development. For example, a child produces all fricative sounds adequately, implying that a relatively late process, stopping of fricatives, has been effectively suppressed. However, at the same time, the child still demonstrates velar fronting ([k] → [t];

[g] → [d]), which is normally suppressed at an earlier age than stopping of [s] and [z]. This early process, which has not yet been suppressed, co-occurs with later developmental speech patterns.

Systematic sound preference pertains to the use of a single phonetic realization for several different phonemes. This sound preference results when both normal developmental processes and idiosyncratic or unusual processes co-occur. Weiner (1981) notes that sound preferences are often limited to replacements for fricatives and operate primarily in initial word positions. An example of systematic sound preference would be the productions of a child who substitutes [d] for [s], [z], [ʃ], [ʒ], [tʃ], [dʒ], and all initial consonant blends.

Unusual or idiosyncratic processes are characterized by patterns that are uncommon in the speech of normally developing children (unusual processes) or processes that seem to be found only in the speech of individual children with phonological disorders (idiosyncratic processes). Grunwell (1987) suggests that the term *idiosyncratic processes* be used very tentatively because these processes can often be found in the speech of normally developing children as well.

The last category, *variable use of processes* denotes two possibilities: (1) a process operating on one target sound may in one context still be active and in another already suppressed, or (2) depending on the context, different processes may be operating on the same target phoneme. A child who uses stopping, realizing [tup] for *soup* and [tʌn] for *sun*, but demonstrates a norm production of [s] in *soap* and *saw* would be an example of the first possibility. The second possibility, the use of different processes for the same target, would be exemplified by a child who employs velar fronting, pronouncing *cake* as [teɪt] and *wagon* as [wædən]. However, when the same target phonemes /k/ and /g/ occur in other contexts, different processes are noted. For instance, final consonant deletion is evidenced when *bake* is pronounced [beɪ], while glottal realization is used when *Maggie* is articulated as [mæʔi]. The speech of children with phonological disorders is characterized by extreme variability of pronunciation patterns. Often, several different realizations are used to represent one phoneme. The variable use of processes may, therefore, be expected frequently in the speech of children with phonological disorders.

Treatment implications of Stampe's theory of natural phonology include suppression of the phonological processes in order to increase the complexity of the child's phonological patterns. While the suppression of these phonological processes occurs naturally in the speech of normally developing children, for children with phonological disorders, treatment must focus on helping to suppress the age-inappropriate processes as well as processes that are not acceptable for the adult language being learned. Typically, several sounds that demonstrate active use of a specific phonological process are selected.

These sounds are trained in close succession to aid the child in suppressing the phonological process. Therapy emphasizes the meaningful use of speech, and words are seen as the smallest units to be contrasted and practiced.

Phonological processes provide a means of classifying error patterns noted in disordered speech and suggest a direct and simple way to handle intervention. Although these processes have been labelled phonological, they are based to a large extent on phonetic production features. For example, substitution processes are named after the differences between the production of the target and the error sound. Phonological processes do not give concrete information about the neutralization of specific phonemic contrasts, nor do they account for phonological rules that might be operating. Even more important, the presence of phonological processes in the speech of an individual does not necessarily indicate the presence of a phonological disorder. In their contemporary usage, phonological processes are descriptive terms; the existence of a particular process neither explains the problem nor denotes its etiology (Butcher, 1990; Fey 1992; Shriberg and Kwiatkowski, 1983; Weismer, 1984). The practice of using phonological processes to *imply* a phonological disorder has been identified by Kamhi (1992) as being the most serious problem associated with this type of analysis.

To summarize, phonological processes, a central aspect of natural phonology, have been extensively used to describe disordered speech patterns and to select treatment goals. The speech of children with disordered phonological systems may show differences in kind and use of phonological processes when compared to the speech of children with normally developing systems. However, caution should be exercised when descriptions of phonological processes are used to imply the presence of a phonological disorder.

CLINICAL APPLICATION

Using Phonological Processes

Lillian, age 5;6, was screened by the speech-language pathologist in her kindergarten class. The classroom teacher said that Lillian was at times hard to understand. The speech-language pathologist summarized her screening results according to phonological processes:

Process	Example	Total Number of Times Used
Velar fronting	[k] → [t] [kʌp] → [tʌp] [d] → [g] [gʌn] → [dʌn]	14 times, all words tested
Final consonant deletion	[beɪk] → [beɪ] [lɑg] → [lɑ]	5 times, only on words ending with [k] and [g]
Cluster reduction	[klaʊn] → [laʊn] [græs] → [ræs]	5 times, only on words with [k] and [g] clusters

First, the therapist realized that this was a case of chronological mismatch. Lillian had suppressed later processes such as stopping of fricatives; however, she was still using the early process velar fronting. In addition, variable use of processes was noted. When [k] or [g] was produced in the word-initial position, fronting was demonstrated. In the word-final position or in consonant clusters containing [k] or [g], the sounds were deleted.

LINEAR VERSUS NONLINEAR PHONOLOGIES

What Are Linear and Nonlinear Phonologies?

Phonological theories, theories of generative phonology included, were based on the understanding that all speech segments are arranged in a sequential order. Consequently, underlying phonological representations and surface phonetic realizations, too, consisted of a string of discrete elements. For example:

Wow, what a test.   [waʊ wʌt eɪ tɛst]

The sequence of segments in this phrase begins with [w] and ends with [st]. All segments in between follow each other in a specific order to convey a particular message. Such an assumption that all meaning-distinguishing sound segments are serially arranged characterizes all linear phonologies. Linear phonologies, exemplified by distinctive feature theories and early generative phonology, can be characterized as follows:

1. emphasis on the linear, sequential arrangement of sound segments
2. assumption that each discrete segment of this string of sound elements consists of a bundle of distinctive features
3. assumption that a common set of distinctive features is attributable to all sound segments according to a binary + and – system
4. assumption that all sound segments have equal value and all distinctive features are equal; thus, no one sound segment has control over other units
5. the phonological rules generated apply only to the segmental level (as opposed to the suprasegmental level) and to those changes that occur in the distinctive features

However, linear phonologies with sound segments (and their smaller distinguishing constituents) as central analytical units fail to recognize and describe larger linguistic units. Linear phonologies also do not account for the possibility that there could be a hierarchical interaction between segments and other linguistic units. Nonlinear or nonsegmental phonologies attempt to account for these factors.

> *Hierarchy* refers to any system in which elements are ranked one above another.

Nonlinear (or what have been termed **multilinear**) **phonologies** are a group of phonological theories understanding segments as governed by more complex linguistic dimensions. The linear representation of phonemes plays a subordinate role. Segments are seen as being governed by more complex linguistic dimensions, for example, stress, intonation, and metrical and rhythmical linguistic factors. These theories explore the relationships among units of various sizes, specifically the influence of larger linguistic entities on sound segments. Therefore rather than a linear view of equal-valued segments (in a left-to-right horizontal sequence), a hierarchy of factors is hypothesized to affect segmental units. Rather than a static sequence of segments of equal value (as in linear phonology), a dynamic system of features, ranked one above the other, is proposed. For example, syllable structure could affect the segmental level. A child may demonstrate the following pattern:

"man"	[mæn]	"window"	[wɪ doʊ]
"dog"	[dɑg]	"jumping"	[dʒʌ pɪ]
"ball"	[bɑl]	"Christmas tree"	[krɪ mə tri]

This child deletes the final consonant of each syllable in a multisyllabic word; however, no final consonant deletion occurs in one-syllable words. In this example, the number of syllables in a word interacts with and affects the segmental level. The number of syllables has priority over the segmental level: it determines segmental features. Nonlinear phonologies would rank syllable structure above the level of sound segments.

Another factor that may affect the segmental level is stress. Children have a tendency to delete segments in unstressed syllables. The following transcriptions demonstrate this:

baˈnana	→	[ˈnænə]
poˈtato	→	[ˈteɪ toʊ]
ˈtelephone	→	[ˈtɛ foʊn]

In these examples, the syllable stress clearly affects segmental realization; word stress has priority over the segmental level. "Instead of a single, linear representation (one unit followed by another with none having any superiority or control over other units), they [nonlinear phonologies] allow a description of underlying relationships that would permit one level of unit to be governed by another" (Schwartz, 1992b, p. 271).

How Do Nonlinear Phonologies Work?

There are many different types of nonlinear/multilinear phonologies. Several new theories have been advanced, while others have been modified. All nonlinear phonologies are based on a belief in the overriding importance of larger linguistic units influencing, even controlling, the realization of smaller ones. Nonlinear phonologies also attempt to incorporate this hierarchical order of linguistic elements into analytical procedures, using so-called *tiered representations* of features.

To describe the many different nonlinear phonologies is beyond the scope of this book. *The New Phonologies: Developments in Clinical Linguistics* (Ball and Kent, 1997) is an excellent source of more detailed information on autosegmental phonology, feature geometry, underspecification theory, dependency phonology, government phonology, grounded phonology, optimality theory, and gestural phonology.

This section will be restricted to an introduction to nonlinear phonologies exemplified by autosegmental phonology, metrical phonology, and feature geometry theories. These theories are in no way superior to other nonlinear phonologies.

Autosegmental Phonology. Autosegmental phonology was proposed by John Goldsmith in 1976. Originally, Goldsmith presented this theory to account for tone phenomena in languages in which segmental features interact with varying tones. Parker (1994) illustrates the essential problem in the following manner: According to the concept of linear (generative) phonology, features extend throughout a segment. Therefore, a segment such as /p/ is considered to be [– voice] throughout its entire segment, while /u/ is [+ voice] throughout its entirety. However, consider the problem posed by affricates. By definition, an affricate begins like a stop and ends like a fricative. The features that differentiate stops and fricatives are + *and* – continuant. This posed a problem for the linear phonologists because one segment cannot be designated as both + and – one distinctive feature. To solve this problem, the linear phonologists constructed the feature of "delayed release" to designate affricates. However, the feature of delayed release violates the construct of distinctive feature theory in that this property does not extend throughout the entire segment.

Autosegmental phonology proposed that changes within the boundary of a segment could be factored out and put onto another "tier." Thus + and – continuant could be placed on another level to indicate the change within the segment boundary. A dia-

Tone languages, which represent well over half of the languages of the world, are distinguished by their ability to change the meaning of a word simply by changing the pitch level at which it is spoken. Thus, phonemic differences can be signalled by distinctive pitch levels known as tones or tonemes (Crystal, 1987). For example, in Mandarin Chinese, four different tones with the identical sound segments [ma] result in words that mean "mother," "hemp," "horse," and "scold." Autosegmental phonology placed these tones on a tier above the sound segments, demonstrating the overriding importance of these tones for the meaning of the word.

gram of an affricate such as /tʃ/ would look accordingly:

As can be seen, a single segment on one tier can be associated with more than one segment on another tier. Using the example of /tʃ/, the + consonantal segment can be associated with + and – continuant on another tier. In fact, the term *autosegmental* refers to the concept that certain segments are autonomous—they do not have a one-for-one match on another level.

As mentioned earlier, Goldsmith's (1976) dissertation addressed tone phenomena in so-called tone languages. This concept was used to explain *one-to-many mappings* (one tone associated with more than one segment) and *many-to-one mappings* (more than one tone associated with one segment). However, this "tiered" organization can demonstrate many characteristics of children's speech as well—relationships between certain syllable types and production of sound segments, for example.

For an understanding of autosegmental phonology, specific terms need to be defined:

Tiers	Separable and independent levels that represent a sequence of gestures or a unified set of acoustic features.
Association lines	Indicators for connections between autosegments on different tiers. Association lines cannot cross.
Linkage condition	Any condition governing the association of units on each tier. A linkage condition states, for instance, that if a segment is not linked to a position on another tier, it will not be phonetically realized.
Skeletal (or CV) tier	A representation of a syllable and its hierarchically related components' onset and rhyme.
Onset	Onset of a syllable. Includes all segments before the nucleus.
Rhyme	Cover term for nucleus (vowel) and coda (the arrest of the syllable).

The following diagram depicts the skeletal tier of a CVC syllable:

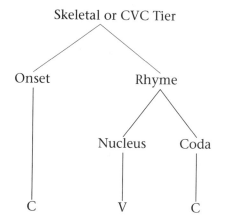

Previously, an example was given of a child who deleted final consonants in two-syllable words. The following diagram illustrates this relationship:

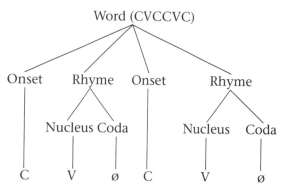

Autosegmental phonology also accounted for *feature spreading*. Certain features such as + and − rounding, for example, can spread to other vowels and consonants. There are two rules for spreading. First, + and − round spreads from a vowel to adjacent consonants. Second, + and − round spreads from a consonant to an adjacent consonant up to a vowel. The following examples demonstrate the two types of feature spreading. The solid line is an inherent feature, while the dotted line represents a spread feature specification:

1. [+ round] spreads from a vowel to adjacent consonant

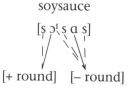

2. [+ round] spreads from a consonant to an adjacent consonant up to a vowel.

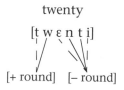

Feature spreading also occurs with such features as [+ voice] and [+ nasal].

To summarize, autosegmental phonology was originally conceived to account for cases in which a single segment is associated with two mutually exclusive features. It has since been expanded to demonstrate relationships between certain syllable types and consonant realizations. Feature spreading accounts for examples in which the feature or property of one segment spreads to adjacent segments.

CLINICAL APPLICATION

Using Autosegmental Phonology to Analyze an Error Pattern

The following autosegmental chart is for a child who produces all initial consonant clusters (two- and three-sound clusters) as [d]:

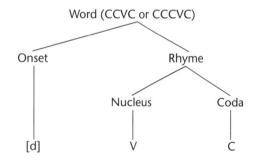

Word (CCVC or CCCVC)

Metrical Phonology. Metrical phonology (Liberman, 1975; Liberman and Prince, 1977) extended a hierarchical-based analysis to stress. In linear phonology, for example, stress is one of the few multivalued features. Stress was not handled in a binary + and – way; rather, there were an infinite number of prominence values that could be assigned to stress. The stress assignment rules of linear phonology produced a relative ordering within any given string of sound segments. This relative ordering can be used (1) to analyze the relative stressing of in-dividual words within a sentence (sentence stress) as well as (2) to analyze the relative stressing of syllables within a word (word stress). The following example demonstrates the linear phonology stress assignment of individual words (word stress) and when these words are placed within a sentence. The numeral 1 indicates the primary stress:

Word stress

a. customer
   1   3   2

b. services
   1   3   2

Sentence stress

c. customer services
       1   2

d. He is the supervisor of customer services.
   4 6 5   1   7   2   3

This system of assigning stress to words within phrases appeared inadequate to Liberman and Prince. First, *customer services* are assigned two different values in examples c and d even though the same words are used. The values of stress, therefore, change with the number of words within an utterance. Second, what do these values actually imply? Is *customer* in example c actually two times more stressed than the same word in example d? Obviously not. Stress assignment rules in linear (generative) phonology were relational and changed depending on the prominence given to the words within a phrase (Hogg and McCully, 1989).

Metrical phonologists proposed another concept for understanding and analyzing stress. "Metrical trees" are used to reflect the syntactic structure of an utterance. To show the relative prominence of each constituent in an utterance, stress patterns are represented by a binary branching of these metrical trees. One branch is labelled S for "stronger" stress and the other W for "weaker" stress. Applying this principle to an example, the following metrical tree can be drawn:

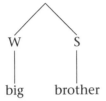

Thus, every tree in metrical phonology must have either a W S or an S W branching. This renders a binary stress representation. If the phrase is expanded, the following stress pattern emerges:

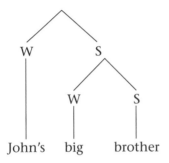

This pattern indicates that *brother* has more prominence than *big* and that the phrase *big brother* is more stressed than *John's*. The same relationship, then, is maintained between *big* and *brother* in both metrical representations.

The second basic concept in metrical phonology pertains to the syllable.

It should be noted that within the field of phonetics and linguistics, there is a long history of attempts to analyze the syllable and to determine syllable boundaries (e.g., Jespersen, 1913; Ladefoged, 1993; Panconcelli-Calzia, 1924; Rosetti, 1959; Scripture, 1927; Sievers, 1901; Stetson, 1936, 1951; Tillmann, 1964; von Essen, 1979). Generative phonologists, then, did not just overlook the syllable; rather, the syllable concept and, especially, determining syllable boundaries remain troublesome.

Although word boundaries are indicated in generative phonology, the syllable structure was not considered. Metrical phonologists indicate not only the number of syllables within a word but also which consonants belong (or are hypothesized to belong) to each syllable. The notation uses the Greek letter sigma (σ) to indicate the individual syllables:

This hierarchical arrangement can also be used to include the morphological representation of the word together with its syllabic divisions. The Greek symbol mu (μ) denotes the morphemes within this word:

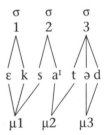

Such an analysis clearly indicates the difference between syllabic and morphological boundaries.

To summarize, metrical phonology is a theoretical construct that extends hierarchical analysis procedures to stress and syllable boundaries. Stress is analyzed according to a binary "strong" and "weak" system rather than to a relational numbering system which was used by earlier phonologists, including the linear (generative) phonologists. This hierarchical analysis has also been used when dividing words into syllables. Syllabic analyses allow for comparisons between syllable and morpheme boundaries.

CLINICAL APPLICATION

Using Metrical Phonology to Analyze an Error Pattern

The following metrical tree demonstrates a child's deletion of unstressed syllables in the two-syllable word *above* and the three-syllable word *umbrella*:

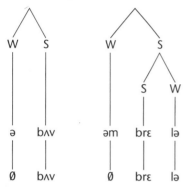

Feature Geometry. Feature geometry represents a group of theories that have adopted the tiered representation of features used in autosegmental phonology. However, feature geometry theories have added a number of other hierarchically ordered feature tiers. Feature geometry attempts to explain why some features (and not others) are affected by assimilation processes (known as *spreading* or *linking* of features) while others are affected by neutralization or deletion processes (known as *delinking*) (Dinnsen, 1997). There are several different tier representations in feature geometry. Figure 4.1 is a feature geometry representation that was provided by Bernhardt and Stemberger (1998) based on the proposals of Bernhardt (1992a, 1992b), Clements (1985), McCarthy (1988), and Sagey (1986).

In accordance with principles of nonlinear phonologies, feature geometry also utilizes hierarchically organized levels of representation, so-called tiers. These tiers interact with one another. Some features are designated as nodes, which means that they may dominate more than one other feature and serve as a link between the dominated feature and higher levels of representation. For example, in Figure 4.1, the Place node serves as a link between the Labial, Coronal, Dorsal, and Radical nodes and the Root node. Features at a higher level of representation are said to dominate other features. The Place node, for example, dominates the different places of articulation (Labial, Coronal, and Dorsal nodes). The Place node must be activated, so to speak, before a specific place of articulation can be chosen. Or, the Laryngeal node as a higher level of representation must be functioning before [+ voice] can be designated. Features that are dominated are considered to be subordinate or at a lower level of representation.

The following is a brief explanation of the different nodes and features, summarized from Bernhardt and Stemberger (1998).

Laryngeal features

1. [+ voiced] sounds produced with vocal fold vibration (e.g., [d], [i]).
2. [+ spread glottis] the vocal cords are spread wide, leading to low-amplitude voice at the glottis (e.g., voiceless aspirated stops [tʰim] are + s.g.).
3. [+ constricted glottis] the vocal cords are pulled together tightly, so that regular periodic vibration is impossible (e.g., all + c.g. segments are – voiced, glottal stops are + c.g.).

Manner features

1. [+ sonorant] sounds in which the pressure above the larynx allows the vocal cords to vibrate continuously, without any rise in pressure above the larynx (e.g., voiced vowels, glides, liquids [r] and [l], and nasals are + sonorant).
2. [+ consonantal] sounds with a narrow constriction in the oral and/or pharyngeal cavities that significantly impede the flow of air (e.g., stops, affricates, nasals, fricatives, laterals, taps, and trills are + consonantal).

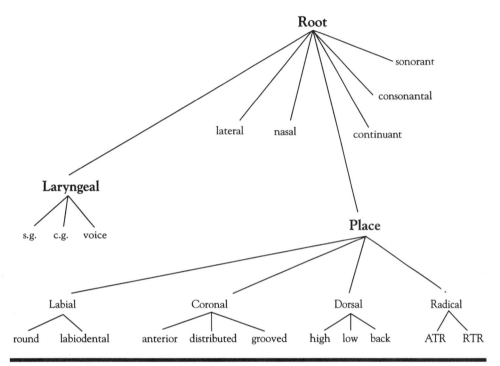

FIGURE 4.1   Feature Geometry of the English Consonant System

Source: From *Handbook of Phonological Development from the Perspective of Constraint-Based Nonlinear Phonology* (p. 92), by B. H. Bernhardt and J. P. Stemberger, 1998, San Diego, CA: Academic Press. Copyright 1998 by Academic Press.

3. [+ continuant] sounds in which air continues to move through the oral cavity (e.g., vowels, glides, liquids, and fricatives).
4. [+ nasal] sounds with the velum lowered so that air moves through the nasal cavity (e.g., nasals).
5. [+ lateral] sounds in which central airflow is blocked in the oral cavity, but in which air is directed over at least one side of the tongue (e.g., laterals).
6. [+ tense] sounds produced with relatively greater "muscular tension" (e.g., tense vowels, voiceless obstruents).

Place features

Lips
1. [Labial] sounds made with more involvement of one or both lips (e.g., bilabials, labiodentals).

2. [+ round] sounds involving protrusion of the lips with narrowing at the corners of the mouth (e.g., all rounded vowels and labialized consonant [kʷ]. Bilabials and labiodentals are – round).
3. [+ labiodental] labial sounds that are made with only one lip (e.g., [f] and [v]).

The tip of the tongue
1. [Coronal] sounds made with raising of the tip or blade of the tongue (e.g., interdentals, dentals, alveolars, palatoalveolars, retroflexes, and palatals, the palatal glide [j] and high front vowels are also included).
2. [+ anterior] coronal sounds made at the alveolar ridge or further forward (e.g., interdentals, dentals, and alveolars are + anterior, – anterior includes palatoalveolars,

alveopalatals, retroflexes, palatals, and front vowels).

3. [+ distributed] coronal sounds made with a wide area of contact between the tip/blade of the tongue and the roof of the mouth or teeth (e.g., interdentals, dentals, palatoalveolars, alveopalatals, and palatals, – distributed sounds include alveolars and retroflexes).

4. [+ grooved] coronal sounds made with a grooved tongue, a narrow channel at or near the midline (e.g., alveolar fricatives, affricates).

The tongue body

1. [Dorsal] sounds made with the back of the tongue (e.g., palatals, velars, vowels, [w], and [j] also dark [l]).

2. [+ back] sounds with the back of the tongue body raised or lowered (e.g., velar sounds, including the dark [l], back and central vowels).

3. [+ high] sounds where the tongue body is raised (e.g., high vowels, glides, velar and palatal consonants).

4. [+ low] sounds where the tongue body is lowered (e.g., low vowels).

The tongue root

1. [Radical] sounds in which the root of the tongue is advanced or retracted (e.g., pharyngeal and pharyngealized consonants, not typical for American English speech sounds).

2. [Advanced Tongue Root (ATR)] sounds in which the tongue root is advanced (e.g., high vowels, [i], [e], [u], and [o], consonants are blank for this feature).

As can be seen from the preceding explanation, the use of features and the definition of certain features are different from those proposed by Chomsky and Halle (1968).

Another nonlinear theory, the *theory of radical underspecification* (Archangeli, 1988; Archangeli and Pulleyblank, 1994; Bernhardt, 1992b; Kiparsky, 1982; Pulleyblank, 1986),

suggests that underlying representations contain only "unpredictable" features. A predictable feature is one that would be commonly associated with that particular segment or class of sounds. For example, nasals are typically voiced (although there are unvoiced nasals in some African languages). Voicing for nasals is, then, predictable and would not be contained in the underlying representation. Or, since all sonorants are voiced, this is again a predictable feature and is not contained in the underlying representation. On the other hand, obstruents can be [+ voice] or [– voice]; therefore, the unpredictable nature of this feature is contained in the underlying representation.

Rules in nonlinear analysis are restricted to two basic operations: *spreading* (known as *linking*) and *deletion* (known as *delinking*) of phonological information from one tier to another. Spreading of features could be exemplified by the production of [gʌk] for *duck*. The coronal place node for /d/ is subject to linking or assimilation from the dorsal place node feature of /k/. Delinking could be exemplified by the production of [dʌ] for *duck*. Under the assumption that the underlying representation is intact, the final consonant slot for that production is delinked from the representation along with the actual features of /k/. Linking and delinking result from, and are constrained by, principles of association between tiers. These principles are outlined in Bernhardt and Stemberger (1998) and could be used as a reference for more detailed analysis procedures.

To summarize, one nonlinear phonology, feature geometry, theorizes that segments are

> The degree of specification of features in the underlying representation in nonlinear phonologies differs from Chomsky and Halle's (1968) distinctive feature notion. In Chomsky and Halle's (1968) concept, both predictable and unpredictable feature values are thought to be a portion of the underlying representation.

composed of multitiered hierarchically organized features. Specific nodes that can dominate other features and link various levels of representation are designated. According to this theory, features can link (assimilate) or delink, causing neutralization or deletion. Principles of association are used to explain occurrences between tiers.

How Did Nonlinear Phonology Develop?

John Firth, Professor of General Linguistics at the University of London, was a key figure in the development of modern linguistics in the United Kingdom. In a way, nonlinear phonology, too, can be traced back to Firth's (1948) so-called prosodic analysis. For the first time, Firth challenged the linguistic one-sided importance of the phonemic units in their consecutive linearity. He advocated the necessity for additional nonsegmental analyses, "prosodies," which represent larger linguistic entities, such as syllables, words, and phrases. He postulated that speech is a manifestation of consecutively ordered units *as well as* a manifestation of larger prosodic units that bind phonemes together into linguistically more comprehensive units. Different analytical systems may need to be set up in order to explain the range of contrasts involved. With this approach, known as *polysystemicism,* the concept of nonlinear phonology was born.

Contemporary nonlinear/multilinear phonologies are an outgrowth of generative phonology. Chomsky and Halle's (1968) major contribution, *The Sound Pattern of English,* was innovative in its description of two levels of representation, a surface phonetic representation and an underlying phonemic representation. Although the idea of distinctive features was taken from the Prague School of linguistics, Chomsky and Halle understood the distinctive feature concept in a different way and modified it accordingly. Nonlinear phonolo-

gies adopt the generative concepts of distinctive features and surface-level and underlying representation. However, these new phonologies understand the surface-level representation in a very different way.

Chomsky and Halle's generative phonology described speech components in a linear manner: It was segment based. The components of any utterance were arranged in a sequence, with one discrete segment following the next. A common set of distinctive features is attributed to all segments and each feature is specified by the assignment of a binary value. This limited the generation of phonological rules in several respects. First, only whole segments could be deleted or added. The only other modifications that could occur in the segment were achieved by changing the + or – values of one or more distinctive features. (Thus, this system analyzes only additions, deletions, or substitutions; analysis of nonphonemic distortions is not possible.) Second, because all segments are equally complex and all distinctive features are equal within this system, there is no reason to expect that any one segment, or any one distinctive feature, might be affected by any given phonological rule. However, many observations and investigations have reported, for example, that certain sounds and sound classes appear to be especially vulnerable to assimilation while others cause assimilation (Dinnsen, 1997). Third, early generative phonology adopted the division between the segmentals and the suprasegmentals which the structural linguists had used to describe and analyze speech events. However, such a division does not allow a vertical, hierarchical understanding of the interaction between segmental units and prosodic features. The nonlinear phonologies represent a challenge to the earlier segment-based approaches. "Nonlinear phonological theory is another step in the evolution of our understanding of phonological systems" (Bernhardt and Stoel-Gammon, 1994, p. 126).

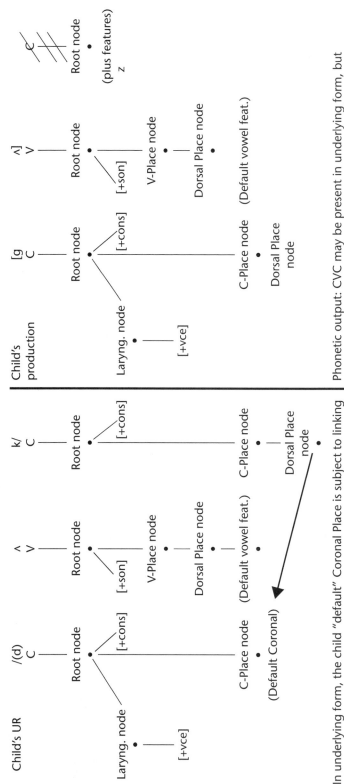

In underlying form, the child "default" Coronal Place is subject to linking (spread of a feature or assimilation) from the specified Dorsal Place feature of /k/. Spread occurs on the consonant tier, hence C-Place and V-Place.

Phonetic output: CVC may be present in underlying form, but articulatory constraints prevent realizations of any final consonant. Deletion (delinking) of C2 skeletal slot and segmental content. Specification of C1 has occurred prior to C2 delinking.

Child's underlying representation of /gʌk/ for *duck*, following spread of Dorsal Place from C₂ of /k/ to C₁ (left) and final consonant deletion rule resulting from articulatory constraints against final consonants: delinking of skeletal slot C and /k/ features of C₂, yielding [gʌ] (right).

FIGURE 4.2 Comparison of a Child's Underlying Representation to the Child's Production Using Feature Geometry

Source: From "Nonlinear Phonology: Introduction and Clinical Application," by B. Bernhardt and C. Stoel-Gammon, 1994, *Journal of Speech and Hearing Research, 37,* p. 132. Copyright © 1994 by the American Speech-Language-Hearing Association. Reprinted by permission.

Nonlinear Phonologies: Clinical Implications

Although contemporary nonlinear phonologies began with Goldsmith's (1976) dissertation on autosegmental phonology, many different nonlinear phonological theories have since been proposed. This section has attempted to briefly introduce three nonlinear approaches: autosegmental phonology, metrical phonology, and feature geometry. However, it should be kept in mind that many other nonlinear phonologies exist.

Several of these nonlinear approaches have been applied to the development of the phonological system in children and to the analysis of disordered phonological systems. For example, Leonard and Brown (1984) and Pollock and Schwartz (1988) demonstrated how disordered phonological systems could be analyzed utilizing autosegmental principles. Bernhardt and Stoel-Gammon (1994) applied principles of grounded phonology (Archangeli and Pulleyblank, 1994) to the analysis of phonologically disordered speech. Stemberger and Bernhardt (1997) used optimality theory (McCarthy and Prince, 1993; Prince and Smolensky, 1993) to develop an intervention plan in a case study of a child. Dinnsen (1997) examined how underspecification theory, more specifically radical underspecification theory (Archangeli, 1988; Kiparsky, 1982; Pulleyblank, 1986), can explain both the normal acquisition of phonological systems and disordered phonology.

Of the three nonlinear phonologies presented in this chapter, feature geometry has been most widely applied to the analysis of phonological disorders in children (Bernhardt, 1990, 1992a, 1992b, 1994; Bernhardt and Gilbert, 1992; Bernhardt and Stemberger, 1998; Bernhardt and Stoel-Gammon, 1994; Chin and Dinnsen, 1991, Von Bremen, 1990). Using feature geometry and the principles of association between tiers, the child's underlying representation is contrasted to the child's production. Figure 4.2 contrasts the child's underlying representation of *duck* to the child's production of [gʌ]. According to Bernhardt and Stoel-Gammon (1994), this child produced [gʌ] for *duck* but [dʌ] for *dumb*. This suggests that the underlying representation of *duck* includes some information from the dorsal place node. Therefore, in the child's underlying representation (framework to the left), C_2 is linked to C_1. The child's actual production is shown in the feature geometry framework to the right. Delinking has occurred at the final consonant slot C (the slashes characterize the delinking of the feature). It must be concluded from these two frameworks that specification of C_1 has occurred prior to C_2.

This method of analysis not only demonstrates the mismatch of features between the underlying representation and the production but also can reveal the hierarchical relationship among features. Feature geometry attempts to provide a more in-depth view of the phonological system of children, which could enhance target selection and intervention strategies.

CLINICAL APPLICATION

More Information—Feature Geometry versus Phonological Processes

In Figure 4.2, an example was provided of a child who says [gʌ] for *duck* and [dʌ] for *dumb*. If phonological processes are assigned to these substitutions and deletions, the following results are noted:

"duck"	[dʌk]	→	[gʌ]	backing [d] → [g]
				final consonant deletion [k] → Ø
"dumb"	[dʌm]	→	[dʌ]	final consonant deletion [m] → Ø

Although these phonological processes are easily identifiable, they give no information about the child's underlying representation. Where to begin in therapy would be a relatively arbitrary choice that would be based on the number of times the processes were observed and the age at which they should be suppressed. Feature geometry demonstrates that the underlying representation for this child includes information about the dorsal place node, that is, about /k/ and /g/. Articulatory constraints, however, prevent realization of final consonants. If this was just a case of final consonant deletion, both *duck* and *dumb* should have been realized as [dʌ]. In the underlying representation, the child might be trying to differentiate between *duck* and *dumb*. This suggests that if the articulatory constraints could be eliminated, the child's g/d substitution (backing) might also be eliminated. The concept of feature geometry and underlying representation provides us with more insight into reasons for the child's output patterns.

Autosegmental and metrical phonologies have not received as much application as other nonlinear theories. Autosegmental phonology was conceived to account for cases in which a single segment is associated with two mutually exclusive features. Although it was originally applied to tone languages, it might also offer some applicability to disordered phonological systems. One important factor that is absent from many phonological theories is the child's production of nonphonemic distortions, for example, a dentalized s-production ([s̪] for /s/). According to generative phonology, this distortion must be classified either as /s/, therefore [+ strident], or as /θ/, [– strident]. It is possible, however, that this single segment [s̪] could share these two seemingly mutually exclusive features of [+ strident] and [– strident]. If so, autosegmental phonology may offer a means of analyzing these types of distortions. Feature spreading within autosegmental phonology is structured to analyze assimilation processes but also offers a means of specifying coarticulatory conditions that might be useful in therapy.

Metrical phonology, which extends hierarchical analysis procedures to stress and syllable boundaries, suggests several possibilities in its application to disordered phonological systems. Stress, both within a word and within a sentence, often plays a decisive role in the production of segments. Metrical phonology offers analysis procedures that emphasize the interrelationships that might exist between stress and segment production. The comparison of syllable and morphological boundaries within metrical phonology provides the potential to link phonological segmental production to other language areas.

To summarize, many different nonlinear phonologies have been developed within the last decade or so. Some of them have been applied to case studies of children with disordered phonological systems. The results seem to indicate that these phonologies promise new insights into, and a deeper understanding of, the phonological system. Future research should document which of these theories can provide the clinician with new possibilities for the assessment and treatment of individuals with impaired phonological systems.

SUMMARY

This chapter first introduced some of the basic terminology and principles underlying contemporary phonological theories. The relationship between the sound form and the sound function (as phoneme) was established as a basis for the understanding of phonological theories. The development of the phoneme concept was traced historically to provide a foundation for the understanding of how phonological theories could evolve from this "new" concept. Clinical application of these basic principles stressed the interrelationship between sound-form and sound-function.

The remainder of this chapter was a summary of several different phonological theories that impact the assessment and treatment of phonological disorders. These theories were enumerated in a historical sequence. The linear phonologies were represented by distinctive feature theory, generative phonology, and natural phonology. The nonlinear phonologies included autosegmental, metrical, and feature geometry. Each phonological theory was discussed in respect to what the theoretical framework stands for, how it developed, how it functions, and its clinical implications.

The field of phonology is constantly evolving. Current phonological theories are an attempt to describe the phonological system with all its complexity in a different manner. While some of the newer models have yet to stand the test of time and research, all offer new insights into the intricate nature of normal and impaired phonological systems.

CHAPTER 5

NORMAL PHONOLOGICAL DEVELOPMENT

CHAPTER OUTLINE

- Aspects of Structural and Functional Development
- Aspects of Perceptual Development
- Prelinguistic Stages: Before the First Words

- Transition from Babbling to First Words
- The First Fifty Words
- The Preschool Child
- The School-Age Child
- Summary

This chapter outlines the prelinguistic behavior and phonological development of children from birth to their school years. **Prelinguistic behavior** refers to all vocalizations prior to the first actual words. **Phonological development** refers to the acquisition of speech sound form and function within the language system. In accordance with current terminology, this is now referred to as phonological development rather than as speech sound development, as it was in the past. To some, this may signal only a difference in wording; however, the concept has actually undergone a fundamental transformation. **Speech sound development** refers primarily to the gradual articulatory mastery of speech sound forms within a given language. Thus, the proficiency of a child to produce adultlike speech sounds is measured. *Phonological development,* on the other hand, implies the acquisition of a functional sound system intricately connected to the child's overall growth in language. *Phonology* refers to the systems and patterns of sounds that occur in a language. Learning to produce a variety of sounds is not the same as learning the contrasts between sounds that convey differences in meaning.

The first goal of this chapter is to explore briefly certain aspects of the structural and functional development that must occur prior to speech sound production in the infant. In addition, the development of specific perceptual skills will be discussed.

The second goal is to examine some of the available information on articulatory and phonological development. Organized according to segmental form as well as prosodic development, this survey ranges from the prelinguistic stages to the near completion of the phonological system during the early school years. In reviewing the literature, an attempt will be made to discuss the various studies so that the reader will become aware of differences in design and purpose, which have often resulted in contrasting outcomes. In addition, it should be noted that much of the literature focuses on the child's acquisition of speech sounds. Very little information is available on the child's gradual development of the phonemic function of these segments within a language. When possible, these studies will also be included.

The third goal of this chapter is to highlight interdependencies between language acquisition and phonological development. Developing phonology cannot be meaningfully separated from other aspects of emerging language; it represents an integral part of the child's total language acquisition process. While cognitive and motor abilities certainly play important roles in the unfolding of phonology, the child's acquisition of semantic, morphosyntactic, and pragmatic skills influences it as well.

Over the years, many investigators have tried to determine approximate ages of individual sound "mastery" in specific groups of children (e.g., Poole, 1934; Prather, Hedrick, and Kern, 1975; Templin, 1957; Wellman, Case, Mengert, and Bradbury, 1931). These guidelines are important when trying to separate normal from abnormal phonological development and when determining therapy goals. However, the role of individual variation and its impact on the child's phonological development must be emphasized. The development of speech sounds and of the phonological system remains an individual process. Although investigations can identify general trends across children, individual variation is more the rule than the exception (e.g., Stoel-Gammon and Cooper, 1984; Vihman, 1992).

ASPECTS OF STRUCTURAL AND FUNCTIONAL DEVELOPMENT

As the infant begins its journey from primarily reflexive crying behavior to babbling and words, important anatomical structures and their development, prerequisites for sound production, need to be taken into consideration. Both the structure and the function of respiratory, phonatory, resonatory, and articulatory mechanisms must advance decisively before any regular articulatory processes can occur. These necessary changes, which continue through infancy and early childhood,

are directly reflected in the transformation from prelinguistic to linguistic sound productions. The following summary from Bosma (1975), Kent (1997), and Kent and Murray (1982) presents a broad outline of the development of the respiratory, phonatory, resonatory, and articulatory systems during this time span.

The shape, size, and composition of the respiratory system are dramatically modified from infancy to adulthood. Newborns and infants are, of course, perfectly able to accumulate enough air pressure against a closed glottis to "phonate" quite impressively. Although small when compared to adults, their lungs are proportionally large for their body structure. Their subglottal pressure is considerable and continues to be so throughout childhood. For example, when comparable loudness levels are contrasted, children demonstrate higher subglottal pressure values than adults (Stathopoulos and Sapienza, 1993). In addition, very few alveoli are present in the lungs of the newborn. It is not until the child is approximately 7 years old that the number of alveoli approaches the adult value (Kent, 1997). Around 7 years of age is also the time when children's respiratory function demonstrates adultlike patterns. Developmental milestones in the respiratory system are summarized in Table 5.1.

The changes in the phonatory and resonatory systems from infancy to childhood are especially impressive. This anatomical-physiological development leads directly to their future secondary physiological function for articulatory purposes. However, in newborns, larynx and vocal tract reflect exclusively primary functions, that is, they are at this time unable to fulfill any articulatory tasks. For example, the oral cavity (with tongue and lips) and the pharyngeal cavity are utilized primarily for sucking and swallowing actions. The tongue, which in young infants fills out the

TABLE 5.1   Developmental Milestones in the Respiratory System

AGE	TYPICAL EVENTS OR PATTERNS
Birth	Diaphragm of newborn has a bellowslike displacement, unlike the pistonlike effect in adults. Rest breathing rate is 30–80 breaths/min. Frequent paradoxing occurs in early infancy; for example, the rib cage makes an expiratory movement as the abdomen performs an inspiratory action. Very few alveoli are present in the lungs of the newborn.
3 yrs	Respiratory function not closely geared to linguistic requirement until this age. Rest breathing rate is 20–30 breaths/min. Functional maturation is especially evident during the period of 3 to 7 yrs.
7 yrs	Essential convergence on adultlike patterns, but children use greater subglottal air pressure than adult for speaking. Number of alveoli is approaching the adult value of about 300,000.
10 yrs	Refinement of respiratory patterns; functional maturation achieved. Rest breathing rate is 17–22 breaths/min.
12–18 yrs	Increase in lung capacity, especially in boys.

Source: From *The Speech Sciences* (p. 97), by R. D. Kent, 1997, San Diego, CA: Singular. Copyright 1997. Reprinted with permission by Singular Publishing Group, Inc.

oral cavity completely, leaves practically no space for the buccal area, the space between the outside of the gums and the inside of the cheeks. In addition, a prenatally acquired "sucking pad," an encapsulated structure of the cheek supporting the lateral rims of the tongue for more effective sucking action, helps to fill out this space entirely. The production of sounds is under these conditions severely restricted. The ability to produce speech sounds is a highly complex process that depends primarily on many anatomical-physiological changes that occur as a product of growth and maturation. Figure 5.1 shows the tongue displacement and the size of several anatomical structures of the newborn infant.

The larynx, too, has to develop structurally before it can effectively contribute to articulation. In newborns, for example, the artytenoid cartilages (and the cricoid lamina) are disproportionately large when compared to an adult larynx (see Figure 5.2). The vocal processes where the vocal folds attach are also large in relationship to the other structures. This means that they reach deeply into the vocal folds, thus stifling their vibratory action. In addition, the infant's larynx sits closely under the angle between neck and chin. This high, semi-fixated position of the larynx does not allow the vocal tract to be effectively elongated in a downward direction. This elongation is indispensable for some resonating effects during vowel articulation, for example.

Stabilization of the pharyngeal airway necessary for an upright position is another significant postnatal development. Anatomical changes include the displacement of the hyoid bone plus larynx downward, away from the base of the skull and the mandible, and the loss of the aforementioned sucking pad. All of these changes must occur as prerequisites for the articulation of speech sounds.

After the child's first words, around the child's first birthday, the speech mechanism

---

To verify the decisive importance of movements of the larynx for normal vowel production, place your index finger lightly on the V-shaped notch of the thyroid cartilage of the larynx with the middle finger and thumb on either side of the lamina. In this position, articulate [i] versus [u]. The downward movement during [u] can easily be felt.

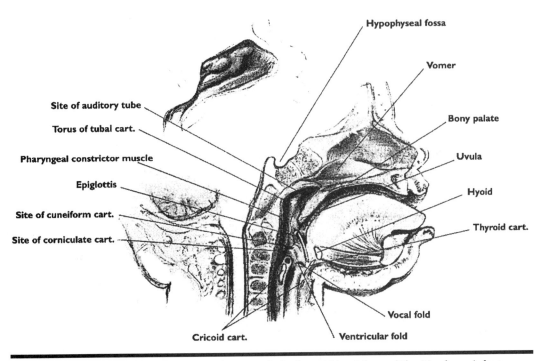

FIGURE 5.1 Paramedian Section of the Pharyngeal, Oral, and Nasal Area of the Newborn Infant
The tongue is displaced slightly downward, away from the palate, and forward. The laryngeal
ventricle and ventricular folds are short, compared with those of the child.
Source: From "Anatomic Physiologic Development of the Speech Apparatus," by J. F. Bosma, in *The
Nervous System, Vol. III: Human Communication and Its Disorders* (p. 470), edited by D. B. Tower, 1975,
New York: Lippincott-Raven Publishers. Copyright 1975 by Lippincott-Raven Publishers. Reprinted with
permission.

undergoes further enlargement and changes in form. Expansions of the laryngeal and pharyngeal cavities are prominent among them. These expansions co-occur with changes in the form and mobility of the arytenoid cartilages, soft palate, and tongue. The following changes characterize this development:

1. The thyroid cartilage enlarges more than the cricoid cartilage.
2. The epiglottis becomes larger and more firm.
3. The arytenoid cartilages, which were relatively large in the early stages of this development, now change little in size; they adapt structurally and functionally to the other laryngeal structures.

4. The vocal and ventricular folds, that is, the "true" and "false" vocal folds, lengthen. This has the effect that less of the vocal fold length is stabilized by the arytenoid's vocal processes or, the other way around, more of the vocal folds' muscular portion is now freed for normal vocal cord vibration.

Skeletal enlargement of the skull and laryngeal areas during childhood occurs mostly in posterior and vertical directions. This allows the velum more room and thus more mobility. However, the oral area is the site of the greatest changes in spatial arrangement and resulting mobility of the anatomical structures. Due to these skeletal changes, the tongue no longer completely fills the mouth. In addition, the tongue and lips become elongated and acquire further mobility. The fine-tuning and coordination of the lip, mandible, tongue, and velar movements for regular voice and speech production are now increasingly acquired.

To summarize, during infancy, we see enormously complex developmental changes. The infant's larynx, mouth, and pharyngeal areas evolve from a mechanism able to serve only respiratory and feeding purposes to a vocal tract that is structurally and functionally ready for the production of speech sounds.

ASPECTS OF PERCEPTUAL DEVELOPMENT

Although it has often been documented that infants are able to discriminate minimal differences in speech sounds within the first months after their births (Eilers, 1980; Eimas, Siqueland, Jusczyk, and Vigorito, 1971; Jusczyk, 1992; Kuhl, 1987), their auditory experiences actually begin even before birth. Using ultrasound technology, researchers have been able to detect fetal eye blink responses to a loud noise between 24 and 28 weeks after conception (Birnholtz and Benacerraf, 1983). Using loudspeakers close to the mothers' abdomens, Lecanuet, Granier-Deferre, and Bushnel (1989) presented the syllables [babi] or

In the study by Birnholtz and Benacerraf (1983), auditory stimulation was provided by an electrolarynx placed several inches from the mothers' abdomens. Using ultrasound, the researchers observed that fetuses aged between 24 and 28 weeks after conception demonstrated notable eye blink behavior approximately half a second after the beginning of the electrolarynx buzz. In this study, 680 fetuses were tested. Only 8 of the 680 did not evidence this eye blink behavior. After birth, it was found that 2 of the 8 infants were deaf and that the remaining 6 had a variety of central nervous system disorders.

FIGURE 5.2 Posterior View of Skeletons of Larynx of Mature Man and of Infant
The infant's larynx is, of course, much smaller than the adult's. The sketches are intended to indicate proportional differences of some laryngeal structures only.
Source: From "Anatomic Physiologic Development of the Speech Apparatus," by J. F. Bosma, in *The Nervous System, Vol. III: Human Communication and Its Disorders* (p. 477), edited by D. B. Tower, 1975, New York: Lippincott-Raven Publishers. Copyright 1975 by Lippincott-Raven Publishers. Reprinted with permission.

[biba] to nineteen women in their last trimester of pregnancy. Changes in fetal heart rate demonstrated that almost all of the fetuses reacted when the syllable stimulation varied, for example, when stimulation changed from [babi] to [biba]. Also, within the first days after birth, infants demonstrate a preference for their own mothers' voices and will actively change their sucking rate to hear this voice more often than another female's voice (De-Casper and Fifer, 1980). And at 4 days of age, babies of French-speaking mothers prefer the sound of French over Russian (Bertoncini, Morais, Bijeljac-Babic, McAdams, Peretz, and Mehler, 1989; Mehler, Jusczyk, Lambertz, Halsted, Bertoncini, and Amiel-Tison, 1988).

These results support the notion that infants start to pay attention and "learn" something about voice and speech probably prior to birth. However, what evidence do we have about the infant's and child's perception and discrimination of speech sounds and phonemic contrasts? The following is an overview of these perceptual skills.

■ *Categorical perception.* **Categorical perception** refers to the tendency of listeners to perceive speech sounds varied along a continuum according to the phonemic categories of their native language. Thus, variations in voice onset time will produce a clear listener distinction between [ba] or [pa], as if an actual boundary divided the two. Based on changes in measured sucking rates, categorical perception for /b/ and /p/ in the syllables [ba] and [pa] has been demonstrated in infants as young as one month of age (Eimas, Siqueland, Jusczyk, and Vigorito, 1971). Infants under 3 months of age can detect differences in place and manner of articulation for consonants (Jusczyk, 1992). It is interesting to note that 2-year-olds needed more variation in voice onset time before they achieved correct categorical perception. By age 4, responses were clearly categorical (Simon and Fourcin, 1978; Zlatin and Koenigsknecht, 1975).

Voice onset time (VOT) refers to the time between the release of an articulatory constriction and the onset of voicing.

■ *Discrimination of nonnative sounds in infants.* If children demonstrate categorical perception at such an early age, it was hypothesized that they might have an inborn ability to make categorical distinctions. In order to test this hypothesis, a task was devised in which the discrimination skills of young infants were tested with unknown minimal phonetic differences exemplified by phonemes of nonnative languages, that is, languages to which they had not been exposed. Although adult nonnative speakers could not discriminate these pairs, results demonstrated that up to approximately 6 to 8 months of age, infants could indeed discriminate between two nonnative sounds that were very similar in their production characteristics

(Trehub, 1976; Werker and Tees, 1983). By 10 to 12 months, this discrimination ability had disappeared and the infants' performance was as poor as that of English-speaking adults (Werker and Tees, 1983). The conclusion drawn was that language experience may result in the loss of this discrimination ability. We do not discriminate between categories that are nonfunctional in our own native language.

■ *Perceptual constancy.* The ability to identify the same sound across different speakers, pitches, and other changing environmental conditions is known as **perceptual constancy.** Perceptual constancy for vowels and consonants in different vowel contexts has been noted in children from 5½ to 10 months of age (Kuhl, 1980).

■ *Perception of phonemic contrasts.* Shvachkin (1973) and Garnica (1973) examined the ability of toddlers from 10 to 22 months to associate nonsense syllables that varied in only one sound element with objects. Could the child learn to differentiate between phonemes that signal word meaning differences? These studies found that in all children, there was a developmental progression in the ability to make these distinctions; that is, some distinctions appear easier to detect than others. However, considerable variability was noted between the children as to which features were discriminated earlier and which later.

■ *Perception of minimal pairs.* Children between the ages of 27 and 35 months were able to discriminate between minimal pair words that contrast most of the later-acquired English speech sounds (Barton, 1976, 1980). It was noted that children responded more accurately if the two were familiar words; error rates were highest when both words in a pair were unfamiliar. Barton suggested that studies of phonemic contrasts using nonsense syllables probably underestimate a child's actual ability to discriminate between minimal pair words.

PRELINGUISTIC STAGES:
BEFORE THE FIRST WORDS

Child language development is commonly divided into *prelinguistic behavior,* vocalizations prior to the first true words, and *linguistic development,* which starts with the appearance of these first words. This division is exemplified by the use of early nonmeaningful versus later meaningful sound productions. Jakobson's *discontinuity hypothesis* (1942/1968) clearly emphasized a sharp separation between these two phases. According to his theoretical notion, babbling is a random series of vocalizations in which many different sounds are produced with no apparent order or consistency. Such behavior is seen as clearly separated from the following systematic sound productions evidenced by the first words. The division between prelinguistic and linguistic phases of sound production, according to Jakobson, is often so complete that the child might actually undergo a period of silence between the end of the babbling period and the first real words.

Research since that time (e.g., Oller, 1980; Oller, Wieman, Doyle, and Ross, 1976; Stark, 1980, 1986) has repeatedly documented (1) that babbling behavior is not random but rather that the child's productions develop in a systematic manner, (2) that the consonant-like sounds that are babbled are restricted to a small set of segments, and (3) that the transition between babbling and first words is not abrupt but continuous; late babbling behavior and the first words are very similar in respect to the sounds used and the way they are combined. It also appears that the child's perceptual abilities are quite developed before the first meaningful utterances. For example, some word comprehension is evident at approximately 7 to 9 months of age (Owens, 1996). The presence of phonemic contrasts in very young children has also been documented (Shvachkin, 1973). Although this ac-

quisition is gradual, more general contrasts begin at approximately 1 year of age. Findings like these suggest that the child's language system starts to develop prior to the first spoken meaningful words.

With this in mind, one could argue that phonological development begins before its manifestation in the use of the first words. But how much before? Only at approximately 6 to 8 months does the child's vocal tract approximate its later adult shape, a prerequisite for sound production as we know it (Bosma, 1975). These physiological changes coincide with the beginning of the *canonical babbling period,* which shows refined perception and production skills similar to those later used in the first fifty words. Sometime during the prelinguistic period, the child's phonological development begins. Therefore, the following represents an overview of the *prelinguistic stages* of production described by Stark (1986). Although these are referred to as stages, there is overlap from one period of development to the next. In addition, individual variation between children necessitates that the ages given are approximates.

> *Stage 1:* Reflexive crying and vegetative sounds (birth to 2 months)
>
> This stage is characterized by a large proportion of reflexive vocalizations. *Reflexive vocalizations* include cries, coughs, grunts, and burps that seem to be automatic responses reflecting the physical state of the infant. *Vegetative sounds* may be divided into grunts and sighs associated with activity and clicks and other noises, for example, which are associated with feeding.

> *Stage 2:* Cooing and laughter (2 to 4 months)
>
> During this stage, *cooing* or *gooing* sounds are produced during comfortable states. Although these sounds are sometimes referred to as vowel-like,

they also contain brief periods of consonantal elements that are produced at the back of the mouth. Early comfort sounds have quasi-resonant nuclei; they are produced as a syllabic nasal consonant or a nasalized vowel (Nakazima, 1962; Oller, 1980). From 12 weeks onward, a decrease in the frequency of crying is noted and most infants' primitive vegetative sounds start to disappear. At 16 weeks, sustained laughter emerges (Gesell and Thompson, 1934).

Stage 3: Vocal play (4 to 6 months)

Although there is some overlap between Stages 2 and 3, the distinguishing characteristics of Stage 3 include longer series of segments and the production of prolonged vowel- or consonantlike steady states. It is during this stage that the infant often produces extreme variations in loudness and pitch. Transitions between the segments are much slower than is the case with children or adults. In contrast to those in Stage 2, Stage 3 vowels demonstrate more variation in tongue height and position.

Stage 4: Canonical babbling (6 months and older)

Although **canonical babbling**—the collective term for the reduplicated and nonreduplicated babbling stages—usually begins around 6 months of age, most children continue to babble into the time when they say their first words. Stark (1986) describes reduplicated and nonreduplicated, or variegated, babbling as follows: **Reduplicated babbling** is marked by similar strings of consonant-vowel productions. There might be slight quality variations in the vowel sounds of these strings of babbles, but the consonants will stay the same from syllable to syllable. An example of this is [əmama]. **Nonreduplicated** or **varie-**

gated babbling demonstrates variation of both consonants and vowels from syllable to syllable. An example of this is [batə]. Smooth transitions can be noted between vowel and consonant productions.

From the previous description, one might conclude that these babbling stages are sequential in nature, a child first going through reduplicated babbling and then later nonreduplicated babbling. This has indeed been documented by Elbers (1982), Oller (1980), and Stark (1986), to mention a few. However, more recent investigators have questioned this developmental pattern. For example, Mitchell and Kent (1990) assessed the phonetic variation of multisyllabic babbling in eight infants at 7, 9, and 11 months of age. Their findings showed that (1) nonreduplicated babbling was present from the time the infant began to produce multisyllabic babbling, not evolving out of an earlier period of reduplicated babbling, and (2) no significant difference existed between the amount of phonetic variation for the vocalizations when the infants were 7, 9, and 11 months old. These and other findings (Holmgren, Lindblom, Aurelius, Jalling, and Zetterstrom, 1986; Smith, Brown-Sweeney, and Stoel-Gammon, 1989) suggest that both reduplicated and variegated forms extend throughout the entire babbling period. At the beginning of this stage, babbling is used in a self-stimulatory manner; it is not used to communicate to adults. Toward the end of this stage, babbling may be used in ritual imitation games with adults (Stark, 1986).

Stage 5: Jargon stage (10 months and older)

This babbling stage overlaps with the first meaningful words. The **jargon stage** is characterized by strings of babbled utterances that are modulated primarily by intonation, rhythm, and pausing (Crystal, 1986). It sounds as if the child is actually attempting sentences but without actual words. Because many jargon vocalizations are delivered with eye contact, gestures, and intonation patterns that resemble statements or questions, parents are convinced that the child is indeed trying to communicate something to which they often feel compelled to respond (Stoel-Gammon and Menn, 1997).

The following section examines the child's segmental productions toward the end of the canonical babbling stage. Because the productions cannot yet be said to be true vowels and consonants of a particular language system, they will be referred to as **vocoids** and **contoids,** respectively. These terms were introduced by Pike (1943) to indicate nonphonemic speech sound productions.

Vocoids

Some of the earliest series of investigations with a large number of children were those carried out by Irwin and colleagues in the 1940s and 1950s (e.g., Irwin, 1945, 1946, 1947a, 1947b, 1948, 1951; Irwin and Chen, 1946; Chen and Irwin, 1946; Winitz and Irwin, 1958). According to the data on fifty-seven children from 13 to 14 months of age, there was a continued predominance of the [ɛ], [ɪ], and [ʌ] vocoids. Thus, front and central vocoids were found to be favored over high and back vocoids. Later investigations (Davis and McNeilage, 1990; Kent and Bauer, 1985) generated similar results.

Contoids

Several authors have investigated the contoids, which predominate in the late babbling stage. Locke (1983) provides an excellent

overview of the results from three major investigations (see Table 5.2). The agreement between these studies is far more striking than the differences. As can be seen from Table 5.2, the most frequent contoids were [h], [d], [b], [m], [t], [g], and [w]. The twelve most frequently produced contoids represent about 95 percent of all the segments transcribed in the three studies (Locke, 1983). These results stand in contrast to earlier statements that babbling consists of a great multitude of random vocalizations. On the contrary, these and other investigations (Locke, 1990; Vihman, Macken, Miller, Simmons, and Miller, 1985) suggest that only a rather limited set of phones is babbled.

Looking at Table 5.2, it appears that there weren't any non-English sound segments utilized by the infants studied. However, this is partially conditioned by the investigative methods employed and by the perceptual limitations inherent in phonetic transcription. As to the investigative methodology, in the Irwin studies, only three non-English sounds were transcribed; the rest were ignored. The Fisichelli study considered exclusively English sounds. The Pierce and Hanna investigation, on the other hand, did document that the infants produced several non-English sounds with some frequency. Other investigations (e.g., Stockman, Woods, and Tishman, 1981) have confirmed the occurrence of non-English sounds in this late babbling period, although not to any high degree.

The phrase *perceptual limitations inherent in phonetic transcription* refers to the difficulty encountered when trying to transcribe non-English sounds. Someone not trained in listening for and transcribing non-English sounds certainly will encounter grave problems recognizing and categorizing them. Locke (1983) summarizes this difficulty appropriately by stating that "there might have been more [non-English sounds] if the listeners were themselves non-English [speakers], or

TABLE 5.2 Relative Frequency of English Consonantlike Sounds in the Babbling of 11- to 12-Month-Old American Infants[1]

MORE FREQUENT CONSONANTS				LESS FREQUENT CONSONANTS			
Sound	A[2]	B	C	Sound	A[2]	B	C
h	31.77	21.0	18.3	v	1.03	1.0	0
d	20.58	30.0	13.5	l	.96	1.0	1.6
b	9.79	5.0	10.0	θ	.85	0	0.4
m	6.69	1.0	7.2	z	.56	0	0
t	4.34	0	3.6	f	.37	0	0.4
g	4.15	12.0	8.4	ʃ	.37	0	0
s	3.45	0	0.4	ð	.34	0	0.8
w	3.39	17.0	8.4	ŋ	.33	1.0	3.2
n	2.65	1.0	4.4	ʒ	.10	0	0
k	2.12	1.0	6.3	r	.10	0	0
j	1.77	9.0	11.6	tʃ	0	0	0
p	1.63	0	1.6	ʤ	0	0	0
Totals	92.33	97.0	93.7		5.01	3.0	6.4

Source: From *Phonological Acquisition and Change* (p. 4), by J. L. Locke, 1983, Orlando, FL: Academic Press. Copyright 1983 by Academic Press. Reprinted with permission.

1. The three investigations represented are: A: Irwin (1947); B: Fisichelli (1950); C: Pierce and Hanna (1974).

2. The A columns total less than 100% because the difference (2.66%) represents several sounds in Irwin's original tabulations that have no phonemic equivalent in American English phonology (e.g., [ʔ ç χ]).

more effectively oriented to non-English sounds and modes of symbolization" (p. 5).

Syllable Shapes

During the later babbling periods, open syllables are still the most frequent type of syllables. In Kent and Bauer (1985), for example, V, CV, VCV, and CVCV structures accounted for approximately 94 percent of all syllables produced. Although closed syllables were present, they were found to be very limited in the repertoires of these infants.

Babbling and Its Relationship to Later Language Development

Jakobson's discontinuity hypothesis denounced any link between babbling and later language development. However, babbling behavior is one aspect of early communication that is emerging as a predictor of later language ability. Several researchers have suggested that both the quantity and the diversity of vocalizations do indeed play a role in later language development.

Attempts have been made to correlate the quantity of vocalizations at a certain babbling age to later language performance (e.g., Camp, Burgess, Morgan, and Zerbe, 1987; Kagan, 1971; Roe 1975, 1977). Here, quantity was defined as the number of vocalizations during a specific time period. Although somewhat different criteria were used in the various studies, the results showed that the amount of prelinguistic vocalizations was positively related to later language measures.

Diversity of vocalizations was measured by (1) the number of different consonantlike sounds heard in the babbling of infants

(Stoel-Gammon and Otomo, 1986; White-hurst et al., 1991), (2) the number of structured CV syllables (Menyuk, Liebergott, and Schultz, 1986; Paul, 1991; Paul and Jennings, 1992), (3) the proportion of vocalizations containing a true consonant (Vihman and Greenlee, 1987), and (4) the ratio of consonantlike sounds to vowel-like sounds (Bauer, 1988; Bauer and Robb, 1989; Whitehurst, Smith, Fischel, Arnold, and Lonigan, 1991). In addition, a Danish investigation (Jensen, Boggild-Andersen, Schmidt, Ankerkus, and Hansen, 1988) utilized both quantity and diversity of vocalizations to predict later language skills. Summarizing the results of these methodologically varying studies, it appears that (1) less language growth is seen in children with more vocoid-babble compared to those with more contoid-babble, (2) greater language growth is related to greater babble complexity, and (3) greater language growth is related to the increased diversity of contoid productions. The future will decide if the quantity and diversity of babbling behavior might be able to predict which toddlers are at risk for language problems.

CLINICAL APPLICATION

Knowledge of Babbling Stages and Diagnostics

Speech-language pathologists, especially those in early intervention services, are often confronted with children who are still within the babbling stages of development. Knowledge of the babbling stages, which includes characteristics and approximate ages of occurrence, can be very helpful in our assessment process. Consider the following information from the parents of Megan, who is 16 months old.

The early intervention program was contacted by Megan's parents, who had been referred by the child's pediatrician. Megan was born four weeks premature and had been followed very closely by both the parents and the pediatrician. She had started to

walk around 11 months of age and the parents reported that all developmental milestones up to that point had been within normal limits. The parents were concerned because Megan did not have any real words. Children of acquaintances had begun to talk when they were 10 to 12 months old.

The speech-language pathologist visited the family home and noted that Megan was a very active toddler who was busy with her toys and enjoyed attention. Occasionally, Megan produced utterances that consisted of single vowels, for example, [a]; CV structures ([ba], [da], [ma]); and CVCV syllables ([mama], [babi], [dada], [dati]). According to the parents, repeated attempts at getting Megan to imitate these babbles had not met with success. It was observed (and the parents verified) that Megan did not use strings of babbles with any intonational patterns, that is, Megan did not produce jargon speech.

Based on these results, we could deduce that Megan is within the canonical babbling stage. However, she has not reached the point where she is imitating these babbles in ritualized games with her parents, nor is she using jargon speech. According to the approximate ages presented, jargon speech begins around 10 months of age. Megan is now 16 months old. This information gives us a general idea of where Megan stands at the moment within the period of prelinguistic development.

Prosodic Feature Development

Vowels and consonants are combined to produce syllables, words, and sentences. At the same time that we articulate these sound segments, our pronunciation varies in other respects. For example, we use a wide range of pitch and loudness variables, which can change the meaning of what is said in a number of ways. Consider the sentence: "You want that.↘" said with a falling tone at the end compared to "You want that?↗" said with a rising tone at the end. (One can even imagine that if *that* is stressed and the vowel prolonged with an excessive rising tone in the second sentence, something incredible is being desired.) The sound segments in these two sentences [ju wʌnt ðæt] relate to *what* we say; *prosodic features* refer to *how* we say it. **Prosodic features** are larger linguistic units, elements occurring across segments, that are used to influence what we say. The linguistically most relevant prosodic features we realize in speech are pitch, loudness, and tempo variations (which include sound duration). They have specific functions and may be analyzed separately. If combined, they constitute the *rhythm* of a particular language or utterance.

The development of prosodic features in infants has gained considerable importance in research in the last years. Current research begins to document their development and supports the hypothesis positing a close interaction between prosodic features, early child-directed speech (motherese), and early language development (Bonvillian, Raeburn, and Horan, 1979; Delack and Fowlow, 1978; Fernald et al., 1989; Hallé, de Boysson-Bardies, and Vihman, 1991; Jacobson, Boersma, Fields, and Olson, 1983; Kent and Murray, 1982; Robb and Saxman, 1990; Stern and Wasserman 1979; Turk, Jusczyk, and Gerken, 1995; Whalen, Levitt, and Wang, 1991). Clearly, far more information is available in the area of sound segment development. However, a better understanding of prosodic features and their development may offer us valuable insights into the transition from babbling to the first words and the close interconnection of segmental and prosodic feature acquisition.

Coinciding with the canonical babbling stage, or starting at approximately 6 months of age, the infant utilizes apparent patterns of prosodic behavior. Certain features are now employed consistently, primarily intonation, rhythm, and pausing (Crystal, 1986). Acoustic analysis shows that falling pitch is the most common intonation contour for the first year of life (Delack and Fowlow, 1978; Kent and Murray, 1982). Prosodic patterns continue to diversify toward the end of the babbling pe-

riod to such a degree that names such as *expressive jargon* (Gesell and Thompson, 1934) or *prelinguistic jargon* (Dore, Franklin, Miller, and Ramer, 1976) have been applied to them. These strings of babbles typically end in a manner that is characteristic of adult General American English intonation patterns, giving the impression of sentences without words.

TRANSITION FROM BABBLING TO FIRST WORDS

Several studies suggest that babbling and early words have much in common (e.g., Boysson-Bardies and Vihman, 1991; Davis and MacNeilage, 1990; Ferguson and Farwell, 1975; Kent and Bauer, 1985; Oller, Wieman, Doyle, and Ross, 1976; Stark, 1980; Vihman, Ferguson, and Elbert, 1986). In fact, they are often so similar that difficulties arise in differentiating between the two. The main characteristics of the transition from babbling to first words include:

1. primarily monosyllabic utterances
2. frequent use of stop consonants, followed by nasals and fricatives
3. bilabial and apical productions
4. rare use of consonant clusters
5. frequent use of central, mid-front, and low-front vowels ([ʌ, ɛ, æ])

In spite of the similarities noted above, data from Vihman et al. (1986) and Davis and MacNeilage (1990) revealed the following distinctions between babbling and first words:

1. A large diversity existed between the children's productions in each of the areas investigated (phonetic tendencies, consonant and vowel inventories, and word selection). The more words the children acquired, the more this diversity seemed to diminish (Vihman, Ferguson, and Elbert 1986).
2. Frequent use of [l] in one child's speech (Davis and MacNeilage, 1990), although

other studies noted that this consonant was not used to any significant degree.

3. The majority of the children utilized voiced stops in babbling but not in words; [g] was the most prominent example of this (Vihman, Ferguson, and Elbert, 1986).

4. Vowels produced during babbling were used as substitutes for other vowel productions in words. The high-front vowel [i] was a frequent substitute (Davis and MacNeilage, 1990).

5. Productions were context dependent. For example, high-front vowels occurred more frequently following alveolars; high-back vowels following velars; and central vowels after labial consonants (Vihman, 1992). However, little evidence of these context dependencies was found in the Tyler and Langsdale (1996) study. The wide range of individual variability could in part explain the differences they encountered.

THE FIRST FIFTY WORDS

Around a child's first birthday, a new developmental era begins: the *linguistic phase.* It starts the moment the first meaningful word is produced. That sounds plain enough, but there are some problems defining the first meaningful word. Must it be understood and produced by the child in all applicable situations and contexts? Must it have an adultlike meaning to the child? What about those utterances that do not resemble our adult representation but are, nevertheless, used as words by the child in a consistent manner?

Most define the **first word** as an entity of relatively stable phonetic form that is produced consistently by the child in a particular context and is recognizably related to the adultlike word form of a particular language (Owens, 1996). Thus, if the child says [ba] consistently in the context of being shown a ball, this form would qualify as a word. If,

however, the child says [dodo] when being shown the ball, then this would not be accepted as a word because it does not approximate the adult form.

Children frequently use "invented words" (Locke, 1983) in a consistent manner, thereby demonstrating that they seem to have meaning for the child. These vocalizations—used consistently but without a recognizable adult model—have been called **proto-words** (Menn, 1978), **phonetically consistent forms** (Dore et al., 1976), **vocables** (Ferguson, 1976), and **quasi-words** (Stoel-Gammon and Cooper, 1984).

The time of the initial productions of words is usually called the *first-fifty-word stage.* This stage encompasses the time from the first meaningful utterance at approximately 1 year of age to the time when the child begins to put two "words" together at approximately 18 to 24 months. Whether this stage is actually a separate developmental entity may be questioned. The first word may be a plausible starting point, but the strict fifty-word cut-off point is, according to several studies, purely arbitrary (Ferguson and Farwell, 1975; Nelson, 1973). Nevertheless, it appears that the child produces approximately fifty meaningful words before the next generally recognized stage of development, the *two-word stage,* begins.

During the first-fifty-word stage, there seems to be a large difference between the production and the perceptual capabilities of the child. For example, at the end of this stage, when children can produce approximately fifty words, they are typically capable of understanding around 200 words (Ingram, 1989a). This fact must have an effect on the development of semantic meaning as well as on the phonological system. It must be clearly understood that by analyzing the child's verbal productions during this stage, we are looking at only one aspect of language development. The child's perceptual, motor, and cognitive growth, as well as the influence of the environment, all play indispensable roles in this stage of language acquisition.

In examining the course of phonological development during this period, we see that it is heavily influenced by the individual words the child is acquiring. Children are not just learning sounds, which are then used to make up words, but, rather, they seem to learn word units that happen to contain particular sets of sounds. Ingram (1976) called this a *presystematic stage* in which contrastive words rather than contrastive phones (i.e., as phonemes) are acquired. The presystematic stage can be related to Cruttenden's (1981) *item learning* and *system learning* stages of early phonological development. In **item learning**, the child first acquires word forms as unanalyzed units, as productional wholes. Only later, characteristically after the first-fifty-word stage, does **system learning** occur, during which the child acquires the phonemic principles that apply to the phonological system in question.

The early portion of the item learning stage is known as the *holophrastic period*, the span of time during which the child uses one word to indicate a complete idea. In addition, the link between the object, its meaning, and the discrete sound segments used to represent the object is not yet firmly established. For example, a child might produce [da] to indicate a dog. The next day, the production might change somewhat to, perhaps, [do]. This time, the production may not refer to a dog alone but also to a cow or horse. According to Piaget (1952), the child is still within the sensorimotor period of development and so has not yet achieved full imitative ability or object permanence. Sounds and meanings drift and change.

Segmental Form Development

Several authors (e.g., Ferguson and Farwell, 1975; Ingram, 1989b) have noted *phonetic variability* and a *limitation of syllable structures*

and *sound segments* during the first-fifty-word stage. **Phonetic variability** refers to the unstable pronunciations of the child's first fifty words. While this has been well documented (Farwell, 1976; Kiparsky and Menn, 1977; Menyuk, Menn, and Silber, 1979; Stoel-Gammon and Cooper, 1984), it appears that some productions are more stable than others. Ferguson and Farwell (1975) call this category of words stable forms. However, the authors do not provide a measure for this stability and, from their examples, it is often not clear why certain words are considered more stable than others. To complicate matters, it seems that some children have a tendency to produce more stable articulations from the beginning of this stage. Stoel-Gammon and Cooper (1984) and French (1989) provide data on children whose phonetic realizations were stable from the first real word.

The second characteristic of this stage is the limitation of syllable structures and segmental productions utilized. From their relatively small repertoire of words, it would seem logical to conclude that children do not produce a large array of syllable structures and sound segments. However, what are the actual limitations during the first-fifty-word stage?

First, certain syllable types clearly predominate. These are CV, VC, and CVC syllables. When CVCV syllables are present, they are full or partial syllable reduplications. This, of course, does not mean that other syllable types do not occur. Looking, for example, at the data from Ferguson and Farwell (1975), French (1989), Ingram (1974), Leopold (1947), Menn (1971), Stoel-Gammon and Cooper (1984), and Velten (1943), these syllables are indeed the most frequently occurring. However, the children produced other syllables as well. Menn's Daniel, for instance, produced CCVC [njaj], Leopold's Hildegard a CCVCV [prɪti], and Ferguson and Farwell's T a CVCVVC [wakuak]. If the individual children are examined to see if patterns emerge, differences can be found. Certain children seem to favor specific types of syllables. For example, some children evidence CVC structures to a moderate degree from the very beginning of this stage. With others, CVC syllables appear only later and do not constitute any major part of the child's phonology until after the first-fifty-word stage (Ingram, 1976).

Second, what are the speech sound limitations that can be observed during the first-fifty-word stage? More specifically, which vowels and consonants are present, and which ones are not? Two studies that have had a large impact on this question are those presented by Jakobson (1942/1968) and Jakobson and Halle (1956). After studying several diary reports of children from various linguistic backgrounds, they concluded that the first consonants are labials, most commonly [p] or [m]; these first consonants are followed by [t] and later [k]; fricatives are present only after the respective homorganic stops have been acquired; and the first vowel is [a] or [ɑ], followed by [u] and/or [i].

CLINICAL APPLICATION

Comparing Jakobson's Results to the First Words of Two Children

The following are the first words of Joan Velten (Velten, 1943) and Jennika Ingram (Ingram, 1974).

	Joan			Jennika	
Age	**Word**	**Actual Production**	**Age**	**Word**	**Actual Production**
;10	up	[ap]	1;3	blanket	[ba], [babi]
	bottle	[ba]		byebye	[ba], [baba]
;11	bus	[bas]		daddy	[da], [dada], [dadi]
	put on	[baza]		dot	[dat], [dati]
	that	[za]		hi	[haⁱ]
1;0	down	[da]		mommy	[ma], [mami], [mama]
	out	[at]		no	[no]
	away	[ˈba ba]		see	[si]
	pocket	[bat]		see that	[siæt]
1;1	fuff	[af], [faf]		that	[da]
	put on	[baˈda]	1;4	hot	[hat]
1;2	push	[bus]		hi	[haⁱ], [haⁱdi]
	dog	[uf]		up	[ap], [api]
	pie	[ba]		no	[nodi], [dodi], [noni]
1;3	duck	[dat]			
	lamb	[bap]			
1;4	M	[am]			
	N	[an]			
	in	[n̩]			

If the month increments are seen as later phases of development, the following order occurs in the first words for Joan and Jennika:

	Joan	Jennika
Vowels	[a] → [u]	[a], [i], [o], [æ], [aⁱ]
Consonants	[p], [b] → [s], [z] → [t], [d] → [f] → [m], [n]	[b], [d], [t], [h], [m], [n], [s] → [p]
Syllable shapes	VC, CV → CVC, CVCV	CV, CVCV, CVC → VC, VCV
	CVCVs are not reduplications	Most CVCVs are reduplications
Phonetic variability	More stable forms	More variability

Both Joan's and Jennika's vowel development follows Jakobson's findings: [a] is followed by, or co-occurs with, [i] and/or [u]. Joan's order of consonant development, though, shows clear differences from the order described by Jakobson. For example, she does seem to use the fricatives [s] and [z] before the homorganic stops [t] and [d]. Both children demonstrate rather late development of specific bilabial sounds that, according to Jakobson, are the earliest consonants: for Joan [m] and for Jennika [p] are later than fricatives.

Over the years, Jakobson's postulated universals have undergone a good deal of scrutiny. Although most of the investigators (e.g., Oller et al., 1976; Stoel-Gammon and Cooper, 1984; Vihman et al., 1986) have concentrated on consonant inventories, Ingram (1976) has attempted to grapple with the acquisition of vowels. Using the data from four case studies (Ingram, 1974; Leopold, 1947; Menn, 1971; Velten, 1943), he compared the vowels in the first fifty words. General trends could be noted, and most children seemed to follow the acquisitional pattern of [a] preceding [i] and [u].

Consonant inventories follow the same pattern. Although certain similarities have been verified, several investigations have pointed out the wide range of variability between individual subjects (e.g., Ferguson and Farwell, 1975; Stoel-Gammon and Cooper, 1984; Vihman, 1992; Vihman et al., 1986). If one wants to generalize, then the marked use of voiced labial and dental stops and nasals has to be underlined. Ferguson and Garnica (1975) make the point that [h] and [w] are also among the first consonants acquired. Findings substantiating these generalizations drawn from five different investigations are summarized in Table 5.3. Table 5.3 compares the consonant inventory of seven children labelled "Stanford" (Vihman et al., 1986) to nineteen other children from research studies noted in the table. As can be seen, all the children have words containing [b] and [m]. Over half of the children in the studies produced [p], [t], [d], [k], [g], [ʃ], [n], [w], and [h] consonants as well.

Longitudinal Findings. Longitudinal research follows a child or a group of children over a specific time frame. It has the advantage of observing the acquisition process of individual children. However, longitudinal research is often limited in that only one child or a small group of subjects is evaluated. Stoel-Gammon (1985) presented a longitudinal investigation

It should be noted that the Vihman et al. (1986) data reduce the individual variation among children considerably. For example, if child A produces two words with word-initial [n] while child B produces forty-three words with [n], both of those children are counted for [n] use in this table. However, the use of this particular sound in the two children's inventories is hardly comparable.

TABLE 5.3 Initial Consonant Productions within the First-Fifty-Word Vocabularies of Seven Stanford Subjects and Nineteen Other English-Speaking Children

	STANFORD	OTHERS			STANFORD	OTHERS[1]
p	×	+		ʃ	+	+
b	×	×		ʒ	0	0
t	×	+		tʃ	−	−
d	×	+		dʒ	−	−
k	×	+		m	×	×
g	+	+		n	×	+
f	+	−		ŋ	−	−
v	−	0		l	−	−
θ	+	−		r	+	−
ð	+	−		w	+	+
s	−	−		j	+	−
z	−	−		h	+	+

Source: From "Phonological Development from Babbling to Speech: Common Tendencies and Individual Differences," by M. M. Vihman, C. A. Ferguson, and M. Elbert, 1986, *Applied Psycholinguistics, 7,* p. 28. Copyright 1986 by Cambridge University Press. Reprinted with permission.

Note: × = all children in study; + = over half but not all children in study; − = more than one but less than half children in study; 0 = none of the children.

1. Data derived from Ferguson & Farwell (1975), Shibamoto & Olmsted (1978), Leonard, Newhoff, and Mesalam, (1980), and Stoel-Gammon and Cooper (1984).

that not only utilized spontaneous speech but also looked at a sizable number of children.

Thirty-four children between 15 and 24 months of age participated in this study. The investigation was constructed to look at meaningful speech only; therefore, the subjects were grouped according to the age when they actually began to say at least ten identifiable words within a recording session. This resulted in three groups of children: Group A children, who had ten words at 15 months; Group B, who had ten words at 18 months; and Group C, who had ten words at 21 months. The resulting data provide information about early consonant development and can be summarized as follows:

1. A larger inventory of sounds was found in the word-initial than in the word-final position.
2. Word-initial inventories contained voiced stops prior to voiceless ones, while the reverse was true for word-final productions.

3. The following phones appeared in at least 50 percent of all the subjects by 24 months of age:

   [h, w, b, t, d, m, n, k, g, f, and s] word-initially
   [p, t, k, n, r, and s] word-finally.

4. The liquid [r] nearly always appeared first in a word-final position.
5. If the mean percentage of norm consonant productions was calculated (Shriberg and Kwiatkowski, 1982b), 70 percent accuracy was achieved. Because there is obviously a large difference between the inventory produced by 2-year-olds and that produced by adults, the author states that this accuracy level suggests that children are primarily attempting words that contain sounds within their articulatory abilities.
6. The order of appearance of initial and final phones was relatively constant across the three groups of children tested. Individual differences in the appearance of

phones related to the classes of fricatives/ affricates and liquids.

Although individual variability was observed in this investigation, the ability to follow the children in a longitudinal manner from the same point (ten identifiable words in a recording session) regardless of their age seemed to reduce the extreme variability noted in other cross-sectional research. Although this study did not contain a large number of subjects, it certainly suggests some clinical implications.

CLINICAL APPLICATION

Developmental Research and Therapeutic Implications

It is often stated that speech-language pathologists follow a developmental model in therapy, that is, sounds or processes that are developmentally earlier are targeted before those that are later. Stoel-Gammon's (1985) data support techniques utilized in therapy:

1. *Sounds first appear in the word-initial position:* In therapy, a newly acquired sound is typically placed in the word-initial position. Developmental data give evidence that this is indeed easier for the child.
2. *Anterior stops and nasals are acquired earlier:* In therapy, this is often used as a guiding principle. These sounds are very early and should, therefore, be in the speech of children. Even most children with phonological disorders have them in their consonant inventories.

There are also some interesting results from this study that are not often employed in therapy:

1. *The liquid [r] nearly always appeared in word-final position:* Based on this finding, words such as *more* and *bear* might be easier than *red* or *rope* for the child with [r] difficulties (assuming that the child has difficulty with the central vowels with r-coloring *and* the liquid [r]).
2. *Word-initial inventories contained voiced stops first; word-final inventories contained voiceless stops first:*

According to this finding, the child with [k] and [g] problems might benefit from first working on [g] in the word-initial position before [k] in the word-final position. (This is based on the earlier result that sounds appear first in the word-initial position followed by later use in the word-final position.)

Due to the limited number of subjects, this application of Stoel-Gammon's (1985) results to therapeutic practice is probably premature. The intent here is to demonstrate how research findings can directly impact therapy.

Individual Acquisition Patterns. Throughout this discussion, individual variability has been stressed. The next question follows automatically: Do children show individual acquisition patterns or strategies? In other words, do children build their phonological inventory around certain sounds? If so, do these sounds represent a child's preference for a particular sound or set of sounds? Ferguson and Farwell (1975) referred to *salience* and *avoidance* factors. *Salience* implies that children will acquire words that contain sounds within their phonological inventories. The **salience factor** is defined as a child's active selection in early word productions of words containing sounds that are important or remarkable (salient) to the child. The **avoidance factor** is defined as the avoidance of words that do not contain sounds within a child's inventory. (This principle seems to apply only to the production of words; investigations relative to comprehension have not produced similar results (see Hoek, Ingram, and Gibson, 1986). Production selection and avoidance have often been observed; for example, Schwartz and Leonard (1982) add experimental support to this claim.

Individual strategies employed may include preferences for certain sounds, certain syllable structures, and/or sound classes or sound features. Individual preference can also refer to those objects and contexts that the child enjoys more than others. The child's preference and environment will most certainly have an effect on which words are acquired and which phonetic inventory is established during the production of the first fifty words.

Prosodic Feature Development

As the child moves from the end of the babbling period to first words, the previously noted intonational contours continue. The falling intonation contour still predominates, although both a rise-fall and a simple rising contour have also been observed (Kent and Bauer, 1985).

An important aspect of communication during the first-fifty-word stage is *prosodic variation*. Examples of children's speech during this time have included pitch variations to indicate differences in meaning. For example, a falling pitch on the first syllable, [da↓ da], as daddy entered the room versus [da↑ da], a rising pitch on the first syllable, was realized when a noise was heard outside when daddy was expected (Crystal, 1986). Prosodic features are also used to indicate differences in syntactical function. Bruner (1975) labels these prosodic units *place-holders*. A demand or question, for example, is often signaled first by prosody; words are added later. For example, a child aged 1;2 first used the phrase "all gone" after dinner by humming the intonation. Approximately a month passed before the child's segmental productions were somewhat accurate (Crystal, 1986). One widely held view is that these prosodic units fulfill a social function. They are seen as a means of signaling joint participation in an activity shared by the child and the caregiver. Several authors suggest that prosodic features are evidence of developing speech acts (Dore, 1975; Halliday, 1975; Menn, 1976). A word with a specific intonation pattern might indicate re-

questing, calling, or demanding, for example. The following prosodic features associated with intentional communication have been observed (Marcos, 1987):

10 to 12 months

first words, naming, labelling

> Begin with a falling contour only. Flat or level contour, usually accompanied by variations such as falsettos or variations in duration or loudness. Example: At 10 and 11 months, Hildegard (Leopold, 1947) lengthened the vowels of words such as [de:] for *there*

13 to 15 months

requesting, attention getting, curiosity, surprise, recognition, insistence, greeting

> Rising contour. High falling contour that begins with a high pitch and drops to a lower one. This is noted in the previous example of [da↑ da].

prior to 18 months

playful anticipation, emphatic stress

> High rising and high rising-falling contour. Example: A child might use a high rising intonation pattern on *ball* to indicate that the game is about to begin.

around 18 months

warnings, playfulness

> Falling-rising contour. Rising-falling contour. Example: A child might use a falling-rising contour on *no* to indicate that he/she has been warned not to do that, that is, to repeat this warning. The same *no* with a rising-falling contour could be used during a game to indicate that daddy is not going to get the ball.

As can be noted, intonational changes seem to develop prior to stress. Although various pitch contours appear earlier than the first meaningful words, contrastive stress is first evidenced only at the beginning of the two-word stage or at the age of approximately 1;6. During the first-fifty-word stage, the observed pitch variations can be said to represent directional sequences (rising versus falling, for example) or range patterns (high versus low within the child's pitch range). For a more detailed analysis of early intonational development, see Crystal (1986).

THE PRESCHOOL CHILD

This section stresses information on the developing phonology of the child from approximately 18 to 24 months, the end of the first-fifty-word stage, to the beginning of the sixth year. It is during this time that the largest growth within the phonological system takes place. However, not only is the child's phonological system expanding but also large gains are seen in other language areas. From 18 to 24 months of age, the child's expressive vocabulary has at least tripled from 50 to 150–300 words (Lipsitt, 1966; Mehrabian, 1970), while the receptive vocabulary has grown from 200 to 1,200 words (Weiss and Lillywhite, 1981). The transition from one-word utterances to two-word sentences, a large linguistic step, is typically occurring at this time. With the production of two-word sentences, the child has entered the period of expressing specific semantic relationships: the beginning of syntactical development.

Around the child's fifth birthday, the expressive vocabulary has expanded to approximately 2,200 words, while about 9,600 words are in the child's receptive vocabulary (Weiss and Lillywhite, 1981). Almost all of the basic grammatical forms of the language—such as questions, negative statements, dependent clauses, and compound sentences—are now present as well (Owens, 1996). More important, the child knows now how to use language to communicate in an effective

manner. Five-year-olds talk differently to babies than they do to their friends, for example. They also know how to tell jokes and riddles, and they are quite able to handle the linguistic subtleties of being polite and rude.

A child's phonological development at 18 to 24 months still demonstrates a rather limited inventory of speech sounds and phonotactic possibilities. At this time, perception seems to precede production somewhat—children can now identify single-segment differences between words. By the end of the preschool period, around the child's fifth birthday, an almost complete phonological system has emerged.

All these changes occur in less than four years. Although this section focuses on phonological development, such a discussion must always be seen within the context of the equally large expansions in morphosyntax, semantics, and pragmatics that occur during this time.

Segmental Form Development: Vowels

One area of sound acquisition that has been widely neglected in most discussions of phonological development is the acquisition of vowels. This neglect has been at least partially justified with the statement that children have acquired all vowels within the English sound inventory by the age of 3 (Templin, 1957). Little information is available on the development of vowels. This section on vowel development in preschool children will utilize the data presented by Irwin and Wong (1983) and Velten (1943). Although several methodological problems with Irwin and Wong's (1983) investigation have been pointed out (see Smit, 1986), it nevertheless examines the vowel productions in spontaneous conversations of children from 18 to 72 months of age. The Velten (1943) data come from a diary study of Joan Velten.

By examining the Irwin and Wong data, it can be seen that the children show the acquisition of [ɑ], [ʊ], [i], [ɪ], and [ʌ] at 18 months if the criterion is set at 70 percent accuracy. For the individual subjects at this age level, the correct production of vowels ranged from 23 percent to 71 percent. By 24 months, the only vowels that did not reach 70 percent group accuracy were [ɝ] and [ɚ]. By the age of 3, all the vowels were accounted for with virtually no production errors. Interestingly enough, at age 4, the accuracy for [ɚ], [u], and [ə] dropped again to less than 90 percent.

These findings generally support Templin's claim that vowels are mastered at age 3. The drop in accuracy at age 4 might indicate that some younger children simply avoided those vowels before.

Another view of vowel acquisition is offered by diary studies. Velten's (1943) data show that prior to the age of 21 months, her daughter utilized the [a] vowel. After a surge in vocabulary at 21 months, the vowel [u] was added. When this child is compared to Irwin and Wong's (1983) data, large discrepancies between the two become obvious. Again, the previously discussed concepts of salience and avoidance may apply to the described differences. Some children possibly select, for the most part, words that consist of sounds within their repertoire, avoiding those words and sounds that are not. Salience and avoidance in conjunction with individual phonetic preference could account for the noted differences.

Far more information is needed in the area of vowel acquisition. From the limited amount of data presently available, it appears that vowels are indeed generally mastered by the age of 3. Whether individual variation plays a large role in this acquisition process still needs to be documented. This is an interesting area of research, especially in light of the deviant vowel systems that are often noted in children with phonological disorders.

Segmental Form Development: Consonants

Cross-Sectional Results. It appears that no chapter on phonological development can be complete without looking at the large sample studies that began in the 1930s (Wellman, Case, Mengert, and Bradbury, 1931) and have continued periodically since. However, it seems appropriate to preface such a discussion with the problems inherent in these studies.

Large sample studies were initiated to look at a large number of children in order to examine which sounds were mastered at which age levels. To this end, they evaluated most of the speech sounds within a given native language. With a few exceptions (Irwin and Wong, 1983; Olmsted, 1971; Stoel-Gammon, 1985, 1987), these studies have used methods similar to articulation tests to collect their data, that is, the children were asked to name pictures and certain sounds were then judged productionally "correct" or "incorrect."

In this type of procedure, general as well as specific problems arise. First, the fact that the child produces the sound "correctly" as a one-word response does not mean that the sound can also be produced "correctly" in natural speech conditions. Practitioners have always been aware of the often large articulatory discrepancies between one-word responses and the same sounds used in conversation. Second, the choice of pictures/words will certainly affect the production of the individual sounds within the word. Not only does the child's familiarity with the word play a role but also factors such as the length of the word, its structure, the stressed or unstressed position of the sound within the word, and the phonetic context in which the sound occurs. These factors help or hinder production. Therefore, strictly speaking, the only conclusion that can be drawn from cross-sectional studies is that the children could or could not produce that particular sound in that specific word.

The third point is a theoretical issue. As stated repeatedly in this textbook, there has been an adoption of certain new concepts and terminology within the field of speech-language pathology. This chapter, for example, is called phonological development, not speech sound development. With the inclusion of the terms *phonology* and *phonological development,* certain conceptual changes have been accepted. These cross-sectional studies are

perhaps indicative of the inventory of speech sounds children typically possess at certain ages, but they are not a documentation of a particular child's phonological system.

Specific methodological differences between various cross-sectional studies are also important factors when interpreting the results. These include the criteria used to determine whether the child has "mastered" a particular sound. Although this has been elaborated upon in several articles and books (e.g., Smit, 1986; Vihman, 1998), it is worth mentioning again. Table 5.4 provides a comparison of several of the larger cross-sectional studies.

TABLE 5.4   Age Levels for Speech Sound Development According to Six Studies

	WELLMAN (1931)	POOLE (1934)	TEMPLIN (1957)	SANDER (1972)	PRATHER (1975)	ARLT (1976)
m	3	3½	3	before 2	2	3
n	3	4½	3	before 2	2	3
h	3	3½	3	before 2	2	3
p	4	3½	3	before 2	2	3
f	3	5½	3	3	2–4	3
w	3	3½	3	before 2	2–8	3
b	3	3½	4	before 2	2–8	3
ŋ		4½	3	2	2	3
j	4	4½	3½	3	2–4	
k	4	4½	4	2	2–4	3
g	4	4½	4	2	2–4	3
l	4	6½	6	3	3–4	4
d	5	4½	4	2	2–4	3
t	5	4½	6	2	2–8	3
s	5	7½	4½	3	3	4
r	5	7½	4	3	3–4	5
tʃ	5		4½	4	3–8	4
v	5	6½	6	4	4	3½
z	5	7½	7	4	4	4
ʒ	6	6½	7	6	4	4
θ		7½	6	5	4	5
ʤ			7	4	4	4
ʃ		6½	4½	4	3–8	4½
ð		6½	7	5	4	5

Looking at age comparisons in Table 5.4, a difference in reported mastery of three years or more can be observed for some sounds. For example, note the difference between the ages of mastery for the [s] in the more recent Prather, Hedrick, and Kern (1975) and in the older Poole (1934) study. The Poole investigation has a mastery age of 7½ years, while the Prather et al. investigation shows an age level of 3 years. A three-year difference can be found for [z] acquisition when the Prather et al. data are compared to the Templin (1957) results. Again, Prather et al. assign a much earlier level of mastery. One question that is often asked in this context is: Does this mean that children are now producing sounds "correctly" at an earlier age? The answer is no; many of these differences are a consequence of the way *mastery* was defined. Poole, for instance, stated that 100 percent of the children must use the sound correctly in each of the positions tested. Prather et al. and Templin, on the other hand, set this level at 75 percent. In addition, rather than using the 75 percent cutoff level for all three positions (initial, medial, and final) as Templin had done, Prather et al. used only two positions (initial and final) for their calculations. This clearly changes the ages to which mastery can be assigned. A shift to earlier acquisition noted in the Prather et al. study could be accounted for by these methodological changes. Also, as Smit (1986) points out, the Prather et al. results are based on incomplete data sets, especially at the younger age groupings. Although Prather et al. began with twenty-one subjects in each age group, several of these children did not respond to many of the words. Thus, at times, only eight to twelve subjects were used to calculate the norms. The children who did

> The lack of response from the younger children could reflect the aforementioned avoidance factor: Words that contain sounds not in the child's inventory will be avoided.

not respond to some words may have been avoiding them because they felt that they could not pronounce them "correctly." This, too, would alter the age norms. Smit (1986) has attempted to compensate for the incomplete data sets of Prather et al. In Table 5.5, the column labelled Complete Data Sets reflects the earliest age all twenty-one children from each age group mastered the sound. The next column, Sets with Data from at Least 14 Subjects, denotes the age of mastery when at least two thirds of the subjects responded. These data are compared to the two-position norms from Templin (1957) that reflect, comparable to the Prather et al. study, a mastery level of 75 percent.

With these adjustments, the Templin and Prather et al. data look suddenly very similar. There are even instances in which the Templin acquisition norms show younger ages than those reported by Prather et al. When the data are realigned in such a way, it becomes clear that children are by no means mastering sounds earlier now.

Ingram (1989a) points out additional problems related to the Templin study and sums them up as follows:

> Templin's study provides a useful descriptive overview of English phonological acquisition.... Here, however, we will conclude with a caution about using large sample data such as these for anything more than the most general of purposes, setting out a series of problems with Templin's study in particular and large sample studies in general. The limitations of such studies need to be emphasized since their results may be inappropriately used both for theoretical and practical purposes, the latter including cases where a child might be misidentified as being speech-delayed because of his performance on a Templin-style articulation test. (p. 366)

TABLE 5.5 Ages of Acquisition of Specific Sounds Determined in Several Different Ways Provided by Prather, Hedrick, and Kern (1975) and by Templin (1957)

	PRATHER, HEDRICK, AND KERN (1975) TWO-POSITION NORMS (I, F)			TEMPLIN (1957)	
Sound	All Data Sets	Complete Data Sets	Sets with Data from at Least 14 Ss	Two-Position Norms (I, F)	Three-Position Norms (I, M, F)
m	≤2;0	4;0	2;4	≤3;0	≤3;0
n	≤2;0	3;8	2;4	≤3;0	≤3;0
h[1]	≤2;0	>4;0	2;8	≤3;0	≤3;0
p	≤2;0	>4;0	2;4	≤3;0	≤3;0
ŋ[1]	≤2;0	4;0	2;4	≤3;0	≤3;0
f	2;4	4;0	2;4	≤3;0	≤3;0
j[1]	≤2;0	>4;0	3;0	3;6	3;6
k	2;4	4;0	2;4	4;0	4;0
d	2;4[2]	3;8	2;4[2]	4;0	4;0
w[1]	≤2;0[2]	4;0	2;8	≤3;0	≤3;0
b	2;8	4;0	2;8	4;0[2]	4;0[2]
t	2;8	3;8	2;8	≤3;0[2]	6;0
g	2;4[2]	4;0	2;4[2]	4;0[2]	4;0[2]
s	3;0[2]	3;8	3;0[2]	4;6	4;6[2]
r	3;4[2]	>4;0	3;4[2]	4;0	4;0
l	3;4[2]	4;0	3;4[2]	6;0	6;0
ʃ	3;8	3;8	3;8	4;0	4;6[2]
tʃ	3;8	3;8	3;8	4;6	4;6
ð	>4;0	>4;0	>4;0	7;0	7;0
ʒ[1]	>4;0	>4;0	4;0	7;0	7;0
dʒ	3;4[2]	>4;0	3;4[2]	7;0	7;0
θ	>4;0	>4;0	>4;0	6;0	6;0
v	>4;0	>4;0	>4;0	6;0	6;0
z	>4;0	>4;0	>4;0	7;0	7;0
hw[1]	>4;0	>4;0	>4;0	>8;0	>8;0

Source: From "Ages of Speech Sound Acquisition: Comparisons and Critiques of Several Normative Studies," by A. B. Smit, 1986, Language, Speech, and Hearing in Schools, 17(3), p. 181. Copyright 1986 by the American Speech-Language-Hearing Association. Reprinted by permission.

Note: The age of acquisition in each case is the earliest stage at which at least 75 percent of children produced the designated sound correctly in each indicated word position.

1. Sound does not occur in all word positions in English.

2. A reversal occurs in older age groups.

What then is the alternative? Several investigators (e.g., Irwin and Wong, 1983; Stoel-Gammon, 1985) have attempted to improve the situation by using spontaneous speech and/or longitudinal investigations. Although spontaneous speech samples are in some respects better than the picture-naming tasks, several problems remain. Their use can also give us a biased picture. We actually probe into only a small portion of the child's conversational abilities and then generalize, assuming that this is representative of the child's overall

> The avoidance factor may also influence spontaneous speech. Words might be avoided that contain sounds that the child cannot say.

performance. Also, factors outside our control might determine which words and sounds the child does produce and which ones he or she does not. As a result, the sample obtained will probably not contain all the sounds in that particular child's phonetic inventory.

Longitudinal data, on the other hand, can give us a real insight into the individual acquisition process, an important aspect missing in cross-sectional studies. The following discussion examines data from longitudinal studies on consonant development in children.

Longitudinal Results. Several longitudinal studies of consonant development exist, but they report on either a single child or a small group of children (e.g., Leopold, 1947; Menn, 1971; Vihman et al., 1985). Therefore, the data cannot be readily generalized. However, Vihman and Greenlee (1987) used a longitudinal methodology to examine the phonological development of ten 3-year-old children with the following results:

1. Stops and other fricatives were substituted for [ð] and [θ] by all subjects.
2. Over half of the subjects also substituted [r] and [l] sounds (gliding) and employed palatal fronting, in which a palatal sound is replaced by an alveolar ([ʃ] becomes [s]).
3. Two of the ten children demonstrated their own particular "style" of phonological acquisition.
4. On average, 73 percent of the children's utterances were judged intelligible by three raters unfamiliar with the children. However, the range of intelligibility was broad, extending from 54 percent to 80 percent. As expected, children with fewer errors were more intelligible than those with multiple errors. Another factor also

played a role: The children who used more complex sentences tended to be more difficult to understand.

This last finding is significant. It documents the complex interaction between phonological development and the acquisition of the language system as a whole. The simultaneous acquisition of complex morphosyntactic and semantic relationships could well have an impact on the growth of the phonological system. It has been hypothesized that **phonological idioms** (Moskowitz, 1971) or **regression** (Leopold, 1947) occurs as the child attempts to master other complexities of language. Both terms refer to accurate sound productions that are later replaced by inaccurate ones. When trying to deal with more complex morphosyntactic or semantic structures, the child's previously correct articulations appear to be lost, replaced by inaccurate sound productions.

CLINICAL APPLICATION

Using Cross-Sectional Mastery Level Charts: Yes or No?

This textbook has pointed out some of the problems inherent in large cross-sectional studies of ages of sound mastery. Should these charts then be discarded? Probably not. Sound mastery charts give useful information about the general ages and order that speech sounds develop. They can provide a broad framework for comparison, especially for beginning clinicians.

Clinicians should remember, however, that varying methodologies and criteria for sound mastery across investigations have produced a wide range of acquisition ages. Differences in ages of mastery for some sounds are often three to four and a half years apart. Based on the results of the Sander (1972) study, a clinician could justify doing [s] therapy with a 3-year-old, but according to the Poole (1934) investigation, a clinician should wait until the child is 7½ years old to work on [s]. These sound mastery charts should never be the single deciding factor for intervention. A colleague once remarked, "When I worked in the public schools, we first decided if the child should be in therapy or not. Then we used the specific sound mastery chart that documented our decision." Clinical decision making involves much more than comparing a child to the mastery ages provided by cross-sectional research.

Phonological Processes

Within the last decade, the study of phonological development has shifted from examining the mastery of individual sounds to the acquisition and ordering of the phonological system. According to natural phonology, there seems to be a time frame during which normally developing children do suppress certain processes. This approximate age of suppression is helpful when determining normal versus disordered phonological systems and can be used as a guideline when targeting remediation goals.

> Definitions and examples of phonological processes are given in the Natural Phonology section of Chapter 4.

The following section will address some developmental aspects of syllable structure, substitution, and assimilation processes.

Syllable Structure Processes. Syllable structure processes are manifestations of the general tendency of young children to reduce words to basic CV structures. They become evident between the ages of 1;6 and 4;0, when there is a rapid growth in vocabulary and the onset of two-word utterances (Ingram, 1989b).

Reduplication is an early syllable structure process. Ingram (1989b) notes that it is a common process during the child's first-fifty-word stage. There was no evidence of this process in the youngest group of children (1;6 to 1;9) in the Preisser, Hodson, and Paden (1988) study.

Final consonant deletion is a relatively early process. Preisser et al. (1988) state that it was extremely rare in the utterances of the subjects in the 2;2 to 2;5 age group. Ingram (1989b) and Grunwell (1987) note the disappearance of this process around age 3.

Unstressed syllable deletion, sometimes called *weak syllable deletion,* lasts longer than final consonant deletion, to approximately 4 years of age (Ingram, 1989b). This is also confirmed by Grunwell's (1987) data. However, Preisser et al. (1988) noted that most of the children in their sample appeared to have suppressed this process by around their second birthday. (Only 3 percent of the twenty children over age 2;2 demonstrated unstressed syllable deletion.)

Cluster reduction is a syllable structure process that lasts for a relatively long time. Haelsig and Madison (1986) noted cluster reductions that still occurred in 5-year-old children, while Roberts, Burchinal, and Footo (1990) evidenced rare instances of this process in their 8-year-old children. In the Smit (1993a) study, there was some evidence of cluster reduction in the 8;0- to 9;0-year-old children for specific initial consonant clusters (approximately 1 to 4 percent of the 247 children for primarily three-consonant clusters). Greenlee (1974) describes four developmental stages of consonant reduction: (1) deletion of the entire cluster: [it] for *treat;* (2) reduction to one cluster member: [tit] for *treat;* (3) cluster is realized but one member is substituted: [twit] for *treat;* (4) norm articulation: [trit]. The Smit (1993a) data support stages 2 through 4, whereas stage 1, complete deletion of a cluster, was very rare even in the 2-year-old subjects.

Epenthesis refers to the insertion of a sound segment into a word, thereby changing its syllable structure. The intrusive sound can be a vowel as well as a consonant, but most often it is restricted to a schwa insertion between two consonants. This schwa insertion, for example [pəliz] for *please,* is used to simplify the production difficulty of consonant clusters. Smit (1993a) and Smit, Hand, Freilinger, Bernthal, and Bird (1990) report that between the ages of 2;6 and 8;0, schwa insertion in clusters is a common process.

Substitution Processes. Stopping refers most frequently to the replacement of stops for fricatives and affricates. Due to the fact that fricatives and affricates are acquired at different ages, stopping is not a unified process but should be broken down into the individual sounds for which this process is employed. Table 5.6 summarizes the ages at which stopping is suppressed for the different fricative sounds.

Fronting denotes the tendency of young children to replace palatals and velars with alveolar consonants. Frequently occurring fronting processes consist of [ʃ] → [s], palatal fronting, and [k] → [t], velar fronting. Palatal fronting may also occur in affricate productions, [tʃ] → [ts] and [dʒ] → [dz]. Lowe, Knutson, and Monson (1985) found velar fronting to be more prevalent than palatal fronting. They also found that fronting rarely occurred after the age of 3;6. Based on the Smit (1993b) data, both velar fronting and palatal fronting were still noted until approximately age 5;0, although the frequency of occurrence is very limited (fewer than 5 percent of the 186 children).

Gliding of [r] and [l] seems to extend beyond 5;0 years of age (Grunwell, 1987; Smit, 1993b) and can be infrequently found even in the speech of children as old as 7 (Roberts et al., 1990; Smit, 1993b).

Assimilation Processes. There are many different assimilation processes that occur in the speech of children. Children at different stages of their speech development tend to

These processes are discussed in some detail in Chapters 2 and 4.

TABLE 5.6 Age of Suppression of Stopping

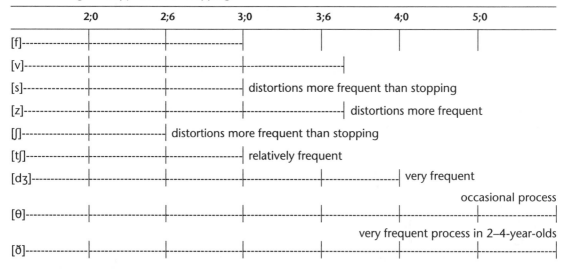

Source: Summarized from "Phonologic Error Distributions in the Iowa-Nebraska Articulation Norms Project: Consonant Singletons," by A. B. Smit, 1993, *Journal of Speech and Hearing Research, 36,* pp. 533–547.

utilize assimilation processes in systematic ways. One of the most frequently occurring assimilatory processes is *velar harmony* (Smith, 1973). Prominent examples are:

[gɔk] for *dog*
[keɪk] for *take*
[kɑk] for *talk*

However, regressive assimilation processes are not limited to velar consonants. Smith (1973) reported similar regressive assimilations in which bilabials influenced pre-

ceding nonlabial consonants and consonant clusters. Among his examples:

[bebu] for *table*
[bɔp] for *stop*
[mibu] for *nipple*

Although not all children display these types of assimilation processes, they may be part of the normal speech development in 1;6- to 2-year-olds. If they persist beyond 3;0, they begin to constitute a danger sign for a disordered phonological system (Grunwell, 1987).

CLINICAL APPLICATION

Diagnostic Implications of Phonological Process Suppression

Approximate ages of suppression have been provided for several common phonological processes. This information can be helpful during our diagnostic assessment. The following phonological processes were identified in Clint, age 3;6.

Word	Production	Phonological Process
house	[haʊ]	final consonant deletion
cup	[kʌ]	final consonant deletion
gun	[gʌ]	final consonant deletion
shovel	[ʃʌbəl]	stopping of [v]
vacuum	[bækju]	stopping of [v], final consonant deletion
vase	[beɪ]	stopping of [v], final consonant deletion
scratching	[krætʃɪŋ]	consonant cluster reduction
skunk	[kʌŋk]	consonant cluster reduction
star	[tɑɚ]	consonant cluster reduction
jumping	[dʌmpɪŋ]	stopping of [dʒ]
jelly	[dɛli]	stopping of [dʒ]
jeep	[dip]	stopping of [dʒ]
that	[dæt]	stopping of [ð]
bath	[bæt]	stopping of [θ]
feather	[fɛdɚ]	stopping of [ð]

Similar processes were also noted in conversational speech.

Which of the noted processes should be suppressed by age 3;6? Final consonant deletion is usually suppressed by around age 3;0, while stopping of [v], [θ], [ð], and [dʒ] extend to age 3;6 or beyond. Consonant cluster reduction is also a process that is suppressed at a relatively late age. Based on these results, the only process that might cause concern at this age would be final consonant deletion. Again, discretion must be exercised when using these approximate ages of suppression as the sole criterion for determining the necessity for intervention.

Developmental Issues: Natural Phonology versus Nonlinear Phonology

Nonlinear phonologies, exemplified by autosegmental theory, metrical phonology, and feature geometry theories, are discussed in the previous chapter. Of the three theories, feature geometry seems to be the one most often applied to both the normal acquisition and the disordered phonological systems. This discussion will concentrate on how feature geometry theory explains the acquisition of children's phonological systems.

First, let's compare the acquisition process when feature geometry is contrasted to Stampe's (1979) generative model of natural phonology. Phonological processes represent surface-level mismatches between the child's and the adult's norm productions. Therefore, if the child says [toᵘp] for *soap*, we say that there is a mismatch in the form, that is, the child has used the natural process of stopping. As the child's phonological system becomes more developed, this process is suppressed, resulting in a norm production of [soᵘp]. However, as a portion of this theory, it is assumed that the child's underlying representation was adultlike. Therefore, although the child says [toᵘp], the child's underlying system is said to be fully intact, that is, the child has the same understanding of the /s/ phoneme as an adult does. One problem with this explanation is that it is highly abstract and lacks empirical data to support the claims about the child's underlying adultlike representation. For example, if the child always produces [t] for [s], what indication do we have that the child's underlying representation matches the adult's? Even if the child can discriminate between [t] and [s], it only indicates that some sort of differentiation has occurred, not that the child actually utilizes the same discrimination categories that adults use. In addition, phonological processes do not explain why

certain substitution processes occur and others do not. Velar fronting is a common phonological process. However, why are velar consonants replaced by alveolars and not bilabials? For this, there is no explanation in the natural phonology construct.

Feature geometries account for the developmental process in a different manner. First, the child is viewed as coming to the language-learning process with a "set of universally determined templates with regard to segmental properties" (Yavaş, 1998, p. 277). In feature geometry, concrete underlying representations can be formulated that are consistent with the child's production while not contradicting properties of the target system. This is done by stating that the underlying representation is *underspecified* for those features that do not contrast in the child's system. If a child replaces [k] with [t], the place features of coronal versus dorsal are underspecified. In the absence of phonemic contrasts in the child's system and the subsequent lack of an underlying specification, so-called default features are formulated. These default features are used to explain the error patterns. The child who replaces all [k]-productions with [t] demonstrates that there is no place of articulation contrast between nonlabial stop-plosives. Dorsal and coronal features have no underlying representation: They are underspecified. However, [t] is seen as the default feature. When either [t] or [k] is needed, [t] is supplied as the default. In the course of development, the child's underlying underspecified features give way to more specified representations that create a match between the child's phonological system and the target system.

Second, the feature geometry tiers represent the general order of acquisition of features (Yavaş, 1998). Thus, higher-level features, those closer to the root node, such as supralaryngeal and laryngeal features, are developmentally earlier than those that are lower or more deeply embedded on the tier, such as coronal, labial, and dorsal place features. As children develop, their phonological mismatches are typically related to features that are lower on the feature geometry tiers. Laryngeal and supralaryngeal features are dominated by the root node. Therefore, according to this framework, early distinctions should develop between nasal versus nonnasal and voiced versus voiceless contrasts. Looking at the developmental patterns of children, we see that these are indeed some of the earliest contrasts—[p], [b], and [m], for example.

In addition, common processes, that is, those that typically occur in the development of children's phonological systems versus idiosyncratic or unusual processes, can be accounted for by using feature geometry's tiered representation. Velar fronting ([k] → [t]) is a common process that involves changes in the place node. On the other hand, an idiosyncratic or unusual process, such as liquid stopping ([r] → [d]) affects a major class feature (sonorant) at the root node. According to the implications of feature geometry, these two "substitutions" would indicate something quite different in the development of the child's phonological system.

Feature geometry is an innovative way to look at phonological development. Although certain hierarchical features and specific theories are still being debated, it has much to offer within the framework of a developing phonological system. For more information on phonological development and nonlinear phonology, the reader is advised to turn to the *Handbook of Phonological Development from the Perspective of Constraint-Based Nonlinear Phonology* by Bernhardt and Stemberger (1998).

Prosodic Feature Development

At the time when children begin to use two-word utterances, a further development in the usage of suprasegmentals occurs: *contrastive stress*. This term indicates that one syllable within a two-word utterance becomes prominent. The acquisition process seems to proceed in the following order.

First, within the child's two-word utterance, a single prosodic pattern is maintained; the two words have a pause between them that becomes shorter and shorter. The next step appears to be the prosodic integration of the two words into one tone-unit. A **tone-unit**, or what is often called a sense-group, is an organizational unit imposed on prosodic data (Crystal, 1986). Such a tone-unit conveys meaning beyond that implied by only the verbal production. When the two words become one tone-unit (i.e., without the pause between them and with one intonational contour), one of these words becomes more prominent than the other, usually louder and associated with an identifiable pitch movement (Crystal, 1986). At the end of this process, there exists a unifying rhythmic relationship between the two items; thus, pauses become less likely. The following developmental pattern could be observed:

> Daddy (pause) eat
> Daddy (pause shortens) eat
> 'Daddy 'eat (no pause, both stressed)
> 'Daddy eat (first word stressed)

The use of contrastive stress in the two-word stage may be used to establish *contrastive meaning* (Brown, 1973). It is assumed that the meaning of the combined one-tone utterance is different from the meaning of the two words in sequence. Later, we see that this contrastive stress is used to signal differences in meaning with similar words. Thus, "'Daddy eat" could indicate that "Daddy is eating," while "Daddy 'eat" could indicate, perhaps, that "Daddy should sit down and eat."

The existing studies of prosodic feature development agree that the acquisition of intonation and stress begins at an early age. Adultlike intonational patterns are noted prior to the appearance of the first word, while the onset of stress patterns seems to occur clearly before the age of 2. However, true mastery of the whole prosodic feature system does not seem to take place until children are at least 12 years old (Atkinson-King, 1973; Malikouti-Drachman and Drachman, 1975).

THE SCHOOL-AGE CHILD

By the time children enter school, their phonological development has progressed considerably. At age 5;0, most of them can converse freely with everyone and make themselves understood clearly to peers and adults alike. However, their pronunciation is still recognizably different from the adult norm. Phonologically, they still have a lot to learn. While their phonological inventory is nearly complete, this system must now be adapted to many more and different contexts, words, and situations. Other phonological features are obviously not mastered at all at this time. Certain sounds are still frequently misarticulated and some aspects of prosodic feature development are only beginning to be incorporated.

Most of the research in child phonology has centered around the development of phonological skills in the first five years of life. However, recent interest in later phonological acquisition has evolved in part due to the established relationship between learning to speak and learning to read.

Segmental Form Development

The development of a child's phonological system includes both perceptual and productional maturation. While the focus of this chapter is on production, it should be emphasized that the school-age child's perceptual skills are still very much in the process of growing. The gradual establishment of pho-

nemic categorization skills, for example, continues well beyond 5 years of age, and it may not be until 14 years of age that children can reliably give categorical responses to certain types of synthetic stimuli (Fourcin, 1978). Tallal, Stark, Kallman, and Mellits (1980) reported that the perceptual constancy of children's phonemic categorizations still changes between 5 and 9 years of age. Also, the recognition of isolated words under quiet and noisy environmental conditions demonstrates improvement until at least age 10 (Elliott et al., 1979). The processing ability of specific continuous speech samples is still measurably slower for fifth-graders than for adults (Cole and Perfetti, 1980), and the ability to understand specifically structured sentences under difficult listening conditions continues to develop until the age of 15 (Elliott, 1979). Perceptually, children are still fine-tuning, certainly during the beginning school years, and in some respects far beyond.

Information on the productional development of the phonological system comes from quite different methodological backgrounds. Most of the information available is based on the results of articulation tests, that is, based on responses to picture naming. If we look at these investigations (e.g., Lowe, 1986, 1996; Templin, 1957), we find that acceptable pronunciation of certain sounds is not achieved until between age 4;6 and 6;0. The most common later sounds are [θ, ð, ʒ] (Sander, 1972). Other findings (Ingram, Christensen, Veach, and Webster, 1980) include one or more of these consonants: [r, z, v]. Based on single-item pronunciation, most investigators agree that children complete their phonemic inventory by the age of 6;0 or, at the latest, 7;0. However, data from the Iowa-Nebraska Articulation Norms (Smit, 1993b) found dentalized [s]-productions in 10 percent of the 9-year-old children tested. Table 5.7 indicates the later developing sounds found in large cross-sectional studies.

TABLE 5.7   Later-Developing Sounds with Approximate Ages of Mastery

SOUND	AGE OF MASTERY	SOURCE
[s]	7½ : 9	Poole (1934); Smit (1993b)[1]
[z]	7½ : 9	Poole (1934); Smit (1993b)
[r]	7½ : 8	Poole (1934); Smit (1993b)
[v]	6½ : 6: 5½	Poole (1934); Templin (1957); Smit (1993b)
[ʃ]	6½ : 5½	Poole (1934); Smit (1993b)
[ʒ]	6: 6½ : 7	Wellman et al. (1931); Poole (1934); Templin (1957)
[θ]	7½ : 6: 6	Poole (1934); Templin (1957); Smit (1993b)
[ð]	6½ : 7: 7	Poole (1934); Templin (1957); Smit (1993b)
[tʃ]	5: 5½	Wellman et al. (1931); Smit (1993b)
[dʒ]	7: 5½	Templin (1957); Smit (1993b)

1. For the Smit (1993b) data, mastery levels were not determined. For the purpose of this table, a sound has been considered mastered if the estimated percentage of acceptable use is approximately 90 percent.

One must keep in mind that most of these results are responses to single-word tasks. To assume, based on this type of task, that these sounds are now "learned" does not take into account the complexity of their use in naturalistic contexts, in new words, and in conversational situations.

Consonant clusters also prove difficult for the school-age child. The acquisition of clusters usually takes place anywhere from about age 3;6 to age 5;6. During this time, the child may demonstrate consonant cluster reduction, lengthening of certain elements of the cluster, for example [s:no], or epenthesis. In epenthesis, the child inserts a schwa vowel between two consonantal elements of a cluster, as in [səno], for example. The Iowa-Nebraska data submitted by Smit (1993a) offer interesting insight into twenty-seven different initial clusters. In this study, 1,049 children between the ages of 2;0 and 9;0 were screened using an articulation test format. The data can be summarized as follows:

1. On fourteen of the twenty-seven initial clusters tested, a small percentage of children in the 8;0- to 9;0-year-old group (N = 247, frequency of occurrence = approximately 2 percent) reduced two consonant clusters to a single element. These clusters included [pl], [kl], [gl], [sl], [tw], [kw], [tr], [dr], [fr], [sw], [sm], [sn], [st], [sk].

2. The consonant clusters [br] and [θr] demonstrated a higher frequency of consonant cluster reduction (5 to 15 percent) for children from ages 5 to 9.

3. For the 5;6- to 7;0-year-olds, the consonant clusters which fell at 75 percent or below group accuracy included [sl], [br], [θr], [skw], [spr], [str], and [skr].

4. Epenthesis, or schwa insertion in consonant clusters, occurs frequently up to age 8;0. The 9-year-olds exhibited schwa insertion rarely.

These data demonstrate that consonant cluster realizations are not adultlike for all children even at age 9.

In addition, the timing of the sounds within consonant clusters is also not yet comparable to adult performance in school-age children (Gilbert and Purves, 1977; Hawkins, 1979). When the temporal relationships between the elements of a cluster were compared for children and adults, it was found that differences, particularly in voice onset time, were still present at 8;0 years of age.

While this information indicates that phonological development extends past the age of 7, most of the available research has focused on the development of the phonological inventory. Unfortunately, other features of the phonological system are still relatively uncharted territory. For example, the development of allophonic variation in older children should also be addressed. How do children learn the acceptable range of phonetic variation in different contexts within their speech community? Local (1983) followed this process as exemplified by the acquisition of one vowel produced by a boy between the ages of 4;5 and 5;6. The variability of sound production and the learning of its acceptable allophonic limitations are decisively important tasks for the developing school-age child.

The intricate interrelation of normal phonological development with other areas of language growth, which has been previously emphasized, demands attention at this point in the child's development as well. The acquisition of vocabulary, for example, is a monumental task to be accomplished in a relatively short time. When children begin kindergarten, they are said to have an expressive vocabulary of approximately 2,200 words (Weiss and Lillywhite, 1981). New sound sequences occurring in words that will now be attained require not only an increased oral-motor control and improved timing skills but also the internalization of new phonological rules. For instance, the conditions under which voiceless stops in English need to be aspirated or not might now become a new achievement.

The acquisition of morphology is also related to phonological growth. The learning of specific morphological structures implies the learning of phonological rules. The child has to understand under which conditions the plural suffix -s is voiced or voiceless, for example. This interconnection between morphology and phonology has been termed **morphophonology**, which refers to the study of the different allomorphs of the morpheme and the rules governing their use. For example, the child's production of [əz] to indicate the plural form for *glass* versus [s] as the plural of *boat* fall within the study of morphophonology as do the rules governing the productional changes from *divide* to *division* and from *explode* to *explosion*. Research findings in this area (e.g., Atkinson-King, 1973; Ivimey, 1975; Myerson, 1978) substantiate that children as old as 17 are still acquiring certain morphophonological patterns. The complex interrelationship between the phonological system and other components of language continues into the child's later school years.

Learning to Speak and Learning to Read

One other important aspect that needs to be addressed in this section pertains to the interconnections between learning to speak and learning to read. Although a general concensus has not been reached as to which variables are indispensable for acquiring reading, there does seem to be a close relationship between early speech and emerging literacy. Thus, a strong correlation between the phonological development, especially segmentation skills, and later reading achievement has been found (e.g., Clarke-Klein and Hodson, 1995; Lundberg, Olofsson, and Wall, 1980). Moreover, early language development, specifically the perceptual processing of sounds, has been found to be one of the strongest predictors of later reading acquisition (Lundberg, 1988). Some of these skills develop during the early school years.

Metaphonological skills are also related to reading. A subcategory of metalinguistics, **metaphonology** involves the child's conscious awareness of the sounds within that particular language. It includes how those sounds are combined to form words. Therefore, metaphonological skills pertain to the child's ability to discern how many sounds are in a word or which sound constitutes its beginning or end. Certain metaphonological abilities seem to be related to the child's acquisition of reading. Although it is not yet clear whether the metaphonological skills are precursors of emerging literacy or a result of the developing reading skills, two factors remain: (1) metaphonology is related to reading performance, and (2) these skills develop at the time when most children start to read, that is, within the age range of 5 to 6 years (Hakes, 1982; Liberman, Shankweiler, Liberman, Fowler, and Fischer, 1977; Read, 1978). Research examining the phonological abilities of schoolchildren with poor reading skills has confirmed the following metaphonological difficulties (e.g., Brady, 1986; Brady and Fowler, 1988; Liberman and Shankweiler, 1985):

Phonological awareness. Poor readers have difficulty analyzing words into syllables and sounds.

Memory storage of phonetic coding. Poor readers are less efficient at creating and maintaining the necessary phonological code for storing verbal information. They can recall fewer items from lists of material. This may contribute to poor phonological awareness tasks.

Phonetic perception in re-creating a phonological code. On repetition tasks, poor readers exhibit clearly greater difficulties if background noise is introduced or if the words to be read are somewhat longer or less familiar. Although these variables affect good readers as well, the group differences are dramatic.

Investigations relating reading and phonological skills have been primarily correlational in nature. Therefore, they do not allow us to say that the previous skills are precursors of reading ability. However, group studies have shown that children with speech and language disorders do significantly poorer than matched normally developing children on phonological awareness tasks (Bird and Bishop, 1992; Marion, Sussman, and Marquardt, 1993; Webster and Plante, 1992). Bird, Bishop, and Freeman (1995) noted that children with persisting speech sound difficulties (beyond the age of 5;6) have problems with phonological awareness tasks and reading. A correlation between speech sound difficulties and literacy skills has been documented in a number of studies (e.g., Bishop and Adams, 1990; Goswami and Bryant, 1990; Hodson, 1994; Hulme and Snowling, 1992; Snowling, Goulandris, and Stackhouse, 1994; Stackhouse, 1993, 1997; Wells, Stackhouse, and Vance, 1996). Children with phonological problems are at risk for developing later problems with learning to read. Several authors have noted that the children with persisting speech difficulties with no obvious medical etiology, that is, those who are identified as having a phonological disorder or developmental apraxia of speech, are most at risk for related and specific literacy problems (Bishop and Robson, 1989; Stackhouse, 1982, 1997).

Prosodic Feature Development

Very little documented research is available on the acquisition of prosodic features in the school-age child. This lack of information is not restricted to our knowledge about prosodic progress during this later developmental period but pertains to the evolution of prosodic features in children in general. Several reasons could account for this gap: (1) the linguistic meaning of the prosodic features is somewhat elusive (Grunwell, 1986); (2) what actually has to be identified is obscured by different methods and analytical frames of reference (Wode, 1980); and (3) the acquisition of prosodic features is often held to be essentially completed by around age 2 (Crystal, 1986). While prosodic features in their variation of pitch, loudness, and duration can be used to signal attitudes and emotions, they can also assume grammatical function. For example, specific intonation patterns have to be employed to differentiate between statements and certain questions in English ("He is coming."↘ versus "He is coming?"↗). Contrasting stress realizations might signal different word classes (*construct* versus con 'struct*). On the sentence level, the combined effects of higher pitch and increased loudness usually convey communicatively important modifications of basic meaning ("This is a 'pen." versus "'This is a pen."). This section examines the grammatical function of prosodic features in school-age children and their relationship to phonological development.

As previously noted, the child begins to use intonational patterns toward the end of the first year of life. As the child's grammatical abilities develop, new uses of intonation emerge. For example, the contrast between rising and falling pitch differentiates the two grammatical functions of a tag question in English ("asking" as in "We're ready, aren't we?"↗ and "telling" as in "We're ready, aren't we!"↘). Differences in intonation patterns like these appear to be learned during the child's third year (Crystal, 1987). However, the learning of intonation goes on for a long time. Studies report that children as old as 12 years were still acquiring some of the fundamental functions of English intonation, especially those for signaling grammatical contrasts (Cruttenden, 1985; Ianucci and Dodd, 1980). As reported by Crystal (1987), even teenagers have been shown to have difficulty understanding sentences in which intonation and pausing are used to differentiate meanings. His example: "She dressed, and fed the baby" (indicating she dressed herself and then fed the baby) versus "She dressed and fed the baby" (indicating she dressed as well as fed the baby). Thus, while certain intonational features seem to be among the earliest phonological acquisitions, others may be some of the last.

Several studies have examined the use of contrastive stress both on the word level ('record versus re'cord) and on the sentence level (determining whom Mary hit in the following sentences: "John hit Bill and then *Mary* hit him" versus "John hit Bill and then Mary hit *him*") (e.g., Atkinson-King, 1973; Chomsky, 1971; Hornby and Hass, 1970; Myers and Myers, 1983). Although the ages differ depending on the type and design of the research, results suggest that children are still learning certain aspects of contrastive stress up until the age of 13.

The acquisition of prosodic features is a gradual process that in some respects extends into the teens. It is closely connected to the new phonological, morphosyntactic, semantic, and pragmatic demands placed on the developing child. As the complexity of the linguistic environment and the child's interaction with that environment increase, so do the subtle intricacies of each of these language levels.

SUMMARY

First, this chapter provided an overview of structural and functional development in infancy and early childhood. At birth, the infant's respiratory, phonatory, resonatory, and articulatory systems are not fully developed. Many changes must occur before the systems are ready to support regular sound and voice production. In addition, the child's perceptual abilities are developing. The second portion of this chapter summarized early perceptual skills, including categorical perception and phonemic awareness. The third section of this chapter traced the segmental form and prosodic feature development of children from vocalizations prior to babbling to the time when their speech sound inventory has reached an adultlike form. The prevalence of certain sounds and syllable shapes was traced from babbling to the first words. As the number of words in children's vocabularies increases, inventory and complexity of syllables grow as well. During this early stage of expansion, the prosodic feature intonation begins to be used to signal different intentions.

The preschool child's development is characterized by a large growth in all aspects of language; the acquisition of new phonological features is a portion of this quickly maturing system. Although cross-sectional studies have attempted to provide so-called mastery ages for sounds, these results cannot be easily generalized. Longitudinal data that document individual variability in sound acquisition among children as well as the influence of other language areas on phonological skills were then summarized. The suppression of many phonological processes is occurring within this time interval as well. Based

on research findings, approximate ages were given for the suppression of several common phonological processes. The differences between natural phonology (the suppression of phonological processes) and the phonological development hypothesized by nonlinear/multilinear phonologies were addressed. When prosodic feature development is examined, contrastive stress is one of the milestones achieved during the preschool years.

Both segmental form and prosodic features continue to mature during the school years. Although the sound inventory is approaching adultlike form, many aspects of the phonological system are still maturing. The child needs to learn morphophonemic variations as well as metaphonological skills. Metaphonological skills were briefly discussed in relationship to the emerging literacy of children. During the school years, phonological development often impacts the child's abilities to learn to read and write. The close interdependencies between phonology, language development, and literacy learning point to the importance of normal phonological development in children.

CHAPTER 6

APPRAISAL
COLLECTION OF DATA

CHAPTER OUTLINE

- Evaluation by the Clinician
- Initial Impression
- Articulation Tests
- Spontaneous Speech Sample
- Evaluation of the Speech Mechanism

- Selection of Additional Assessment Measures
- Special Considerations
- Summary of the Data
- Summary

The last chapters have provided a foundation that can now be applied to the diagnosis and treatment of impaired articulation and phonology. Two important considerations before our diagnosis begins are (1) What information do we actually need? and (2) How should we gather that information? Consider a child coming to us whose parents are concerned because the child's speech is virtually unintelligible. Or consider an adolescent who seeks therapy because of a somewhat conspicuous [s] production. These two individuals present completely different situations, different ages, different degrees of impairment, and differences in the information we would need to evaluate the situation effectively. How, then, do we assess these diverse situations? Let's begin by looking at the various parts of an assessment.

Assessment is one of the most important tasks a clinician will perform; it is the basis for treatment decisions. **Assessment**, the clinical evaluation of a client's disorder, can be divided into two phases: appraisal and diagnosis (Dar-

ley, 1991). **Appraisal** refers to the collection of data, while the **diagnosis** represents the end result of studying and interpreting these data. Therefore, the appraisal portion of our assessment would answer the two questions previously stated concerning what information we actually need and how we gather that information. Appraisal is a very important aspect of our assessment. The collection of too little or unspecific information will not provide enough data for an adequate diagnosis. At the other extreme, collecting too much or unnecessary data is wasting the client's and clinician's valuable time. Therefore, professional assessment demands qualified (and verifiable) decisions throughout the appraisal process.

This chapter deals with the appraisal portion of assessment. Its first goal is to identify the constituent parts of an appraisal, that is, the different types of data needed for a comprehensive diagnosis. These parts will be identified and procedures outlined for each of the appraisal methods. The second goal is to emphasize the clinician's role in choosing among available measures, that is, the clinical decision-making process leading to the selection of instruments serving each individual client maximally. Because the selection of appraisal instruments will necessarily influence the interpretation of the collected data, every appropriate choice will lead to a more complete diagnosis. Effective assessments are essential for clinical procedures; they lead us through the entire diagnostic and therapeutic process.

The collection of data pertains to at least four different areas: (1) the case history, (2) interviews with parents and other professionals, (3) school and medical records, and (4) the evaluation by the clinician. Procedures and information important for the first three areas are covered in many texts. Selected sources are given in Box 6.1. This chapter will cover only the fourth and most specific task, the evaluation by the clinician.

EVALUATION BY THE CLINICIAN

Clinicians collect data in two different ways: through a procedure known as screening or through a more comprehensive evaluation. A **screening** consists of activities or tests that identify individuals who merit further evaluation. A screening procedure does not collect nearly enough data to establish a diagnosis, it only demonstrates the need for further testing. Screening measures can be formal or informal. Formal measures include elicitation procedures, which often have normative data and cut-off scores. Informal measures are typically devised by the examiner and may be directed toward a particular population or age level. Screenings are typically used to give the clinician an initial impression of a large group of children. For example, public schools may screen all kindergarten and first grade children. Screenings are beneficial for those individuals who "fail" the procedure and are later

Box 6.1_____

Interviewing and Obtaining Case History Information: Bibliographical Sources

Emerick, L. L. (1969). *The parent interview.* Danville, IL: Interstate Press.

Emerick, L. L., & Haynes, W. O. (1986). *Diagnosis and evaluation in speech pathology* (3rd ed.). Englewood Cliffs, NJ: Prentice-Hall.

Haynes, W. O., Pindzola, R. H., & Emerick, L. L. (1992). *Diagnosis and evaluation in speech pathology* (4th ed.). Englewoods Cliffs, NJ: Prentice-Hall.

Hutchinson, B. B., Hanson, M. L., & Mecham, M. J. (Eds.). (1979). *Diagnostic handbook of speech pathology.* Baltimore: Williams and Wilkins.

Meitus, I. J., & Weinberg, B. (1983). *Diagnosis in speech-language pathology.* Baltimore: University Park Press.

Peterson, H. A., & Marquardt, T. P. (1990). *Appraisal and diagnosis of speech and language disorders* (2nd ed.). Englewood Cliffs, NJ: Prentice-Hall.

Schulman, E. D. (1991). *Intervention in human services: A guide to skills and knowledge* (4th ed.). New York: Merrill.

Shipley, K. G. (1992). *Interviewing and counseling in communicative disorders: Principles and procedures.* New York: Merrill/Macmillan.

Shipley, K. G., & McAfee, J. G. (1992). *Assessment in speech-language pathology: A resource manual.* San Diego: Singular.

Stewart, C. J., & Cash, W. B. (1991). *Interviewing: Principles and practices* (6th ed.). Dubuque, IA: William C. Brown.

more comprehensively evaluated. Screenings are not always reliable in that some individuals may "pass" the procedure but still demonstrate impairments. Screenings were not devised to serve as a database for a diagnosis; they are too limited in their scope. In contrast, a **comprehensive evaluation** is a series of activities and tests that allow a more detailed and complete collection of data. A *comprehensive phonetic-phonemic evaluation* is the core of the appraisal for articulatory/phonological impairments. It includes data from the following sources:

- an articulation test and stimulability measures
- conversational speech assessment in varying contexts
- hearing testing
- speech mechanism examination
- the possible selection of additional measures such as language testing, perceptual performance, contextual testing, and/or cognitive assessment (Bankson and Bernthal, 1998; Lowe, 1994).

The following section will examine each of these portions of the appraisal process, beginning with an initial impression and its usefulness in the collection of data.

INITIAL IMPRESSION

Clinicians can start collecting data even before the formal appraisal actually begins—for example, by closely observing the conversation between the caregiver and the child, the teacher and the child in a classroom situation, or the child communicating with his or her peers. This initial contact will provide an important first impression. The task is to notice certain features of the conversation and put them onto a simple form like the one in Figure 6.1. Although more and other variables have to be considered later, this record of the initial impression is meant to aid in planning and organizing the remainder of the assessment.

If the initial impression is that the child is partly or totally intelligible, then the next step, the appraisal within the scope of an articulation test, could be initiated. If, on the other hand, the initial impression yields an unintelligible child, additional measures for data collection may need to be considered, especially for the spontaneous speech sample.

Very young children, dialect speakers, and individuals with English as a second language will all require additional considerations. Guidelines for these populations are found later in this chapter.

ARTICULATION TESTS

Some Advantages and Disadvantages of Articulation Tests

Articulation tests are typically designed to elicit spontaneous naming based on the presentation of pictures. Most consonants of General American English are tested in the initial, medial, and final positions of words.

There are several advantages to using an articulation test. First, these tests are relatively easy to give and score; the necessary time expenditure is usually minimal. This is an attractive feature for those who feel limited in the time they can spend with appraisal procedures. Second, the results provide the clinician with a quantifiable list of "incorrect" sound productions in different word positions. This is clearly relevant to further assessment and planning of therapy. Third, several of the tests provide standardized scores. These scores allow the clinician to compare the individual client's performance with the performance of other children of a similar age. In addition, these scores could be used to document the client's need for, and progress in, therapy.

There are, however, also several problems inherent in articulation tests. Many of them have already been discussed (see Chapter 2 and Chapter 5) and can be summarized as follows:

1. An articulation test examines sound articulation in selected isolated words. However, eliciting sounds based on single-word responses can never give adequate information on the client's production realities in connected speech. Sound articulation within selected words may not be

FIGURE 6.1   Sample Form for the Initial Impression

Name _____   Age _____

Conversational partner _____   Date _____

Intelligibility

Good _____   Partly intelligible _____   Unintelligible _____

Single-word responses and continuous speech show comparable intelligibility _____

Single-word responses are more intelligible than continuous speech _____

General overview of misarticulations

Affects consonants _____

Affects consonants and vowels _____

Noted misarticulations _____

_____

_____

Other factors affecting intelligibility (for example, hyper- or denasality, vocal loudness or quality, rate of speech)

_____

Caregiver's/teacher's/peer's response to misarticulations

No response _____   Asks for repetition _____   Tries to correct_____

Child's response to parent's/caregiver's intervention _____

_____

_____

representative of the child's ability to produce a particular sound under natural speech conditions.

2. Articulation tests do not give enough information about the client's phonological system. Articulation tests are measures of speech sound production; they are phonetic tests. As such, they were never meant to provide enough assessment data for a phonological analysis. Although some spontaneous naming measures analyze sounds in error according to phonological processes, the information they provide is not enough for a comprehensive phonological analysis.

3. Articulation tests do not test all sounds in all the contexts in which they occur in General American English. While this would admittedly be a rather large task, some articulation tests do not even test all of the speech sounds of General American English. If scored according to the directions provided, most articulation tests do not test vowels, for example, and very few consonant clusters are sampled.

4. The sounds actually tested do not occur in comparable phonetic contexts, that is, they are not context-controlled. For example, the sounds before and after the tested consonants are different from word

to word. The words used are also of varying lengths and complexities. This presents to the child a task that changes in its production difficulty from word to word.

5. Articulation tests, like all standardized tests, are selected probes into rather limited aspects of an individual's total articulatory behavior and/or abilities. An articulation test examines only a very small portion of that child's articulatory behavior—it explores the child's speech performance with particular test items, on a certain day, in a unique testing situation. To generalize that such limited results represent a reliable measure of the client's articulatory abilities, let alone the client's phonological system, would be an obvious mistake.

Factors to Consider When Selecting a Measure of Articulation

When selecting a measure of speech sound competency, several factors are important. In addition to the test's construct and its technical characteristics, the following should be considered: (1) the test's appropriateness for the age or developmental level of the client, (2) the test's ability to supply a standardized score, (3) the test's analysis of the sound errors, and (4) the test's inclusion of an adequate sample of the sound or sounds relevant to the individual client at hand.

Appropriateness for the Age or Developmental Level of the Client. Although the age ranges vary, most tests can be administered to children from approximately 3 years to school age. Selection becomes a troublesome issue for very young and for older adolescent or adult clients. Younger clients, and this may include 2-year-olds or delayed 3- and 4-year-olds, may not respond well to a formal articulation test. Some younger children might react better to those tests that contain large colored pictures. For other children, the naming of actual ob-

jects or spontaneous speech may be the only way to assess sound production skills. For the evaluation of adolescent or adult clients, two problems exist.

> Later in this chapter, the section on Special Considerations will examine alternative ways to assess younger clients with emerging phonological systems.

First, many of the tests are not standardized for children beyond the ages of 12 or 13. In addition, most articulation tests are oriented toward a much younger population. This may prove demeaning for older adolescents and adults and is, therefore, inappropriate. Certain articulation tests contain printed sentences that can be read by clients. Although the sentence content and the reading level are designed for early school-age children, articulation tests that provide sentences to be read might prove less of a problem for older clients.

Ability to Provide a Standardized Score. Some articulation tests are not standardized, that is, standardized scores are not available as outcome measures. Therefore, the results obtained from a client cannot be compared to the performance of other children of a similar age. If it is important that the results of an articulation test yield standardized scores, tests should be selected correspondingly.

Analysis of the Sound Errors. There are many different tests to choose from. Some are labelled articulation tests, while others purport to be tests of *phonology*. Articulation tests and tests of phonology do not differ in their examination format (both use the same format: spontaneous picture naming) but in their analysis of the results. Typically, tests of phonology categorize misarticulations according to phonological processes. Although the clinician could go through any articulation test noting the number and type of phonological processes used, those tests that already contain such a procedure will probably allow the clinician a more expedient assessment.

CLINICAL APPLICATION

Using Articulation Tests to Examine Phonological Processes

The evaluation of phonological processes is a portion of several articulation tests (e.g., Assessment Link between Phonology and Articulation (ALPHA), Lowe, 1996; Bankson-Bernthal Test of Phonology, Bankson and Bernthal, 1990; Khan-Lewis Phonological Analysis, which uses the responses from the Goldman-Fristoe Test of Articulation, Khan and Lewis, 1986).

Phonological processes can be determined from the results of any articulation test. The clinician examines the results of the articulation test and notes the phonological processes employed. The following is an example from the PAT: Photo Articulation Test (Pendergast, Dickey, Selmar, and Soder, 1984):

Word	Child's Response	Phonological Process
saw	[tɑ]	stopping [s] → [t]
pencil	[pɛnθəl]	fronting [s] → [θ]
house	[haʊ]	final consonant deletion [s] → ø
spoon	[pun]	consonant cluster reduction [sp] → [p]
skates	[keɪtθ]	consonant cluster reduction [sk] → [k]
		consonant cluster substitution [ts] → [tθ], fronting
stars	[tɑɚ]	consonant cluster reduction [st] → [t]
		final consonant deletion [z] → ø*
zipper	[dɪpɚ]	stopping [z] → [d]

*In this example, the production is characterized as a final consonant deletion because [ɑɚ] is considered a centering diphthong. If the r-sound is viewed as a rhotic, transcribed as [stɑr], then this would be a consonant cluster reduction [rz] → [r].

Based on the results, the clinician could determine which phonological processes were operating and how often they occurred.

Test's Inclusion of an Adequate Sample of the Sound or Sounds Relevant for the Individual Client. Articulation tests typically contain words that sample the sound inventory of General American English. Thus, most of the consonants of General American English are tested within the test. However, most articulation tests do not sample the most frequently misarticulated sounds in a large number of different contexts. For example, the [s] may be tested in only two or three different words. An adequate number of words containing the sound in various word positions is often not available. While supplemental testing with additional words can always be achieved later, a test that provides adequate goal-directed

material for individual clients uses our diagnostic time more efficiently.

Assessment Procedures to Supplement Articulation Tests

Which assessment strategies, then, can be employed to minimize the previously mentioned shortcomings of articulation tests?

1. *If a word contains any aberrant vowel or consonant productions, transcribe the entire word.* This gives valuable additional information about the client's sound production skills. For example, assume that the tested word is *yellow,* that the initial [j] is being evaluated, and

Articulation tests are often referred to as citation-form testing. The citation form refers to the spoken form of a word produced in isolation, as distinguished from the form it would have when produced in conversational speech. Both citation-form testing and spontaneous speech sampling should be used to collect data for a comprehensive evaluation.

that the child says [jɛwoᵘ]. According to the scoring instructions, the initial [j] would be noted as being "correct" and the clinician would continue on to the next item. However, if the entire word has been transcribed, the clinician can later evaluate the [l] production and compare it to the other words on the test that contain [l]. (In addition, some articulation measures test only sounds in the initial and final word positions; however, some clients demonstrate difficulties with medial productions.) Transcribing the entire word complements the test information considerably and supplies insights into vowels and consonant cluster productions as well.

2. *Supplement the articulation test with additional utterances that address the noted problems of the client.* The target sound(s) should be sampled in various vowel contexts and word positions, for example. There are several ways to do this. One is to develop a list of words containing the needed sound(s). This has the advantage of narrowing the supplemental materials to fit the client's needs. One could also use commercially prepared materials. Two examples are McDonald's Deep Test of Articulation (McDonald, 1964) or Secord's Clinical Probes of Articulation Consistency (C-PAC) (Secord, 1981a). McDonald's deep test uses pictures to elicit a compound word, such as *hot* + *dog* = *hotdog*. The words formed are not typical compound words of General American English; however, a variety of phonetic contexts can be sampled this way. The C-PAC assesses the targeted consonant before

and after various vowels (in one-syllable words, consonants initiating and terminating the word), in consonant clusters, in sentences, and during storytelling. For children who cannot read, the elicitation mode is imitative. These commercially available protocols have the advantage of assessing a sound in a variety of contexts without any preparation on the part of the clinician.

3. *Always sample and record continuous speech.* Although it has been well documented that production differences exist in children between single-word tasks (citing) and spontaneous speech (talking) (e.g., Andrews and Fey, 1986; Dubois and Bernthal, 1978; Faircloth and Faircloth, 1970; Morrison and Shriberg, 1992; Shriberg and Kwiatkowski, 1985; Stoel-Gammon and Dunn, 1985), many practitioners continue to use articulation tests as the sole basis for their analysis procedures. Morrison and Shriberg (1992) state that "citation-form testing yields neither typical nor optimal measures of speech performance" (p. 271). An articulation test is not good enough for the appraisal and diagnosis of clients with phonetic and/or phonemic disorders. See the section on spontaneous speech sampling for further information.

4. *Determine the stimulability of the error sounds.* This task can be easily and relatively quickly accomplished at the end of an articulation test. See the following section on stimulability testing.

Organizing Articulation Test Results: Describing the Error

Most articulation tests include a form that can be used to record the client's responses. By completing this form, the clinician obtains information about the accuracy of the sound articulation and the position of this sound within the test word. Each articulation test gives directions on how to record accurate and inaccurate sound realizations. To describe sound errors, there are at least three different scoring systems (Shriberg and Kent, 1995). The following scoring systems are available:

Two-Way Scoring. A choice is made between a production that is "right" (accurate articulation of the sound in question) and "wrong" (inaccurate articulation). Two-way scoring can be used effectively to give feedback to the client and to document therapy progress. It can also be used in a screening protocol. However, because of its limitations and its inability to render any usable information about the kind of aberrant articulation taking place, the two-way scoring system is inappropriate for the scoring of articulation tests.

Five-Way Scoring. This system uses a classification based on the type of error. "Correct," or norm productions, constitute one category. The other four categories are (1) deletion or omission, that is, a sound is deleted completely; (2) substitution—a sound is replaced by another sound; (3) distortion—the target sound is approximated but not closely enough to be considered a norm realization; and (4) addition—a sound or sounds are added to the intended sound. The five-way scoring system is commonly suggested in the manuals of articulation tests. However, this system has several inherent problems.

First, most articulation tests do not define, or give examples of, sound articulation within normal limits. There are many dialectal and contextual variations that could result in a somewhat different but entirely acceptable pronunciation. For example, the alveolar flap [ɾ] is a common pronunciation for [d] in *ladder*. Should this variation be considered "correct" if the medial d-sound is being tested? Clinicians should be aware of these common variations and how they may impact their scoring. Second, the category of de-

letion or omission may include the presence, rather than the absence, of a sound. Normally, deletion implies that a sound segment has been eliminated, as in [mu] for *moon*, for example. However, Van Riper and Irwin (1958) include glottal stops, unvoiced articulatory placements, and short exhalations under omissions as well. If the production of [wæʔən] for *wagon* is considered, according to these authors, the [g] would be classified as a deletion. Actually, it would be more accurate to label this as a substitution of a glottal stop for [g]. This ambiguous definition of deletion can detract from the accuracy of the results when sound realizations are later analyzed. Third, the terms *substitution* and *distortion* have a long history of definitional unclarity. Some authors (Van Riper, 1978; Van Riper and Irwin, 1958; Winitz, 1975) state that a more precise way of considering distortions is to regard them as substitutions of non-English sounds. For example, a child produces [ʃ] in which the organ and place of articulation is too far back, that is, rather than prepalatal, it has a palatal placement. There is a palatal fricative, transcribed as [ç], which is a regular speech sound in many languages. Therefore, this palatal [ʃ] production could be designated either as a distortion of [ʃ] or as a substitution of [ç] for [ʃ]. Such vagueness in regard to what constitutes a distortion versus a substitution can also impact the scoring of many articulation tests.

Phonetic Transcription. Transcription systems describe speech behavior. The goal of any phonetic transcription is to represent spoken language by written symbols. Of the three scoring systems mentioned, phonetic transcription requires the highest degree of clinical skill. The goal is not to *judge* specific misarticulations but to *describe* them as accurately as possible. Phonetic transcription has several advantages over the other two systems: (1) it is far more precise; (2) it gives more information about the misarticulation, which is helpful for both assessment and intervention; and (3) among professionals, it is the most universally accepted way to communicate information about articulatory features. Phonetic transcription uses broad transcription of the speech sounds of General American English and narrow transcription, diacritics which further delineate the characteristics of the sounds produced. Both broad and narrow transcription are indispensable for a comprehensive evaluation. This scoring system will be used for the following analyses of citation articulation tests as well as of spontaneous speech sampling.

Stimulability Testing

Stimulability testing refers to testing the client's ability to produce a misarticulated sound in an appropriate manner when "stimulated" by the clinician to do so. Many variations in this procedure exist, but commonly, the clinician asks the client to "watch and listen to what I am going to say, and then you say it." (Bankson and Bernthal, 1998a). Although there is no standardized procedure for stimulability testing, an isolated sound is usually first attempted. If a norm articulation is achieved, the sound is placed within a syllable and subsequently in a word context. The number of models provided by the clinician typically varies from one to five attempts (Diedrich, 1983).

For many clinicians, stimulability testing is a standard procedure concluding the administration of an articulation test. It gives a measure of the consistency of a client's performance on two different tasks: the spontaneous naming of a picture and the imitation of a speech model provided by the clinician. Such information is very helpful in appraising the articulatory capabilities of a client.

Children's articulatory stimulability has been used to determine therapy goals and to predict which children might benefit more from therapy. In the past, it has been suggested that sounds that were more stimulable would be easier to work on in therapy; therfore, highly stimulable sounds would be targeted first (Newman and Creaghead, 1989). When used as a means of predicting which children might benefit from therapy, high stimulability was correlated with more rapid therapeutic success (Newman and Creaghead, 1989). It was also proposed that high stimulability might mean that children were on the verge of acquiring the sounds and would not even need therapeutic intervention (Bankson and Bernthal, 1998b). However, after an extensive review of the literature on stimulability, Diedrich (1983) concluded that stimulability testing *cannot* be used (1) to absolutely predict which error sounds will improve in therapy, (2) to make definite decisions about the level (isolated sound, syllable, word) at which to begin therapy, and (3) to predict which children do not need therapy. Although there is a positive relationship between stimulability and responsiveness to therapy, these relationships are not strong enough to predict these factors for an individual client accurately.

There appears, nevertheless, to be a close relationship between the stimulability of a client and speech improvement. Clinicians can be reasonably sure that speech sounds that show a high degree of stimulability have a better chance of responding to therapy (Newman and Creaghead, 1989). Stimulability testing might also be used to suggest a hierarchy of error sounds that can be selected for treatment (Diedrich, 1983).

As a portion of the data collected in a client's appraisal, stimulability testing gives useful information. However, stimulability testing should not be the only source when deciding whether a client receives services or which therapy sequence to choose.

SPONTANEOUS SPEECH SAMPLE

Over the years, numerous authors have documented the differences that exist in children's speech when single-word citing responses are compared to spontaneous speech (e.g., Andrews and Fey, 1986; Campbell and Shriberg, 1982; Dubois and Bernthal, 1978; Healy and Madison, 1987; Hoffman, Schuckers, and Daniloff, 1989; Klein, 1984; Menyuk, 1980). However, assessment and treatment protocols continue to be based primarily on the results of citation articulation tests. Some clinicians may argue that they don't have time to complete the transcription and analysis of a spontaneous speech sample. However, these samples can serve many different functions. For example, conversational speech samples can supply additional information about the language, voice, and prosodic capabilities of the client. Specific semantic, morphosyntactical, and pragmatic analyses could supplement additional language testing when required. The conversational speech sample is not optional, but rather a basic necessity for every professional appraisal.

Although any conversational speech sample is more representative of a client's production capabilities than a one-word sample, the type of sampling situation also plays a role. Several authors have found an increase or decrease in errors depending on the production task required. First, more complex linguistic contents generally cause an increase in misarticulations (Panagos, Quine, and Klich, 1979; Panagos and Prelock, 1982; Schmauch, Panagos, and Klich, 1978). Second, different communicative needs can also influence production accuracy. For example, Menyuk (1980) reported the improvement of speech patterns in five children when they were trying to relate information that was important to them.

To obtain the most representative sample, clinicians should carefully select a variety of talking situations. This could include describing pictures, storytelling, describing the function of objects, or problem solving in addition to a normal conversation about school or the last vacation. Varying communicative situations could also include conversations with siblings, parents, or classmates before or after the assessment session. None of these talking events needs to be lengthy, but the variety will certainly aid in documenting the client's production realities.

Organizing the Continuous Speech Sample

A continuous speech sample should be planned and executed in a systematic manner in order to minimize the time investment and maximize the results. Here are some suggestions.

Begin with the Articulation Test. One goal of a continuous speech sample in a comprehensive assessment is to compare the child's productions on a single-word citation task to those in continuous speech. Errors that have been noted in single words can be helpful in planning the continuous speech sample. For example, if the child demonstrates error productions for [s], [ʃ], [tʃ], [dʒ], and [l] on the articulation test, or if the articulation test does not sample particular sounds, these could be targeted.

Provide Objects or Pictures that May Elicit Targeted Sounds. Objects and pictures containing the targeted sounds can then become a portion of the spontaneous speech procedure. Comparability between citing and talking tasks could be increased by attempting to trigger some of the same words that were in the articulation test.

Plan the Length of the Sample. There has been a lot of discussion about which sample length furnishes adequate information for a comprehensive assessment. Grunwell (1987) states that "100 different words is the minimum size of an adequate sample; 200–250 words is preferable" (p. 55). On the other hand, Crary (1983) found that 50-word samples for process analysis provided as much information as 100-word speech samples. Unfortunately, this problem does not have an easy solution. While 50 words seems more palatable, a sample of that size might not give the needed information.

It should be kept in mind that in normal conversation, children articulate between 100 and 200 syllables per minute (Culatta, Page, and Wilson, 1987). Therefore, three minutes of conversational speech will render approximately 450 syllables or, depending on the length of each word, about 200 words. In most cases this will probably constitute an adequate sample. If allowances are made for nonspeech events, interaction with the clinician, and deletion of certain portions due to lack of intelligibility, a 200- to 250-word sample should take no more than ten to fifteen minutes to record. With most children, much of the transcription can be attained spontaneously. Assuming that another ten to fifteen minutes is required later to transcribe portions of the sample from tape, the total recording and transcribing time amounts to around thirty minutes. In light of the gains in needed information for goal-directed therapy, this is not a large time investment. Perhaps a lack of the necessary transcription skills deters clinicians more than the actual time involvement.

Plan Diversity into the Sample. Various communicative situations should be a portion of the recorded speech sample. A variety of situations will ensure that the sample adequately represents the phonetic and phonemic skills of the client. This may include several different talking situations, such as picture description, storytelling, describing the function of objects, or problem solving. Communicative diversity could also include the client talking with caregivers or siblings. The recording time for each different sample needs to be only two to three minutes. Varying communicative situations will also allow for articulatory differences that occur between pragmatically and linguistically diverse samples.

Recording the Continuous Speech Sample

Recording the continuous speech sample has several advantages. It allows later transcription if certain portions cannot be spontaneously transcribed. In addition, it can be used to document production changes over time or before and after a certain interval of therapy. Attaining a high quality recording is a basic necessity. The very purpose of this assessment procedure will be jeopardized if the quality of the recording does not accurately mirror the productions of the client. Also, many additional hours will be spent trying to transcribe a mediocre or poor recording. Again, with very little time investment in the planning stage, considerable time can be saved in the later analysis.

Audio and/or Video Recording. There are advantages and disadvantages to both audio and video recordings. While video systems have become more prevalent in recent years, certain prerequisites must be fulfilled before a video recording should be considered. Video systems do provide one important advantage over audio recordings in that they visibly document the client's articulation patterns. However, this may not be particularly helpful if the sound quality is poor. This problem may be partially solved by the use of an external microphone connected to the video camera.

Sometimes, the choice of audio or video equipment may lie simply in the availability of one or the other. Many clinicians do not have access to video equipment within their working environments. But, an audio tape recorder need not be a second-class alternative; many relatively inexpensive tape recorders provide good sound quality. In fact, a good portable tape recorder is probably one of the best investments a clinician can make. When choosing audio equipment, information on its technical specifications needs to be considered.

Use of an External Microphone. One necessity for a video or audio recording is the use of an external microphone. Built-in microphones are seldom good enough to allow a reliable transcription of the often minimal but important changes in sound quality. Microphones are relatively inexpensive but, again, should be tailored to the needs at hand.

Accurately Position the Microphone. To obtain a first-class recording, one must position the microphone properly. If it is too close to the

---

Unidirectional microphones, while excluding a considerable amount of room noise, are what their name implies—accurate in one direction. If the goal is to tape just one child, they are probably the microphones of choice. Omnidirectional microphones, on the other hand, allow more recording potential from a larger area of the room. When recording a small group of children they may, therefore, be more effective than unidirectional microphones. However, background and other ambient room noises will also be recorded. A third option is a lavaliere microphone, a device that can be pinned to, or hung from, the child's clothes. Lavaliere microphones can be wireless or attached to a small cord that plugs into the recording equipment. Wireless lavaliere microphones, while costly, are of relatively good quality, easy to handle, and inconspicuous. However, disadvantages (aside from the cost) must also be considered. Any movement by the child or touching of the microphone will seriously distort the signal.

Two important technical specifications of a tape recorder should be considered: the signal-to-noise ratio and the frequency response. The signal-to-noise ratio can be expressed as the difference between the amplitudes of the highest and lowest recordable signals. A signal-to-noise ratio that is too small will result in a machine-noise component interfering with the signal. Tatham and Morton (1997) state that the minimum signal-to-noise ratio should be 50 dB. The frequency response of the tape recorder refers to the machine's ability to record and replay a frequency range without distorting the amplitude relationships. The frequency range should be wide enough to include the frequencies of the speech spectrum, which basically range from 50 to 10,000 Hz (Denes and Pinson, 1963). In addition, the recorder's ability to maintain this amplitude should be stated. A typical specification of a modern recorder is 45 to 18,000 Hz (Tatham and Morton, 1997).

---

child, speech sounds can be easily distorted. For example, popping sounds may be heard on plosives and an overriding noise component on fricative consonants. If the microphone is too far away, the signal may not be strong enough for accurate discrimination. In this case, the common tendency is to turn the input volume level up. Although this will increase the overall volume, background and internal machine noises of the recorder will be increased at the same time.

For portable microphones, the best distance from the child is approximately six to eight inches. The microphone should be slanted slightly toward the client's nose to eliminate distortions due to the expiratory release components of certain consonants.

Select an Appropriate Environment for Recording. The room in which the recording is made should be as quiet as possible. If the therapy room cannot provide this, look for another spot that does. If the final recording has signal-distorting background noises, much time will later be spent with the analysis.

Check Your Equipment before Beginning. *Always* check your recording equipment before actually beginning. Clients can say their names and the date on the recording, for example. This trial recording should be played back immediately so that the quality can be evaluated. Not only will this simple procedure secure that the equipment is actually working but also any volume or placement difficulties will be detected.

Monitor Your Recording and Gloss Any Utterances that Might Later Be Difficult or Impossible to Understand from the Taped Recording. Constant monitoring will ensure that the quality of the recording remains constant. This can mean anything from readjusting the microphone if the client moves to asking the client to repeat an utterance if it is not completely intelligible. It is helpful and often necessary to gloss the word or phrase, especially if later transcription difficulties are anticipated. **Glossing** means repeating with normal pronunciation what the client has just said for easier identification later. This can be done quite naturally so that it will not interfere with the structured situation.

Try to Transcribe As Much of the Spontaneous Speech Sample As Possible during the Recording. Live transcriptions have the advantage of capturing phonetic detail that may be lost with a tape recording. They also decrease the subsequent transcription time. In addition, listening to one or two minutes of conversation before transcribing may dramatically increase transcription effectiveness due to the clinician's adjustment to the client's pronunciation patterns. Unintelligible utterances should be clearly marked (language sampling techniques use a series of *X*s to note unintelli-

gibility). It is not necessary to spend a considerable amount of time trying to decipher these responses. Instead, it is better to gloss the utterance whenever the intelligibility of the response might be later questioned.

EVALUATION OF THE SPEECH MECHANISM

An evaluation of both the structure and the function of the client's speech mechanism is a prerequisite for any comprehensive appraisal. Its intent is to assess whether the system appears adequate for regular speech sound production. At first glance, the examination of the speech-motor system looks like a relatively simple procedure which has often been described. However, the interpretation of the results is not necessarily as straightforward as it would seem.

To aid our evaluation, let's view the results of the evaluation of the speech mechanism along a continuum in which one end indicates normal structure and function while the other end indicates grossly deviant structural and/or functional inadequacies. At the normal end of the continuum, assume that the client has passed all required procedures. This is commonly the case, and no further speech-motor testing appears to be necessary—the client has passed the oral-speech assessment. But does stating that the client has passed actually mean that structural or functional inadequacies do not play any role in his or her aberrant productions? Phonetic disorders are defined as motor production difficulties. Therefore, although the client passed all requirements, the assumption is that some subtle peripheral-motor inadequacies are causing the disorder in question. In some ways, then, the speech-motor assessment may not give information adequate for further clinical work.

At the other end of the continuum, results could show such a pronounced structural or functional aberration from norm that an organic cause of the speech difficulties needs to be concluded. If organicity is noted, further testing by the clinician and/or referral to a medical expert are warranted.

Between the endpoints of this continuum exists a broad range of structural and functional deviations that may or may not directly impact the adequate production of speech sounds. Often, clinicians will find minor structural and/or functional inadequacies that don't appear severe enough to be considered "organic," yet certainly do not qualify as "passing." Interpreting such results is often difficult. Our evaluation of the speech mechanism is actually just a screening measure requiring more testing and possible referral when any functional and/or structural inadequacies are found. One possible screening form for the evaluation of the speech-motor system is summarized in Appendix 6.1.

What to Look for When Evaluating the Speech Mechanism

Examining the Head and Facial Structures. One of the first impressions is provided by simply observing the client's face and head. Sitting opposite the client, first evaluate the size and the shape of the head. Relative to the body size, the head should appear normal—not too large and not too small. In addition, the shape should be considered. The relationship between the cranium (the upper portion of the skull containing the brain) and the facial skeleton (the lower portion of the skull containing, among other structures, the articulators) should be evaluated. The cranial portion should not appear too large nor the facial area too small or vice versa. Micrognathia, for example, is marked by an unusually small jaw. Next, the symmetry of the facial features should be inspected. Do the right and left sides of the face appear fairly similar both in proportion and in overall ap-

pearance? *Proportion* refers to the structures on both sides being on corresponding planes and their dimensions being similar on both sides. For example, right and left eyes are level and both appear to be about the same size. *Appearance* refers to the overall shape of the structures in question and to the normal state of resting muscle, that is, to the muscular tone. Oddly shaped eyes, nose, or mouth would be a deviancy within this category. In addition, any drooping of the structures or lack of muscle tone on one side of the face should be noted. At rest, the right and left sides of the lips should be even, the red of the lips, or vermilion, forming a smooth curve. Appearance and proportions of the nares (the nostrils), the nasal septum (the structural division of the nose, dividing the nasal cavity into right and left halves), the philtrum (the vertical groove between the upper lip and the nasal septum), and the columella (the vertical ridges on either side of the philtrum) should be evaluated. In short, any striking features of the head and face should be noted. This would include a fairly common syndrome called adenoid facies. Adenoid facies is the result of chronic or repeated infections that lead to enlarged adenoids, mouth breathing, a shortening of the upper lip, and an elongated face (Zemlin, 1988).

Examining Breathing. Respiration can be indirectly observed by examining breathing patterns. The clinician should observe and evaluate the client's breathing patterns at rest (silent breathing) and during speech. During silent breathing, the client's mouth should be closed with no noticeable clavicular breathing (excursions in the clavicular area that cause the shoulders to move up and down during breathing). In addition, during silent breathing, the amount of time between the inspiratory and expiratory phases should be fairly equal. Therefore, an approximately one-to-one relationship exists between the time for inspiration and for expiration. During speech production, the normal time relationship between inspiratory and expiratory phases is somewhere between one and two+, that is, depending on the length of the utterance, the expiratory phase should be at least twice as long as the inspiratory. Any irregularities in breathing patterns should be noted. This includes irregular breathing patterns, muscular jerks or spasms during breathing, forced inhalations or exhalations, or any other (especially recurrent) conspicuous respiratory movements.

Examination of the Oral and Pharyngeal Cavity Structures. The structures involved in this area of the speech mechanism examination include the teeth, the tongue, the palate, and pharyngeal areas.

The Teeth. First, the occlusion of the teeth is important. Normal occlusion (Class I) is characterized by the lower molars being one-half of a tooth ahead of the upper molars. There are several different types of malocclusions, including Class II malocclusion (overbite), Class III malocclusion (underbite), open bite, and cross bite. (Definitions of these malocclusions are given in Appendix 6.1.) Next, the clinician should check to see if all teeth are present and whether the spacing and their axial orientation appear adequate. The *axial orientation* of the teeth refers to the positioning of the individual teeth. Abnormalities in this respect would pertain to irregularly "tipped" or rotated teeth. Malocclusions of the teeth and missing teeth may affect the production of specific speech sounds.

The Tongue. First, examine the size of the tongue in its relationship to the size of the oral cavity. Does it appear too large, overfilling the oral cavity (macroglossia), or does it

seem too small for the cavity size (microglossia)? Both of these conditions would signal a deviancy. In addition, the tongue's appearance is examined to see if the color appears normal and if the muscular dorsum of the tongue demonstrates a healthy muscle tone. Any "shriveled" tongue appearance might signal a paralytic condition. Next, the surface of the tongue needs to be observed. It should be relatively smooth. Any fissures (grooves or cracks in the dorsum of the tongue), lesions (wounds or abrasion), and fasciculations (any visible "bundling" of muscles) would indicate a deviancy. Finally, the tongue needs to be examined in its resting position. It should look symmetrical without any muscular twitching or movements.

The Hard and Soft Palate. Up until this point, the clinician has just observed structures. Examination of the hard and soft palate goes beyond observation. It necessitates feeling structures with your finger and evaluating structures within the pharyngeal cavity. Therefore, it is necessary that the clinician wear examining gloves and be equipped with a small penlight to carry out the task. The hard palate's color, the size and shape of the palatal vault, and the presence or absence of clefts, fissures, and fistulas (openings or holes in the palate) are determined. The midline of the hard and soft palates is usually a pink and whitish color; a blue tint may suggest a submucous cleft. To exclude this possibility, the clinician should feel along the midline of the hard palate to ensure that the underlying bony structure is intact. The uvula should be examined and its length and any structural abnormalities noted. A bifid uvula (a uvula that is split into two portions), for example, may indicate a submucous cleft. Finally, the fauces (the passage between the oral and the pharyngeal cavities) and the pharyngeal area itself need to be assessed. Excessive redness or a swollen appearance of the tonsils and/or adenoids might indicate an inflammation and warrants medical referral.

Functional Assessment of the Speech Mechanism. The functional integrity of the speech mechanism is as important as adequate structures. In this portion of the assessment, the function of the lips, mandible, tongue, and velum is examined. For the purpose at hand, proper function means not only that the client can move the structures on command but also that the range, smoothness, and speed of the movements are adequate. As the client is performing the various tasks, the clinician should pay attention to the following:

1. Can the client adequately perform the task?
2. Is the range of movements adequate?
3. Are the movements integrated and smooth?
4. Given the age of the client, is the speed of movement within normal limits?

If the client cannot move individual structures on command but movements are noted during involuntary tasks—for example, the client cannot stick out the tongue when asked to do so but can stick out the tongue to lick a postage stamp—this could indicate an apraxic condition. Further testing becomes necessary. The major goal of this portion of the assessment is to determine whether the function of the articulators appears adequate. Isolated functional deviancies do not necessarily translate into an inability to articulate certain speech sounds. They only suggest motor problems. Such functional difficulties should be evaluated in light of the client's articulatory performance,

> The sections on developmental apraxia of speech and apraxia of speech in adults in Chapter 10 will offer further suggestions in this area.

articulatory limitations, and intelligibility. Several different functional tasks for lips, mandible, tongue, and velum are indicated in Appendix 6.1.

SELECTION OF ADDITIONAL ASSESSMENT MEASURES

Approximately 80 percent of the clinical population with "delayed speech" have associated language problems (Shriberg, 1991; Shriberg, Kwiatkowski, Best, Hengst, & Terselic-Weber, 1986; Shriberg, Kwiatkowski, and Rasmussen, 1990). Therefore, language testing is recommended for every child who has a phonetic and/or phonemic disorder. In addition, a hearing screening is essential. Other measures may include the testing of specific auditory discrimination skills and an appraisal of the cognitive abilities of the client. Selection of additional tests will largely depend on an evaluation of the background information, medical and/or school records, and the clinical impression of the individual client.

Hearing Screening

A hearing screening is a portion of every assessment procedure. According to the revised set of "Guidelines for Identification Audiometry" (American Speech-Language-Hearing Association [ASHA], 1985) and the "Guidelines for Audiologic Screening" (ASHA, 1997), the following procedures should be a portion of the audiologic screening:

1. taking a history, which includes noting recent episodes of ear pain (otalgia) and/or ear discharge (otorrhea)
2. visual inspection to determine the presence of structural defects, and ear-canal and eardrum abnormalities
3. identification audiometry
4. acoustic immittance measurements.

TABLE 6.1   Referral Criteria for Audiologic Screening

HISTORY INFORMATION

Recent history of earaches, ear pain (otalgia)   ⟶   Refer
Recent history of ear discharge (otorrhea)   ⟶   Refer

VISUAL INSPECTION OF THE EAR

Structural defect of the ear, head, or neck   ⟶   Refer
Ear canal abnormalities, including blood or effusion, occlusion, inflammation,   ⟶   Refer
  excessive cerumen, tumor, and/or foreign material
Eardrum abnormalities, including abnormal color, bulging eardrum, fluid line or   ⟶   Refer
  bubbles, perforation, retraction

IDENTIFICATION AUDIOMETRY

Procedure: Air conduction screening at 20 dB HL at 1,000, 2,000, and 4,000 Hz.*

Failure to respond at one frequency in either ear   ⟶   Refer

TYMPANOMETRY

Procedure: Static admittance, equivalent ear-canal volume, and tympanometric width
are used in the screening protocol.

Flat tympanogram and equivalent ear canal volume (V_{ec}) outside normal range   ⟶   Refer
Low static admittance (Peak Y) on two successive occurrences in a 4–6 week interval   ⟶   Refer
Abnormally wide tympanometric width (TW) on two successive occurrences in a 4–6   ⟶   Refer
  week interval

Source: Summarized from *Guidelines for Screening for Hearing Impairments and Middle Ear Disorders,*
1990. Copyright 1990 by the American Speech-Language-Hearing Association.

*According to ASHA (1985, 1997), these criteria may require alteration for various clinical settings and
populations.

Referral criteria for each are included in Table 6.1.

Especially with children, the clinician should have knowledge of any developmental history that could affect the child's hearing status. This would include a history of episodes of otitis media, "earaches," or the placement of tubes. Shriberg and Kwiatkowski (1982a) verified that one third of children enrolled in speech or language intervention had histories of recurrent middle-ear disease. Although controversy exists surrounding the exact role chronic otitis media plays in the acquisition of phonology, it may at least interact with other risk factors in some children.

This interaction could easily lead to a greater risk of delayed or impaired communication skills.

Language Testing

Due to the high percentage of language problems in children with speech disorders, language screening belongs to the evaluation process. This can be done using formal, standardized assessment measures or informal evaluations. For example, the previously recorded speech sample could be analyzed to determine if morphosyntactic and semantic skills are age-appropriate. As with any screen-

Selected Language Screening Measures for Preschool and School-Age Children

BIRTH TO 3 YEARS SCREENING MEASURES

Bzoch, K., & League R. (1991). *Receptive-expressive emergent language scale* (2nd ed.). Austin, TX: PRO-ED.

Coplan, J., Gleason, J. R., Ryan, R., Burke, M., & Williams, M. (1993). *Early language milestone scale* (2nd ed.). Austin, TX: PRO-ED.

Furuno, S., O'Reilly, K., Inatsuka, T., Husaka, C., Allman, T., & Zeisloft-Falbey, B. (1991). *Hawaii early learning profile.* Palo Alto, CA: VORT.

Glover, M., Preminger, J., & Sanford, A. (1978). *Learning accomplishment profile for infants (Early LAP).* Winston-Salem, NC: Kaplan Press.

Rogers, S., Donovan, C., D'Eugenio, D., Brown, S., Lynch, E., Moersch, M., & Schafer, S. (1981). *Early intervention developmental profile* (rev. ed.). Ann Arbor: The University of Michigan Press.

Sparrow, S., Balla, D., & Cicchetti, D. (1984). *Vineland adaptive behavior.* Circle Pines, MN: American Guidance Service.

PRESCHOOL, SCHOOL-AGE SCREENING MEASURES

Fauthier, S., & Madison, C. (1983). *Kindergarten language screening test.* Austin, TX: PRO-ED.

Fluharty, N. (1978). *Fluharty preschool speech and language screening test.* Austin, TX: PRO-ED.

Morgan, D., & Guilford, A. (1989). *Adolescent language screening test* (3rd. ed.). Austin, TX: PRO-ED.

Reid, D., & Hammill, D. (1991). *Test of early language development* (2nd ed.). Austin, TX: PRO-ED.

Semel, E., Wiig, E., & Secord, W. (1989). *CELF-3 screening test.* San Antonio, TX: The Psychological Corporation.

Speech-Ease Associates (1985). *Speech-Ease screening inventory (K–1).* Austin, TX: PRO-ED.

ing tool, if the client does not pass the procedure, further testing becomes necessary.

Several language screening measures are available for children of all ages. Box 6.2 gives a few examples of standardized and non-standardized language screening measures for preschool and school-age children.

Specific Auditory Perceptual Testing

For many years, the appraisal of auditory perceptual skills, specifically speech sound discrimination testing, was a standard procedure for all clients with speech sound difficulties. The reasoning was that faulty speech sound perception often caused, or was linked to, the production problems. This was promoted by earlier works such as Van Riper's (1939b) *Speech Correction,* in which discrimination training was seen as a necessary portion of every therapy sequence.

Investigations into the relationship between auditory discrimination abilities and the production of speech sounds have extended over half a century (e.g., Anderson, 1941; Aungst and Frick, 1964; Cohen and Diehl, 1963; Hall, 1938; Kronvall and Diehl, 1954; Lapko and Bankson, 1975; Locke, 1980b, 1980c; Mase, 1946; Monnin and Huntington, 1974; Prins, 1963; Travis and Rasmus, 1931; Williams and McReynolds, 1975; Winitz, 1969; Winitz, Sanders, and Kort, 1981). The results of these and many other studies were inconclusive: some investigators found a positive relationship between auditory discrimination and articulation skills but others did not. Several reasons for why these results varied have been suggested (Schwartz and Goldman, 1974; Sherman and Geith, 1967; Weiner, 1967; Winitz, 1984). These different outcomes, however, did not support the cause–effect relationship earlier hypothesized. As a result of these findings, auditory discrimination testing seemed to lose much of its value as a standard assessment procedure.

Currently, speech sound discrimination testing is typically done only with those clients who demonstrate a collapse of two or more phonemic contrasts into a single sound

(Bankson and Bernthal, 1998). If a child substitutes [w] for [r] and [l], this would exemplify the collapse of three phonemic contrasts into a single sound: /w/, /r/, and /l/ would all be represented by the phoneme /w/. Auditory discrimination testing is a means of ascertaining whether clients who do not utilize phonemic contrasts might also not perceive the difference between these contrasts.

Within the last few years, auditory discrimination testing has departed from the testing of general discrimination skills. General tests of auditory discrimination would include measures such as the Auditory Discrimination Test (Wepman, 1973) or the Goldman-Fristoe-Woodcock Diagnostic Auditory Discrimination Test (Goldman, Fristoe, and Woodcock, 1970). Although these tests are designed to measure general auditory deficiencies, they do not give enough information about the discrimination skills of specific phonemic collapses noted in individual clients. Both Locke (1980c) and Winitz (1984) advocate the use of specific auditory discrimination testing that (1) is tailored to the individual client, (2) considers the client's speech sound difficulties or the collapse of the particular phonemic contrasts, and (3) includes the productionally problematic phonetic environment as well as uses these words in more meaningful sentence contexts.

Speech Production Perception Task (Locke, 1980c). This task utilizes selected stimuli based on the child's aberrant productions. The clinician first identifies these productions. For example, the child says [wæmp] for *lamp*. The norm production [læmp] and the child's production [wæmp] are now used to construct the perception task. The norm production is identified as the *stimulus production* (SP) and the child's aberrant production as the *response production* (RP). A perceptually similar third phoneme, the *control production* (CP), is also used when constructing the task.

In this case, [ræmp] could be selected. Next, the clinician presents a picture of the stimulus production, in this example a picture of a lamp. The child is then asked "Is this a _____?" The three stimuli—stimulus production, response production, and the control production—are presented in a random order. Figure 6.2 exemplifies this perception task.

Discrimination Testing and the Phonological Performance Analysis (Winitz, 1984). Winitz offers additional suggestions that could be incorporated into the assessment of auditory discrimination skills of clients:

1. *The test items should be relevant and client-oriented.* General auditory discrimination tests are not a good measure of the client's difficulties. If a child produces [r] incorrectly, for example, tasks should concentrate on the child's discrimination of [r] and not of [l] or [t].
2. *The specific aberrant productions of the client should be targeted.* The client's production should be contrasted to the norm production of the sound in question. If a child lateralizes [s], the child's abilities to discriminate between a lateral [s] and a regular [s] should be examined. Therefore, the clinician must be able to replicate any of the client's distortions.
3. *The phonetic context in which the incorrect productions occur must be considered.* The clinician must know whether the client's production occurs in the word-initial, -medial, or -final position; in singletons or in consonant clusters; or with specific vowels, for example. If a child evidences deletion of [z] at the end of a word, the discrimination testing should emphasize the presence versus the absence of [z] in this position—for example, *toe* versus *toes*. Similarly, a child who produces an unrounded [ʃ] preceding front vowels should

FIGURE 6.2 Speech Production Perception Task

| Child's Name _____ | Sex: M F | Birthdate: _____ |
| | | Age: _____ |

Date _____	Date _____	Date _____
Production Task		
Stimulus · Response*	Stimulus · Response	Stimulus · Response
[læmp] · [wæmp]	[ ] · [ ]	[ ] · [ ]
SP /l/ · RP /w/ · CP /r/	SP / / · RP / / · CP / /	SP / / · RP / / · CP / /
Stimulus · Response	Stimulus · Response	Stimulus · Response
1. [ræmp] · yes NO	1.	1.
2. [wæmp] · yes NO	2.	2.
3. [læmp] · YES no	3.	3.
4. [læmp] · YES no	4.	4.
5. [wæmp] · yes NO	5.	5.
6. [ræmp] · yes NO	6.	6.
7. [ræmp] · yes NO	7.	7.
8. [læmp] · YES no	8.	8.
9. [wæmp] · yes NO	9.	9.
10. [læmp] · YES no	10.	10.
11. [wæmp] · yes NO	11.	11.
12. [ræmp] · yes NO	12.	12.
13. [wæmp] · yes NO	13.	13.
14. [læmp] · YES no	14.	14.
15. [ræmp] · yes NO	15.	15.
16. [wæmp] · yes NO	16.	16.
17. [læmp] · YES no	17.	17.
18. [ræmp] · yes NO	18.	18.
RP____ CP____ SP____	RP____ CP____ SP____	RP____ CP____ SP____

Source: From "The Inference of Speech Perception in the Phonologically Disordered Child, Part II: Some Clinically Novel Procedures, Their Use, Some Findings," by J. L. Locke, 1980, *Journal of Speech and Hearing Disorders, 45,* p. 447. Copyright 1980 by the American Speech-Language-Hearing Association. Reprinted by permission.
*The correct response is in uppercase letters.

be tested with words with front vowels—for example, *ship, sheep,* and *sheet.*

Winitz (1984) also proposes that a phonological performance analysis supplement the aforementioned auditory discrimination tasks. The purpose of such an analysis is to determine whether children perceive the distinction between contrastive sounds that they misarticulate. Although the previous suggestions are guidelines for appraising all clients with speech sound difficulties, the phonological performance analysis is appropriate for those who demonstrate the collapse of two (or more) phonemic contrasts. Minimal pairs containing the respective phoneme contrasts are embedded in sets of three identical sentences with a somewhat connected topic. Each set of sentences has an appropriate illustrative picture. After reading one set of sentences, the clinician tells the child to select the picture that best represents the meaning of the sentences. At a later point in the assessment process, the child is read the second set of sentences and again asked to pick the appropriate picture. Figure 6.3 represents sets of sentences and pictures used to appraise the /w/ and /r/ contrasts. Although

the phonological performance analysis attempts to test minimal pairs in connected sentences rather than in isolated word productions, the development of such a battery for each child not only would be time-consuming but also would probably tax a clinician's artistic and creative skills. To aid in this task, several examples of sentences contrasting commonly substituted sounds in minimal pairs are contained in Chapter 8.

Cognitive Appraisal

Speech-language pathologists are not qualified to perform formal IQ testing. However, the results of a cognitive appraisal may be im-

Phonological Performance Analysis Test

He said to put the rings on.
I didn't want to put the rings on.
But he said the rings should be put on.

He said to put the wings on.
I didn't want to put the wings on.
But he said the wings should be put on.

FIGURE 6.3 Example of a Phonological Performance Task

Source: From *Treating Articulation Disorders: For Clinicians by Clinicians* (p. 36), by H. Winitz, 1984, Baltimore: University Park Press. Copyright 1984 by Harris Winitz. Reprinted with permission.

portant when developing further assessment and treatment goals. IQ testing might then be initiated by referring the client to appropriate professionals. Often, such test results may be obtained through medical, school, or client records.

Caution should be exercised, though, when interpreting the results of IQ measures of children demonstrating phonetic-phonemic disorders. First, a large percentage of children with speech disorders also demonstrate language difficulties. Some cognitive assessment tools use tasks very similar to those used to assess language. Therefore, IQ scores may be affected by the child's language incompetencies. This is particularly a problem with full-scale IQ scores (Nelson, 1998). For this reason, some authors have suggested using nonverbal cognitive measures (Paul, 1995), although tests designed to evaluate nonverbal cognitive skills may appraise only a limited aspect of cognition (Johnston, 1982; Kamhi, Minor, and Mauer, 1990). Second, intelligibility may play a role in the assessment of children with moderate to severe phonemic difficulties, particularly if verbal IQ measures are used. Nonverbal measures would be helpful with the unintelligible child, however, as previously noted, these tests appear somewhat restricted. Third, cognitive measures, similar to other standardized tests, do not adequately reflect the abilities of children from culturally and linguistically diverse backgrounds. Although the sample used to norm a particular test typically contains a percentage of children from culturally and linguistically diverse backgrounds (usually the same percentage as these minorities are represented within the U.S. population), this percentage is so small that the inherent test bias for these populations is not eliminated. The presence of language and/or phonetic-phonemic impairments may further compound the interpretation of IQ scores of children from culturally or linguistically diverse backgrounds.

Although the results of a cognitive appraisal may give helpful guidelines for planning subsequent assessment and remediation strategies, the interpretation of the results is not without its problems. Clinicians should be aware of the type of cognitive assessment instrument used to appraise the individual (e.g., verbal versus nonverbal) and the limitations of each measure. *Extreme care should be exercised when interpreting the scores of children from linguistically and culturally diverse backgrounds.*

CLINICAL APPLICATION

How Much Time Does a Comprehensive Appraisal Require?

A comprehensive phonetic-phonemic appraisal seems to involve a considerable amount of time. However, gathering data could be distributed over several therapy sessions. The following sequence is possible if a clinician is limited to twenty minutes of data collection per setting.

Time #1	Impression of intelligibility. Hearing screening. Speech-motor screening.
Time #2	Articulation test + stimulability measures.
Interim planning	Analyze articulation test and plan spontaneous speech sample.
Time #3	Spontaneous speech sample in at least two different settings. Could include sample with family, siblings, classmates.
Time #4	Supplemental testing, if necessary. This could include additional word lists to supplement articulation test, specific auditory discrimination testing, language screening, etc.

SPECIAL CONSIDERATIONS

The Child with Emerging Phonology

The period of **emerging phonology** is the time span during childhood in which conventional words begin to appear as a means of communication. Although this level of development usually occurs when children are toddlers, it may also occur in older children with more severe deficits in language learning. Within the assessment process, special consideration must be given to the child with an emerging phonological system. Both the diagnostic procedures themselves and the analysis of the results will be different for this population.

Characteristics of Children with Emerging Phonological Systems. Children with emerging phonology are referred for speech-language services for several reasons. First, some may have been born with known risk factors. Identifiable developmental disorders include Down syndrome and other genetic disorders, known hearing impairments, and cerebral palsy. Second, some children will have early acquired disorders secondary to diseases or trauma such as encephalitis, closed head injury, or abuse. Third, children will be brought by parents who are concerned about the child's development: Parents might have observed differences in the expressive communication abilities and/or intelligibility of their child compared to other children of a similar age. Fourth, children will be referred through various sources because they are "late talkers" and their expressive language is slow to emerge.

The group of children with developmentally delayed emerging phonology is typically characterized by small expressive vocabularies showing a reduced repertoire of consonants and syllable shapes (Paul and Jennings, 1992). Often, their words are unintelligible. The lim-

ited phonological system may also impact further semantic and morphosyntactic development. Therefore, it is important to appraise the phonological system within the broader framework of the child's developing language system. In addition to hearing screening, assessment procedures should always include language testing for this group of children.

Procedural Difficulties with These Children. Previously noted assessment procedures encompass several different tasks that provide useful and necessary information. However, for children at this level of development, several of these tasks may be difficult to complete.

1. *Articulation tests and stimulability measures:* Depending on the client's developmental level, the administration of standardized articulation tests and stimulability measures might not be possible because these children are not yet skilled at following directions or with imitation tasks. An alternative method might include the naming of objects. However, due to the limited expressive vocabulary of most of these children, this adaptation may have severe limitations.

What to Do?

With the caregivers' help, one can usually procure a fairly complete sample of words the child is using. Based on the production of these words, the child's consonant and vowel inventory as well as syllable shapes can be established. Such words can be obtained in a number of ways. The following possibilities are given as suggestions:

1. Have the family tape-record the child saying specific spontaneous and elicited words at home.
2. Have the caregiver bring from home a few objects that the child can name.
3. Have the caregivers keep a log of the intended words that the child can produce

as well as the approximate way in which each word was pronounced.

While a tape recording is a good idea, the quality must be secured so that the productions can be accurately evaluated. Based on personal clinical experience, asking the caregiver to bring familiar objects from home and keeping a log of utterances usually provide more diagnostic information than tape recordings. Bringing in familiar objects from the home environment is especially productive in the initial session. For a young child in an unfamiliar setting, this might provide a small comfort zone that will open communication doors. Caregiver logs of the child's spoken words become a necessity when attempting to appraise the shy child who does not communicate at the first or even second meeting. Clinicians need to keep in mind that caregivers are not skilled in phonetic transcription, so they will be limited in their abilities to write down how the child pronounced a certain word. Explanations and examples should be given to the caregiver on how to proceed with this task.

2. *Spontaneous speech sample:* Children with emerging phonological systems who are being evaluated for a possible communication disorder probably do not talk a lot. When they talk, utterances may contain only one or two words and what they say may be partially unintelligible. Collecting a spontaneous speech sample may, therefore, be a challenge. However, spontaneous samples not only provide data for establishing sound and syllable inventories but also establish communicative situations that elicit spontaneous utterances. If the child is using primarily single words, a one-word utterance analysis such as Bloom's (1973) or Nelson's (1973) will quantify the types of words the child is using. As mentioned earlier, a child's emerging phonological system should be examined and evaluated within the broader parameters of the child's emerging language as a whole.

What to Do?

Techniques described in the previous section on articulation testing can also be used to obtain a conversational speech sample. With the shy child who does not respond in an unfamiliar setting, observations of the child's communicative interaction with the caregivers before or after the session may give valuable information.

3. *Examination of the oral-facial structures and the speech-motor system.* Important diagnostic information will be gained if a relationship can be verified between the speech-motor abilities and the slow speech development of these children. However, the assessment of the structure and function of the speech-motor system is often very difficult to obtain from younger children. This is in part due to their intolerance of the procedures needed to complete an intraoral examination as well as to their limitations in imitating sounds and movements on command.

What to Do?

Several fun situations can be initiated to assist in this process. Paul (1995) suggests pretending to make clown or fish faces together, letting the child first look inside your mouth with a small flashlight, and then pretending to look for a dinosaur or elephant in the child's mouth. However, even with the best ideas, clinicians will often fail to get the cooperation of a young child. One possibility would be to wait until the child becomes better acquainted with the clinician and then attempt the procedure again. A second possibility is to gather information about the child's feeding and babbling behaviors. Questions about the child's feeding behavior might help discover related developmental

> The relationship between babbling and language development was discussed in Chapter 5.

disorders. Box 6.3 contains some sample questions about feeding that could be used to gather information about the speech-motor system of the child indirectly. Babbling history could attempt to establish the quantity and diversity of the child's babbling. Both quantity and diversity of babbling behaviors have been correlated to measures of language.

4. *Hearing screening:* A hearing screening is indispensable for children with emerging phonological systems for a number of reasons (the high prevalence of otitis media and its impact on hearing is only one). Speech-language specialists equipped with a portable audiometer typically use a screening procedure that has the client signalling, by raising a hand, for example, when a tone is heard. This type of screening procedure may not be possible with children at this age. However, conditioned response audiometric screening may yield results.

What to Do?

If screening attempts have failed, the child needs to be referred for a comprehensive audiological evaluation.

5. *Additional tests.* It is well documented that children with phonological disorders often have language problems as well (e.g., Shriberg, 1991; Shriberg et al., 1986; Shriberg,

---

Box 6.3

Questions to Assess the Feeding Behavior in the Child with an Emerging Phonological System

During sucking of liquids, did any of the following occur?

- Tongue thrusting (abnormally forceful protrusion of the tongue from the mouth)
- Lip retraction (drawing back of the lips so that they form a tight line over the mouth)
- Jaw thrusting (abnormally forceful and tense downward extension of the mandible)
- Lip pursing (a tight purse-string movement of the lips)
- Jaw clenching (abnormally tight closure of the mouth)
- Tonic bite reflex (abnormally strong jaw closure when the teeth or gums are stimulated)

During swallowing, did/do any of the following occur?

- Drooling
- Excessive mucus present

- Coughing, choking, gagging
- Hyperextension of head or neck

During biting and chewing, do any of the following occur?

- Abnormal movements of the jaws, lips, and tongue with solid foods of different consistencies.
- Munching versus chewing motions (munching is the earliest form of chewing and involves a flattening and spreading of the tongue combined with up-and-down jaw movement, whereas chewing is characterized by spreading and rolling movements of the tongue and rotary jaw movements).
- Abnormal patterns

Source: Summarized from "Feeding At-Risk Infants and Toddlers," by M. Jaffe, 1989, *Topics in Language Disorders, 10*(1), pp. 13–25.

Kwiatkowski, and Rasmussen, 1990). Therefore, the language abilities of these children need to be assessed. For younger children between 2 and 3 years of age, the language assessment instrument must be selected with care. Because of these children's limited attention span, difficulties in following directions, and their relatively poor imitation skills, even some standardized language tests normed for these ages may not be successfully administered.

> The reader is referred back to Language Testing in this chapter for selected language measures that can be used for the birth to 3 population.

What to Do?

There are numerous developmental tests that rely partially or totally on the information supplied by the caregiver about the child's level of functioning. The analysis of language in naturalistic contexts can also be used to assess the child's pragmatic, morphological, syntactical, and semantic competencies. See, for example, Lund and Duchan (1992).

Analyzing the Child's Emerging Phonological System. Several authors suggest that an independent analysis be used with children who are at this level of phonological development (Bankson and Bernthal, 1998a; Paul and Jennings, 1992; Stoel-Gammon and Dunn, 1985). An **independent analysis** takes only the client's productions into account; they are not compared to the adult norm model. Because only a relatively limited number of consonants and vowels are typically present in the child's inventory, a comparison to the adult norm model would not be helpful for later assessment and intervention. At this stage of the child's development, more information can be gained by seeing which sounds and syllable shapes *are* present. The child's inventory must

first be expanded before comparisons to the adult model can be made.

Three kinds of data are collected for the independent analysis: the inventory of speech sounds, the syllable shapes the child uses, and any constraints noted on sound sequences. The inventory of speech sounds includes all vowels and consonants found in the accumulated word productions of the child. Data on syllable shapes would pertain to single sound productions to signify a word (V, C) and to the use of both open and closed syllable forms (CV, CVCV, CVC). Sound production constraints would include any sound or sound combinations that are used only in certain word or context positions. Examples of this category would include [p] used only word-initially or [d] used only in CVCV structures.

CLINICAL APPLICATION

Inventory of Speech Sounds, Syllable Shapes, and Constraints

Ted is a 1:8-year-old Down syndrome child who is being followed in the early intervention program. These twelve words have been recorded by his mother and the speech-language pathologist.

"yes"	[jɛ]	"pig"	[pɪ]
"mom"	[mʌm]	"hug"	[hʌk]
"daddy"	[dædi]	"bike"	[baɪ]
"hello"	[hoʊ]	"duck"	[dʌk]
"grandpa"	[dapa]	"truck"	[tʌk]
"bye"	[baɪ]	"cow"	[daʊ]

Vowel inventory: [i, ɪ, ɛ, æ, a, oʊ, aɪ, aʊ, ʌ]

Consonant inventory: [m, p, b, t, d, k, j, h]

Syllable shapes: CV, CVC, CVCV

Constraints: [k] is used only in a postvocalic position after the central vowel [ʌ].

An Index of Severity. For children with emerging language skills, Paul and Jennings (1992) suggest a procedure used to obtain an index of severity of phonological delay. This index is based on the number of different consonants and the syllable shapes represented in the child's productions. For both indices, data from normally developing children were compared to those of children with small expressive vocabularies. Table 6.2 describes the procedures and subsequent results which can be used to examine the severity of phonological delay.

TABLE 6.2   An Index of Severity of Phonological Delay (Paul and Jennings, 1992)

TOTAL NUMBER OF CONSONANTS

Procedure: The gathering of words for the analysis is based on a 10-minute communications sample. The total number of different consonants are counted.

Results:

Children	Age	Average Number of Consonants
Norm	18–24 mos.	14
Small expr. vocab.	18–24 mos.	6
Norm	24–36 mos.	18
Small expr. vocab.	24–36 mos.	10

The child's average number of different consonants can be compared to see if they are closer to the number produced by the norm children or to those with small expressive vocabularies.

SYLLABLE STRUCTURE LEVEL (SSL)

Procedure: This analysis is based on 20–50 vocalizations.
It examines intelligible words and nonconventional vocalizations.
Based on the syllable shape, each utterance is assigned a certain level.
The ratings given to each vocalization are added together and divided by the total number of vocalizations rated.

Levels: Level 1: vocalization is composed of only a voiced vowel (V syllable shape [ɑ], [u]), a voiced syllabic consonant (C syllable shape [l̩], [m̩]), or CV syllable in which the consonant is a glottal stop, glide, or [h] ([wi], [hɑ]). The following are examples of Level 1 vocalizations: [i], [oʊ], [l̩], [m̩], [n̩], [hɑ], [wa], [ʔa], [ja], [ju].

Level 2: vocalization is composed of a VC ([ʌp], [ɪk]), CVC with a single consonant ([bab], [mam]), or a CV shape that contains consonants other than those noted at Level 1 ([tu], [mu]). Voicing differences are disregarded; therefore, [bip] or [toʊd] would be considered Level 2. The following are examples of Level 2 vocalizations: [ʌk], [um], [ab], [papa], [baba], [noʊ], [tɛdi], [kaka], [lala].

Level 3: vocalization is composed of syllables with two or more different consonant types ([dɑli], [kɪti]). Voicing differences only would be considered Level 2. The following are examples of Level 3 vocalizations: [bati], [boʊmo], [dʌk], [hɛlo], [jʌki], [hat], [koʊt].

Results: Norm children at 24 months of age   SSL = 2.2
Children with small expressive vocabularies at 24 months of age   SSL = 1.7

The child's SSL average can be compared to see whether it is closer to the average for children in the norm group or to the average for children with small expressive vocabularies.

CLINICAL APPLICATION

Index of Severity

Further utterances were gathered from Ted, who was presented in the previous Clinical Application. The syllable structure level is noted for each vocalization.

"yes"	[jɛ]	Level 1	"pig"	[pɪ]	Level 2
"mom"	[mʌm]	Level 2	"hug"	[hʌk]	Level 3
"daddy"	[dædi]	Level 2	"bike"	[baɪ]	Level 2
"hello"	[hoʊ]	Level 1	"duck"	[dʌk]	Level 3
"grandpa"	[dapa]	Level 3	"truck"	[tʌk]	Level 3
"bye"	[baɪ]	Level 2	"cow"	[daʊ]	Level 2

Additional nonconventional vocalizations:

[ha]	Level 1	[oʊ]	Level 1
[dɪdɪ]	Level 2	[bubu]	Level 2
[pu]	Level 2	[i]	Level 1
[bæbæ]	Level 2	[pabi]	Level 2
[bʌpi]	Level 2	[ja]	Level 1
[m̩]	Level 1	[ʌ]	Level 1

Total Number of Consonants: 8

Syllable Structure Level: 1.83

Ted is 20 months of age. His total number of consonants is much closer to the average found for the children with small expressive vocabularies. Although Ted's syllable structure is higher than those found in children with small expressive vocabularies, it is still closer to the average for that group when compared to the norm children at 24 months of age.

The Unintelligible Child

The speech of unintelligible children is so disordered that the speaker's message cannot be understood. Unintelligible children are not limited to any specific age group. For example, Hodson and Paden (1981) report children who at 8 years of age were considered unintelligible.

Characteristics of Unintelligible Children. Hodson and Paden (1981) evaluated the speech of sixty unintelligible children ranging from 3 to 8 years of age. All of these highly unintelligible children evidenced varying degrees of difficulty with the production of liquids, stridents, and consonant clusters. Prevalent phonological processes in the speech of these children were cluster reduction, stridency deletion, stopping, gliding and vocalizations of liquids, and labial and nasal assimilations. Hodson (1984) notes that the least intelligible children were those who omitted entire classes of sounds. A few of the children produced no obstruents, either before or after the vowel nucleus (*bed* was realized as [ɛ] or [wɛ]), and a small number of the children did not produce sonorants (*run* was pronounced [ʌ]).

Procedural Difficulties with Unintelligible Children. Children 3 years and older will usually not have difficulties completing an articulation test, stimulability testing, or the speech-motor assessment. Even with reduced intelligibility, a single-word articulation test will probably render transcribable results which can be used for a phonetic/phonemic analysis. The major difficulty for the clinician when evaluating unintelligible children is being able to understand and transcribe a spontaneous speech sample. This may present a task that cannot always be successfully completed, but with careful structuring, an understandable spontaneous speech sample may be possible even with unintelligible children.

What to Do?

1. *Choose the topic and attempt to structure the situation as much as possible.* If the context is unknown, that is, if the unintelligible child is talking about a self-generated topic, the clinician will have even more difficulty understanding the sample. Scripts of action events, routine events, and scripted events (Lund and Duchan, 1992) will give structure and predictability to the conversation. Scripts of action events depict everyday occurrences with predictable elements. Therefore, if children are asked to explain what they do at McDonald's to get a hamburger, the predictability of the events should aid comprehension. *Routine events* begin, progress, and end in essentially the same way each time they occur. If the topic is baseball and the child should explain what the person coming up to bat must do, the known progression of events will again help the clinician understand the conversation. *Scripted events* are activities that have been performed previously and, therefore, all participants have expectations of how they will progress. For example, a child and clinician could fix the wheel on a broken toy truck. The clinician would then ask the child to explain what they had just done. If the clinician models sentences, for example, "First, we saw that the truck had a missing wheel. Next, we looked for the wheel," the child might use similar sentence patterns. Again, the predictability of the utterances should increase the clinician's ability to understand what the child is attempting to say.

2. *Gloss the utterances the child says as much as possible.* Any utterances that may later be difficult to understand from the tape recording should be glossed by the clinician. Glossing means repeating the child's utterance according to norm pronunciation. If the child says [aɪ oʊ oʊm] for "I go home," the clinician repeats the utterance in a regular manner so that it is recorded together with the sample.

The Dialect Speaker

A **dialect** is a language variation spoken by the members of a particular regional, cultural, or social community. Dialect use *is not* a speech-language disorder; it is merely a *difference* in pronunciation or language use based on the individual's geographical location or cultural background. It is very important that every clinician be aware of dialectal changes that may impact the phonological system of the individual. They are relevant to both assessment and (possible) intervention measures.

Regional dialects represent a set of linguistic features, pronunciation prominently included, that are utilized by individuals from a specific geographical area. The systematic study of regional dialects—known as dialectology, dialect geography, or linguistic geography—is a highly detailed and complex endeavor to categorize linguistic changes, including word usage and pronunciations for dozens of geographic regions within the United States, for example. Geographical dialect information is far too detailed for the purpose at hand. However, it is important to note that every geographical area has its own distinct set of pronunciation patterns. These

TABLE 6.3   Regional Dialects with Notable Changes in Pronunciation

DIALECT	GEOGRAPHICAL AREA
New York	Metropolitan New York
New England	Upper Maine, the Narragansett Bay region, and metropolitan Boston
Southern	Coastal plains from Virginia to eastern Texas; includes most of North Carolina, South Carolina, Georgia, Alabama, Mississippi, and Louisiana
Ozark English	Northern Arkansas, southern Missouri, and northwestern Oklahoma
Appalachian English	Areas of Kentucky, Tennessee, Virginia, North Carolina, and West Virginia (southern Appalachians, Ozarks, Bluegrass area of Kentucky, and Nashville basin area)

Source: Carver (1987); Christian, Wolfram, and Nube (1988).

may include both vowel and consonant variations. Regional dialects that demonstrate notable changes of pronunciation are contained in Table 6.3.

The most prevalent *cultural dialect* within the United States is African American English, which is also known as African American Vernacular, Black English, and Ebonics. This dialect is spoken by many, but not all, African Americans. African American English may also be influenced by regional pronunciations. Table 6.4 summarizes some major phonological features noted in these regional and cultural dialects.

CLINICAL APPLICATION

African American Dialect: More than Phonological Changes

Although several phonological features of African American dialect have been introduced in this section, semantic, morphosyntactic, and pragmatic variations are also a part of this dialect (see for example van Keulen, Weddington, DeBose, 1998 or Terrell and Terrell, 1993). Children may use these dialect features during language assessment; it is therefore important that the clinician be aware of these variations. The following is a summary of African American dialect features noted in the grammatical structure of preschoolers (Washington and Craig, 1994).*

Morphological and Syntactic Form	Examples
Zero copula or auxiliary *Is, are,* and modal auxiliaries *will, can,* and *do* are not consistently used.	"the bridge out" "how you do this"
Subject-verb agreement A subject and verb that differ in either number or person is used.	"what do this mean"
Fitna/sposeta/bouta Abbreviated forms for "fixing to," "supposed to," and "about to."	*fitna:* "she fitna a backward flip"
Ain't *Ain't* is used as a negative auxiliary.	"why she ain't comin?"
Undifferentiated pronoun case Nominative, objective, and demonstrative cases of pronouns occur interchangeably.	"him did and him"
Multiple negation Two or more negative markers in one utterance.	"I don't got no brothers"
Zero possessive Possession coded by word order so that the possessive -s marker is deleted or the nominative or objective case of pronouns is used rather than the possessive.	"he hit the man car" "kids just goin' to walk to they school"

*While other morphological and syntactic variations were noted, these forms were used by at least one third of the children in the study.

TABLE 6.4 Specific Phonological Features of Regional and Cultural Dialects

PHONOLOGICAL FEATURE	EXAMPLE		DIALECT
Changes in r-Sounds			
Loss of r-coloring on central vowels	"bird" "father"	= [bɜd] = [fɑðə]	New York, New England, Southern, African American English
Neutralization of [r] in postvocalic clusters	"farm"	= [fɑm]	New York, New England, Southern
Neutralization of [r] in an intervocalic word position	"Carol"	= [kɛəl]	African American English, Appalachian English, Ozark English
Neutralization of [r] after a consonant	"throw"	= [θoᵘ]	Appalachian English, Ozark English
Changes in Individual Consonants			
Initial [w] reduction	"will"	= [ɪl]	Appalachian English, Ozark English
Substitution of t/θ and d/ð initiating a word	"that" "think"	= [dæt] = [tɪŋk]	Appalachian English, Ozark English, African American English
Substitution of f/θ and v/ð intervocalic and in final word position	"bathtub" "mouth"	= [bæftʌb] = [maᵘf]	African American English
Aspirated vowels initiating a word, sounds like an [h] sound	"it"	= [hɪt]	Appalachian English, Ozark English
Intrusive [t]	"cliff"	= [klɪft]	Appalachian English
Devoicing of final [b], [d], and [g]	"lid"	= [lɪt]	African American English
Changes in Consonant Clusters			
Epenthesis	"ghosts"	= [gostəs]	Appalachian English, Ozark English
Metathesis	"ask"	= [æks]	African American English
Word final reduction of consonant cluster (especially prominent if one of the consonants is an alveolar)	"test"	= [tɛs]	African American English
Deletion of [l] in word-final consonant clusters	"help"	= [hɛp]	African American English, also noted in Appalachian English and Ozark English before labial consonants
Deletion of word-final consonants with nasalization of preceding vowels	"man"	= [mæ̃]	African American English

Source: Summarized from Christian, Wolfram, and Nube (1988); Fasold and Wolfram (1975); Seymour and Miller-Jones (1981); and Wolfram (1994).

Implications for Appraisal. For the dialect speaker, several issues need to be considered during the assessment process. The first and foremost is determining which phonological characteristics constitute dialectal differences. When contrasted to General American English, the noted variations in pronunciation of the dialect speaker may be dialectal differences and not signs of a disordered phonological system.

What to Do?

1. Be sensitive to local dialect patterns and to any regional or cultural dialects that may impact the client's speech. Any unbiased as-

sessment of the individual's phonology accounts for the norms of the particular dialect. In other words, are these phonological variations also represented in individuals with whom this client interacts? In addition, in a society in which the mobility level is high, clinicians should expect that certain regional dialects will appear outside of their associated geographical areas.

2. Choose assessment instruments that account for dialectal variations or consider dialect features when scoring any standardized measure. Some articulation tests—the Goldman-Fristoe (Goldman and Fristoe, 1986) and Fisher-Logemann (Fisher and Logemann, 1971), for example—have guidelines for scoring certain dialect features. However, many instruments do not. The clinician's knowledge of dialect features (see Table 6.4) will be helpful in scoring these measures.

3. Evaluate not only the presence of specific dialect features but also their frequency of occurrence. The results of research indicate that a judgment of disordered versus different phonological systems is often influenced by the relative frequency rather than just the categorical presence or absence of certain patterns (Bauman-Waengler, 1993a, 1993b, 1994, 1995, 1996, Kercher and Bauman-Waengler, 1992; Seymour, Green, and Hundley, 1991; Stockman, 1996; Wolfram, 1994).

4. Assess the client's communicative effectiveness in the regional or cultural dialect. If unfamiliar with the dialect, ask other professionals or members of the community about the client's communication skills. The client's teachers are often a good source of information.

The Speaker of English as a Second Language

The United States has a large influx of immigrants from a variety of cultural and linguistic backgrounds. Children of these immigrants typically grow up learning two languages,

their native language and General American English. If English is acquired after the native language, as is usually the case, the phonological system of the native language can impact the pronunciation of the second language. Knowledge of the vowel and consonant differences between the inventories of the native language and General American English will aid the clinician in assessment and when trying to determine whether the client has a phonological disorder. It is also the basis for accent reduction if that is the therapeutic goal.

Speakers of Spanish make up by far the largest number of immigrants to the United States. Spanish has become the second most common language spoken in the United States, with more than 11 million people speaking it (Iglesias and Goldstein, 1998). However, Spanish, like American English, has several different dialects. It is estimated that six major dialects of Spanish are spoken within the United States (Dalbor, 1980). The second largest group of immigrants is Asians, who include Pacific Islanders (U.S. Bureau of Census, 1990). These individuals speak a variety of languages, including several different dialects of Japanese, Mandarin Chinese, Vietnamese, and Cantonese, to mention just a few. It is beyond the scope of this book to consider all the language varieties spoken in the United States. For more information on this issue, see Cheng (1991, 1993), Goldstein (1995), Ruhlen (1976), So and Dodd (1994), and Wang (1990), for example. For the purpose at hand, only the phonological inventories of Spanish, Japanese, Mandarin, and Vietnamese will be contrasted to General American English in Tables 6.5, 6.6, 6.7, and 6.8.

Implications for Appraisal. The native language may impact the client's acquisition of English to varying degrees. Therefore, it is quite possible that the client's irregular pronunciations may be a consequence of native language interference. If so, the differences

TABLE 6.5   Phonological Inventory: A Comparison of Spanish to General American English (GAE)

SPANISH VOWELS	VOWEL DIFFERENCES: SPANISH AND GAE
[i, e, u, o, a]	■ [ɪ, ɛ, æ, ʊ, ʌ, ə, ɝ, ɚ] and diphthongs are not present in Spanish. ■ Spanish speaker may substitute similar vowels in GAE, e.g., *could* → [kud] ■ Spanish speaker may substitute [er] for [ɝ], *bird* → [berd]
SPANISH CONSONANTS	**CONSONANT DIFFERENCES: SPANISH AND GAE**
[p, t, k, b, d, g]	■ Because voiceless stops are unaspirated in Spanish, speaker may produce GAE voiceless stops as unaspirated. ■ In Spanish, [t] and [d] are dentalized productions.
[f, χ, s] ([χ] is a voiceless uvular fricative)	■ [v, z, ð, θ, ʃ, ʒ] not present in Spanish.
[tʃ]	■ [dʒ] not present in Spanish.
[w, j, l, ɾ, r,]	■ [r] is produced as a trilled vibrant production in Spanish.
[m, n, ŋ]	■ [n] is a dentalized production in Spanish. ■ [ŋ] is palatalized in Spanish.

Source: Goldstein (1995); Perez (1994); Ruhlen (1976).

TABLE 6.6   Phonological Inventory: A Comparison of Japanese to General American English (GAE)

JAPANESE VOWELS	VOWEL DIFFERENCES: JAPANESE AND GAE
[i, e, o, u, a]	■ [ɪ, ɛ, æ, ʊ, ʌ, ə, ɝ, ɚ] and diphthongs are not present in Japanese. ■ Japanese speaker may substitute similar vowels in GAE, e.g., *bed* → [bed] ■ [u] vowel in Japanese is unrounded; may use this unrounded vowel for [u] in GAE.
JAPANESE CONSONANTS	**CONSONANT DIFFERENCES: JAPANESE AND GAE**
[p, t, k, b, d, g]	■ [t] and [d] are produced as dentalized sounds in Japanese. ■ intervocalic [b] and [d] are often perceived and produced as [β] (a voiced bilabial fricative) and [ɣ] (a voiced velar fricative) in the Japanese speaker of GAE.
[s, z, ʃ, ʒ]	■ [f, v, ð, θ] do not exist in Japanese. ■ [f, v] may be produced as bilabial fricatives in Japanese speakers of GAE. ■ Japanese speakers of GAE often have distributional problems with other fricatives.
[tʃ, dʒ]	■ Japanese speakers of GAE often have distributional difficulties with affricates.
[w, j, l, ɾ]	■ [r] is a tap production in Japanese. ■ Many Japanese speakers of GAE do not recognize [l] and [r] as two different phonemes.
[m, n] Japanese is a tone language.	■ [ŋ] is not present in Japanese.

Source: Conly, Bauman-Waengler, and Waengler (1989); Ruhlen (1976).

TABLE 6.7 Phonological Inventory: A Comparison of Mandarin to General American English (GAE)

MANDARIN VOWELS	VOWEL DIFFERENCES: MANDARIN AND GAE
[i, u, o, e, a, y] ([y] is a rounded high front vowel)	■ [ɪ, ɛ, æ, ʊ, ʌ, ə, ɝ, ɚ] and diphthongs are not present in Mandarin.
	■ Mandarin speakers of GAE may substitute similar vowels, e.g., *will* → [wil]
MANDARIN CONSONANTS	**CONSONANT DIFFERENCES: MANDARIN AND GAE**
[p, t, k]	■ [b, d, g] do not exist in Mandarin.
	■ In Mandarin, phonemic oppositions are signalled by the presence and absence of aspiration; may have distributional difficulties with aspirated and unaspirated productions in GAE.
	■ In Mandarin, phonemic oppositions are signalled by dentalized and retroflexed productions of [t] and [s].
	■ The Mandarin speaker of GAE may have difficulty with [t] and [s] sounds.
[f, s, ç, χ] [ç] is a voiceless palatal fricative	■ [v, z, ð, θ, ʃ, ʒ] do not exist in Mandarin.
[w, j, l, r]	■ In Mandarin, there are two variations of [r], a uvular trill production and a retroflex production.
[m, n, ŋ] Mandarin is a tone language.	■ No consonant blends in Mandarin.

Source: Cheng (1994); Ruhlen (1976).

TABLE 6.8 Phonological Inventory: A Comparison of Vietnamese to General American English (GAE)

VIETNAMESE VOWELS	VOWEL DIFFERENCES: VIETNAMESE AND GAE
[i, u, e, ɛ, o, ɔ, ʌ, æ, ɐ, ɯ, ɤ] ([ɯ] is a high back vowel without lip rounding; [ɤ] is a mid-back vowel without lip rounding; [ɐ] is a low central vowel.)	■ [ɪ, ʊ, ɝ, ɚ] and diphthongs do not exist in Vietnamese.
	■ Vietnamese speaker may substitute similar vowels in GAE, e.g., *hit* → [hit]
VIETNAMESE CONSONANTS	**CONSONANT DIFFERENCES: VIETNAMESE AND GAE**
[p, ɓ, t, ɗ, k, g/ʔ] ([ɓ] is a bilabial implosive; [ɗ] is an alveolar implosive.)	■ Cheng (1994) notes the presence of [g] in Vietnamese; Thompson (1965) describes it as a glottal stop.
[f, s, z, x, ɣ] ([x] is a velar fricative.)	■ [v, ʃ, ʒ, ð, θ] do not exist in Vietnamese.
	■ [tʃ, dʒ] do not exist in Vietnamese.
[j, w, l]	■ r-sounds exist only in some dialects of Vietnamese.
[m, n, ŋ, ɲ] [ɲ] is a palatal nasal.	■ Final consonants are limited to [p, t, k, m, n, ŋ].
Vietnamese is a tone language.	■ No consonant blends in Vietnamese.

Source: Cheng (1994); Ruhlen (1976).

TABLE 6.9 Considerations When Collecting Data

Hearing Screening	
Does not pass screening ⟶	Referral
Examination of Speech Mechanism	
Not passing, deviancies ⟶	Additional testing, referral
Initial Impression	
Poor intelligibility ⟶	Need careful planning of further evaluation, especially spontaneous speech sample; see section on the unintelligible child
Articulation Test	
Few errors ⟶	Stimulability, contextual testing
Many errors ⟶	Attempt stimulability
Speech Sample	
Poor intelligibility ⟶	Choose topic, structure situation, gloss utterances
Language Screening	
Not within normal limits ⟶	Do more extensive language testing
Auditory Discrimination Testing	
Noted collapse of phoneme oppositions ⟶	Do auditory discrimination testing
Cognitive Appraisal	
Necessary ⟶	Referral, obtain records

between the sound inventory, phonemic values, and phonotactic constraints of the native language, on the one hand, and of General American English, on the other, will provide guidelines for accent reduction. A second possibility is that the client may evidence a phonological disorder in both the native language and General American English. To decide this, tests that assess the phonological systems of both languages should be used. For many of the languages, however, such standardized assessment tools will not be available or the clinician's knowledge of the foreign language will not be adequate enough to administer the test. In this case, other professionals with knowledge of the language and/or family members can be a valuable portion of the appraisal process.

SUMMARY OF THE DATA

Tables 6.9 and 6.10 can be useful in organizing your data for later analysis.

SUMMARY

First, this chapter summarized the various areas of data collection in the appraisal portion of the assessment process. These include (1) an articulation test, (2) spontaneous speech sampling, (3) evaluation of the oral mechanism, and (4) additional measures exemplified by a hearing screening, auditory perceptual testing, language screening, and cognitive appraisal. Methods and goals for each of these areas were discussed together with limitations that might be inherent in

TABLE 6.10 Checksheet for Data Collection

Hearing Screening	Pass _____ Not Passing _____
Examination of Speech Mechanism	Pass _____ Not Passing _____
	Noted deviancies _____
	_____

Initial Impression

Intelligibility

Good _____ Fair _____ Poor _____

Error productions noted

_____

Articulation Test

Error productions noted

_____

Stimulability testing

Sound _____

Sound level: Yes _____   No _____

Syllable level: Yes _____   No _____

Word level: Yes _____   No _____

Sound _____

Sound level: Yes _____   No _____

Syllable level: Yes _____   No _____

Word level: Yes _____   No _____

Sound _____

Sound level: Yes _____   No _____

Syllable level: Yes _____   No _____

Word level: Yes _____   No _____

Contextual Testing

Sound _____

Word contexts that elicit norm production

_____

Sound _____

Word contexts that elicit norm production

_____

Sound _____

Word contexts that elicit norm production

_____

(continued)

TABLE 6.10   Continued

Speech Sample	Intelligibility
	Good _____ Fair _____ Poor _____
	Error productions noted
	_____
Language Screening	Pass _____ Not passing _____
Auditory Discrimination Testing	Sound _____
	Does _____ Does not _____ discriminate
	Sound _____
	Does _____ Does not _____ discriminate
Information on Cognitive Appraisal	Necessary _____ Not necessary _____

the procedures. For example, an articulation test provides a relatively time-efficient way to evaluate articulation skills; however, it does not provide the clinician with any information about the client's abilities to use these skills in naturalistic contexts. In the second portion of this chapter, special assessment considerations were examined for the child with an emerging phonological system, the unintelligible speaker, the dialect speaker, and the speaker with English as a second language. Each of these groups of clients presents the clinician with challenges that will necessitate changes in the appraisal process and the evaluation of the results. This chapter is seen as a guide to assist the clinician in the selection of appraisal procedures that will maximize clinical decision making within the diagnostic process.

APPENDIX 6.1_____

FIGURE 6.4 Speech-Motor Assessment Screening Form

Each of the following parameters is assessed using the following system:

Pass   Within normal limits

Deviant   Deviant from norm, divided into "slight" or "marked" deviancy

Not passing   Clearly outside of normal limits

STRUCTURE

Head/Face				
Sitting opposite the client, evaluate head and facial structures according to the categories provided.	**Pass**	**Deviant** **Slight**	**Marked**	**Not Passing**
Size, shape of head				
Symmetry of facial features:				
Left half vs. right half				
Absence of drooping or spasticity				
Mandible/maxilla relationship				
Appearance of lips (contact at rest; vermilion)				
Appearance of nose (septum; nares)				
Appearance of philtrum/columella				
Absence of any striking features (e.g., adenoid facies, facial dimensions)				
Comments:				

Breathing				
Observe and evaluate the client's breathing behavior (as "structural" prerequisite for speaking and voice production) during normal (silent) breathing during speaking. During silent breathing the client's mouth should be closed and no clavicular movement should be noticeable.	**Pass**	**Deviant** **Slight**	**Marked**	**Not Passing**
Silent breathing				
Mouth closed (mouth open would indicate a deviancy)				
Relationship for the time of inspiration versus expiration is about 1:1				
Lack of clavicular breathing				

(continued)

FIGURE 6.4   Continued

Breathing	Pass	Deviant Slight	Deviant Marked	Not Passing
Breathing during speaking				
Breathing through nose (exclusive mouth breathing is a deviancy)				
Relationship for the time of inspiration versus expiration is 1:2+				
Lack of clavicular breathing				
Comments:				

Oral/Pharyngeal Cavity

The head should be bent back slightly for inspection of the palatal areas. A few reminders:

Missing frontal teeth might have a direct effect on sibilant production.
Dentition:
    Class I (normal) occlusion: lower molars (or canine for children without molars) half a tooth ahead of upper molars.
    Class II malocclusion (overbite): Maxilla protruded in relation to mandible, measured by the positions of the first (maxillary and mandibular) molars.
    Class III malocclusion (underbite): Mandibular molar more than half a tooth ahead of maxillary molar.
    Open bite: Gap between biting surfaces. Especially frontally open bites might influence articulation negatively.
    Cross bite: Misalignment of the teeth characterized by a crossing of the rows of teeth.
Macroglossia = tongue appears too large
Microglossia = tongue appears too small
Shrinkage, i.e., a "shriveled" tongue area, might indicate a paralytic condition.
The midline of the hard and soft palates appears normally pink and white; a blue tint suggests a submucous cleft.
Redness of fauces and pharynx might indicate inflammation.

	Pass	Deviant Slight	Deviant Marked	Not Passing
Dentition				
Front teeth present				
Spacing of teeth adequate				
Axial orientation of teeth is adequate				

Oral/Pharyngeal Cavity	Pass	Deviant Slight	Deviant Marked	Not Passing
Dentition				
Class I normal occlusion				
If a malocclusion is noted, indicate the type:				
Tongue				
Normal size in relationship to oral cavity				
Normal color				
No shrinkage				
Absence of fissures, lesions, fasciculations				
Normal resting position				
Palate (hard and soft)				
Normal color				
Normal width of vault				
Absence of fistulas, fissures				
Absence of clefts				
If cleft, circle one: Repaired Unrepaired				
Normal uvula				
If abnormal, circle one: Bifid Other deviations				
Normal length of uvula				
Appearances of fauces, pharynx				
Comments:				

FUNCTION

For older children and adults these tasks can be elicited by asking the client to complete the task. For younger children (preschool age and below) imitation may be required.

Head/Face	Pass	Deviant Slight	Deviant Marked	Not Passing
Eyes/facial appearance				
Raising of eyebrows is symmetrical				
Can smile, frown on command				
Smiling, frowning symmetrical				

(continued)

FIGURE 6.4   Continued

Head/Face	Pass	Deviant Slight	Marked	Not Passing
Lips				
Can protrude lips with mouth closed				
Can protrude lips with mouth slightly open				
Can protrude lips to left/right side				
Can protrude and spread lips ([u]–[i])				
Demonstrates rapid lip movements				
("pa-pa-pa")				
Mandible				
Can lower mandible on command				
Can move mandible to left/right side				
Comments:				

Oral/Pharyngeal Cavity	Pass	Deviant Slight	Marked	Not Passing
Tongue				
Can stick out tongue				
Can move tongue upwards (try to touch nose with tip of tongue)				
Can move tongue downwards (try to touch chin with tip of tongue)				
Can move the tip of the tongue from the left to the right corner of the mouth				
Can move the tongue quickly and smoothly from the right to the left corner of mouth				
Can move tongue smoothly around the vermilion of lips (lick around lips) clockwise and counterclockwise				
Can move the tongue from left to right on the outside/inside of the upper teeth				
Can move the tongue from left to right on the outside/inside of the lower teeth				

Oral/Pharyngeal Cavity	Pass	Deviant		Not Passing
		Slight	Marked	
Tongue				
Can say "pa-pa-pa" quickly, smoothly				
Can say "ta-ta-ta" quickly, smoothly				
Can say "ka-ka-ka" quickly, smoothly				
Can alternate between quick repetitions of "pa-ta" and "ta-pa"				
Can alternate between quick repetitions of "pa-ta-ka," "ka-ta-pa," and "ta-pa-ka"				
Velopharyngeal function				
During short, repeated "ah" phonation adequate velar movement is noted				
Can puff up cheeks				
Can maintain intraoral air (puffed cheeks) when slight pressure is applied to cheeks				
Absence of nasal emission				

Breathing	Pass	Deviant		Not Passing
		Slight	Marked	
Silent breathing				
During quick inspiration breath intake is through nose				
During quick inspiration breath intake is thoracic/abdominal				
Breathing during speaking				
Can sustain "ah" for 5 seconds				
Comments:				

DIAGNOSIS
PHONETIC VERSUS
PHONEMIC EMPHASIS

CHAPTER OUTLINE

- Preliminary Analysis: Inventory and Distribution of Speech Sounds
- Decision Making: Primarily Phonetic Emphasis

- Decision Making: Primarily Phonemic Emphasis
- Measures of Intelligibility and Severity
- Summary

In Chapter 6, different means of appraisal were outlined that would inform the clinician about the client's articulatory-phonological abilities in several areas. These means included both citation form and spontaneous speech sound performance as exemplified by the gathering of data from an articulation test and a spontaneous speech sample. Supplemental tests that would screen the adequacy of the oral mechanism, hearing, language, auditory perception, and cognitive abilities were also suggested. The next step in the assessment process is to *organize, analyze, and interpret the collected data.* The end product of this assessment portion not only provides the clinician with a solid foundation for diagnostic decisions but also leads directly to treatment goals.

One of the first diagnostic decisions facing a clinician concerns *how* to organize and analyze the available data. There are many possibilities, which all lead to somewhat different interpretations. It is important to choose the organization and analysis that best suit the individual client. Above all, the client's type and degree of speech sound difficulties will play a major role in this selection process.

The first goal of this chapter is to present some general organizational methods that can be used to give the clinician an overview of the speech sound problems noted on the articulation test and spontaneous speech sample. This organization is suitable for any of our clients, regardless of age or the type and degree of impairment. The chapter's second goal is to provide an analysis procedure that will aid the clinician in determining whether the client has primarily a phonetic disorder, an impairment of speech sound form, or a phonemic disorder, that is, deficiencies in phonemic function. This analysis will first take into account the preservation or collapse of phonemic contrasts in the client's speech. Although a clear division into phonetic versus phonemic disorder is not always possible (a client may demonstrate characteristics of both), the clinician needs to be aware of the important differences between the two. A tentative decision as to primarily phonetic versus phonemic impairment will guide the clinician in further analyses and intervention decisions. The third goal of this chapter is to present additional analysis procedures for children with a primarily phonetic versus a primarily phonemic disorder. For the client with a primarily phonetic disorder, suggestions will be offered for further testing and guidelines will be given on integrating diagnostic results into beginning therapy goals. For the client with a primarily phonemic disorder, a phonological assessment battery will be introduced. Organizational categories for this battery include (1) the inventory and distribution of sounds, (2) syllable shapes and constraints, (3) phonological contrasts, and (4) phonological rules or patterns. Analyzing the patterns or phonological rules of a particular client's speech can be achieved in a number of ways. Several contemporary methods for this analysis will be described.

It should be emphasized that the overall aim of this chapter is to provide information that will aid in clinical decision making. There are no prescribed answers. Based on all assessment data collected, each clinician will need to determine for each and every individual client which analysis procedures need to be completed for a valid diagnosis. This chapter is seen as an aid to making those decisions.

PRELIMINARY ANALYSIS: INVENTORY AND DISTRIBUTION OF SPEECH SOUNDS

One way to organize the results of the articulation test and spontaneous speech sample is to look at the inventory and distribution of speech sounds. The **inventory of speech sounds** is a list of speech sounds that the client can articulate within normal limits. However, for many clients, this is not a simple dichotomy between norm and aberrant productions. Some will show a regular production of a speech sound in one context but not in another. This is exemplified by a child who substitutes [t/s] within a word and at the end of a word but realizes the target sound correctly when the word begins with [s]. Such inconsistencies should be duly noted because they provide important clinical information. In addition, some clients realize a sound normally in contexts where it does not belong but consistently mispronounce it in contexts where it should be used. For example, an analysis revealed that a child had no accurate productions of [s] in all words which contained s-sounds. However, in the word *brush,* [ʃ] was replaced by an accurate [s]. This phenomenon has often been reported (Fey, 1992; Pollack and Rees, 1972; Smith, 1973) and frequently occurs in children with phonemic disorders (Fey, 1992). Examples like these demonstrate that norm articulation of the sound in question is within the client's capabilities; however, the client does not seem to understand the language-specific function and/or organization of speech sounds as phonemes. Such information aids considerably in determining which clients show evidence of a phonemic disorder.

The **distribution of speech sounds** refers to where the norm and aberrant articulations occurred within a word. Articulation tests often categorize according to three word positions: initial, medial, and final. As previously noted, *word-medial position* is an imprecise term. This lack of precision has bothered many practitioners who were interested in a closer look at the client's error patterns.

> Some of the problems inherent in using the term *medial* to refer to all sounds in between the first and last sounds of a word were discussed in the Syllable Structure section of Chapter 2.

In an attempt to introduce more structure and to reflect the hierarchical relationship of the syllable to the word, Grunwell (1987), for example, adopted a categorization that divides each multisyllabic word into its syllables. The sounds within the syllable are then further classified according to whether they initiate or terminate syllables. Although this system is clearly superior to the three-position one used by most articulation tests, dividing words into syllables poses its own problem: where to place the syllable boundaries. There is no clear-cut way to predict where a particular speaker will divide up the syllables of a word. For example, does one say "Ap-ril" or "A-pril"? Ask several people how *telephone* is divided: *te-le-phone* or *tel-e-phone*? The problem of where and how to syllabify words is not a new one. For decades, many scholars have wrestled with the problem (e.g., Jespersen, 1913; Ladefoged, 1993; Rosetti, 1959; Scripture, 1927; Sievers, 1901; Stetson, 1936, 1951). To date, it still cannot be said with any certainty exactly where syllables begin and end.

More recently, syllabication guidelines for General American English have been offered (e.g., French, 1988; Grunwell, 1987; Lowe, 1994). These guidelines are based on where the majority of a given set of normal speakers syllabified specific words. However, they are often based on subjective feelings of where syllables can and cannot be divided. Although most syllabication guidelines contain the warning that syllable divisions may vary from speaker to speaker, they do not solve the problematic aspects of the syllable and its division.

Therefore, the following analysis procedure is based not on where the syllable supposedly begins and ends but rather on where the consonants occur relative to the vowel nuclei. This procedure eliminates the neces-

sity of establishing syllable divisions and can be used on words from an articulation test or from a spontaneous speech sample. The consonants can be divided into three categories:

1. *Prevocalic consonants.* Consonants that occur before a vowel. These may be singletons (i.e., single consonants) or consonant clusters at the beginning of the word or utterance.
2. *Postvocalic consonants.* Consonants that occur after a vowel. These may be singletons or consonant clusters at the end of a word or utterance.
3. *Intervocalic consonants.* Consonants that occur between two vowels. These may be singletons or consonant clusters at the juncture of two syllables.

Using a Matrix to Examine the Inventory and Distribution of Speech Sounds

Figure 7.1 is a matrix that can be used to record the utterances from both articulation tests and spontaneous speech samples. The entire word is written in the left-hand column. Next, the word is divided into individual sound realizations. Using phonetic transcription, the intended production (Int.) and the actual realization (Prod.) should be recorded for each sound within the word: When applicable, prevocalic, syllable nucleus, and postvocalic sounds are recorded for one-syllable words, while multisyllable words would contain intervocalic sounds. Let's use the word *Christmas* [krɪsməs], for which the client says [kwɪməs], to demonstrate the process.

It seems plausible that children with phonological difficulties may syllabify words quite differently from what is normally the case. By imposing predetermined syllabication guidelines on words, which may or may not be accurate in a specific case, any subsequent analysis could be faulty and could lead to wrong conclusions.

Word: Christmas

Prevocalic		Nucleus		Inter-/Post-vocalic		Nucleus		Inter-/Post-vocalic	
Int.	Prod.	Int.	Prod.	Int.	Prod.	Int.	Prod.	Int.	Prod.
kr	kw	ɪ	ɪ	sm	øm	ə	ə	s	s

In this example, the symbol ø is used to indicate deletions. In addition, any type of

Word	Prevocalic		Nucleus		Inter-/postvoc.		Nucleus		Inter-/postvoc.		Nucleus		Inter-/postvoc.		Nucleus		Inter-/postvoc.	
	Int.	Prod.	Int.	Prod.	Int.	Prod.	Int.	Prod.	Int.	Prod.	Int.	Prod.	Int.	Prod.	Int.	Prod.	Int.	Prod.

FIGURE 7.1 Preliminary Matrix for Recording Utterances

aberrant productions could be circled by the clinician.

This information is then transferred to the matrix for summarizing phones according to pre-, inter-, and postvocalic word positions, found in Figure 7.2. For the purpose at hand, a check mark (✓) will be used to indicate a norm realization, a ø to record deletions, and the appropriate phonetic symbols with diacritics to document substitutions and distortions. Therefore, this matrix is used to record both the norm and the aberrant productions of the client. As can be noted in Figure 7.2, singleton consonant productions are recorded separately from clusters. Using the *Christmas* ex-

ample from above, [kw] would be recorded in the prevocalic matrix under clusters ([kr] → [kw]), [øm] would be recorded under intervocalic clusters ([sm] → [øm]), and a check mark would be placed in the [s] postvocalic box. If the clinician would like to consolidate the results even further, Figure 7.3 depicts a matrix that could be used to record pre-, inter-, and postvocalic realizations on a single form. Results from Figures 7.2 and 7.3 will give the clinician (1) the inventory of consonants, (2) the distribution of phones, and (3) the number of times each consonant occurred.

In order to demonstrate how each of these matrices could be clinically utilized,

FIGURE 7.2 Matrix for Recording Phones According to Pre-, Inter-, and Postvocalic Word Positions

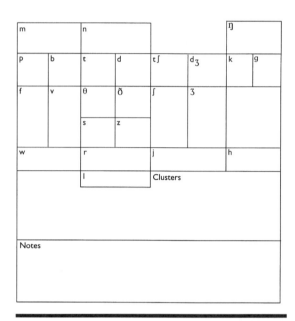

FIGURE 7.3 Matrix for Recording the Overall Inventory of Phones

Table 7.1 presents the results of the Goldman-Fristoe Test of Articulation (Goldman and Fristoe, 1986) for H. H., a 7;4-year-old child. The entire word has been transcribed for each of the utterances. Although spontaneous speech results should also be included in the assessment, for simplification, this introduction will only analyze the results of the articulation test. A spontaneous speech sample that could be analyzed according to these procedures is contained in Appendix 7.1. Figures 7.4, 7.5, and 7.6 (pages 172 and 174) are examples of how these matrices could be

used to record the responses for H. H. A more detailed analysis for H. H. is contained in Appendix 7.1.

Phonemic Contrasts: Differentiating Phonetic from Phonemic Disorders

Clients with phonemic disorders are characterized by impaired phonemic systems; they show difficulties using phonemes contrastively to differentiate meaning. Therefore, if two or more phonemes are represented by the same sound production, this indicates that the contrastive phonemic function has not been maintained. The emphasis in this phase of the analysis is on the contrastive use of sounds, not on their accurate production. Fey (1992) gives the example of a child who distinguishes between fricative and nonfricative sounds by substituting [ts] for all fricatives. Although this is clearly not the regular way of signalling these differences, it does indicate that the

TABLE 7.1 Single-Word Responses to Goldman-Fristoe Test of Articulation for Child H. H.

TARGET WORD	CHILD'S PRODUCTION	TARGET WORD	CHILD'S PRODUCTION
1. house	[haʊ]	22. carrot	[tɛwə]
2. telephone	[tɛfoʊ]	orange	[oʊwɪn]
3. cup	[tʌp]	23. bathtub	[bætʌ]
4. gun	[dʌn]	bath	[bæ]
5. knife	[naɪ]	24. thumb	[bʌm]
6. window	[wɪnoʊ]	finger	[bɪnə]
7. wagon	[wædən]	ring	[ɾɪn]
wheel	[wi]	25. jump	[dʌmp]
8. chicken	[tɪtə]	26. pajamas	[dæmi]
9. zipper	[tɪpə]	27. plane	[beɪn]
10. scissors	[tɪtə]	blue	[bu]
11. duck	[dʌt]	28. brush	[bʌs]
yellow	[jɛwoʊ]	29. drum	[dʌm]
12. vacuum	[ætu]	30. flag	[bæ]
13. matches	[mætət]	31. Santa Claus	[tænə dɑ]
14. lamp	[wæmp]	32. Christmas	[tɪtmə]
15. shovel	[dʌvə]	tree	[ti]
16. car	[tɑə]	33. squirrel	[twɜə]
17. rabbit	[wæbɪ]	34. sleeping	[twipɪn]
18. fishing	[bɪdɪn]	bed	[bɛd]
19. church	[tɜ]	35. stove	[doʊ]
20. feather	[bɛdə]		
21. pencils	[pɛntə]		
this	child would not say		

child uses some type of contrast to signal fricative versus nonfricative sounds. Such contrastive use proves that the client somehow differentiates between two groups of phonemes on the production level. On the other hand, the neutralization of contrasts, that is, when one phone is used to represent two or more phonemes, signals a clear lack of phonemic contrasts. Loss of phonemic contrast is the central problem of clients with phonemic, that is, phonological impairments.

Depending on the client, the neutralization of specific phonemic contrasts can be consistent or inconsistent. A consistent loss is indicated by a substitution occurring every time in the client's realizations. *Consistent loss* of a phonemic contrast can be exemplified by the child who, regardless of the position of the

sound in the word, realizes all [s] sounds as [t]. The child has neutralized the contrast between /s/ and /t/. Also, the child who always deletes the intended phoneme would demonstrate a consistent loss of phonemic contrast as well. *Inconsistent* realizations refer to substitutions or deletions that occur only in certain contexts. The sounds produced by a child who prevocalically realizes [t] for [s] but produces [s] accurately in specific words in postvocalic positions would be indicative of an inconsistent loss of the phonemic contrast. In addition, the sounds produced by a child substituting one sound for another in the pre- and intervocalic position but deleting the sound in the postvocalic position would demonstrate an inconsistent realization. The final decision on which speech sounds are indeed

Word	Prevocalic Int.	Prevocalic Prod.	Nucleus Int.	Nucleus Prod.	Inter-/postvoc. Int.	Inter-/postvoc. Prod.	Nucleus Int.	Nucleus Prod.	Inter-/postvoc. Int.	Inter-/postvoc. Prod.	Nucleus Int.	Nucleus Prod.	Inter-/postvoc. Int.	Inter-/postvoc. Prod.	Nucleus Int.	Nucleus Prod.	Inter-/postvoc. Int.	Inter-/postvoc. Prod.
house	h	h	aᵘ	aᵘ	s	∅												
telephone	t	t	ɛ	ɛ	l	∅	ə	∅	f	f	oᵘ	oᵘ	n	∅	unstressed syllable deletion - 2nd syllable			
cup	k	t	ʌ	ʌ	p	p												
gun	g	d	ʌ	ʌ	n	n												
knife	n	n	aɪ	aɪ	f	∅												
window	w	w	ɪ	ɪ	nd	n∅	oᵘ	oᵘ										
wagon	w	w	æ	æ	g	d	ə	ə	n	n								
wheel	w	w	i	i	l	∅												
chicken	tʃ	t	ɪ	ɪ	k	t	ə	ə	n	∅								
zipper	z	t	ɪ	ɪ	p	p	ɚ	ɚ										
scissors	s	t	ɪ	ɪ	z	t	ɚ	ɚ	z	∅								
duck	d	d	ʌ	ʌ	k	t												
yellow	j	j	ɛ	ɛ	l	w	oᵘ	oᵘ										
vacuum	v	∅	æ	æ	kj	t	u	u	m	∅								

FIGURE 7.4 Example of Preliminary Matrix for Recording Utterances for Child H. H.

employed as contrastive phonemes will often necessitate that the clinician check sound oppositions through minimal pairs, for example.

What to Do?

The analysis of phonemic contrasts can begin with the matrices presented in Figures 7.2 and 7.3. These provide an overview, which can be used to fill out Figure 7.7, the Neutralization of Phonemic Contrasts Summary Form (page 175).

1. Look for those sounds that are *consistently* used for another phoneme. For example, [k] was consistently realized as [t] in H. H.'s productions (see Figures 7.5 and 7.6). There were no instances (including consonant clusters) in which [t] was not substituted for /k/.

2. Look for those sounds that are *inconsistently* used, that is, occurring only in certain contexts. Inconsistencies are exemplified by (1) norm productions in some instances and the collapse of the phoneme contrast in others, (2) the production of two or more different sound realizations for one phoneme, or (3) the use of substitutions in certain contexts together with sound deletions in other contexts. For H. H., [f] shows an inconsistent loss of a phonemic contrast. In the prevocalic position, [f] → [b]; postvocalically, [f] is deleted; the intervocalic production was accurately articulated. Also, check to see if

---

CLINICAL APPLICATION

For H. H., the following neutralization of phonemic contrasts for singleton consonants was established:

1. Consistent neutralization of contrasts: [k] → [t]

   [dʒ], [ð] → [d]

2. Inconsistent contrast neutralization: [tʃ], [z], [s] → [t] (note: [tʃ], [z], and [s] are deleted in the postvocalic position)

   [ʃ] → [s] (note: occurs in postvocalic position)

   [g] → [d] (note: [g] is deleted in the postvocalic position

   [ʃ] → [d] (note: occurs in pre- and intervocalic positions)

   [f], [θ] → [b] (note: [f] is realized correctly one time in intervocalic position)

   [r] → [w] (note: [ɚ] is produced as [ə] in the postvocalic position)

   [l] → [w] (note: [l] is deleted in the postvocalic position)

3. Sound preferences: [d] is used to represent four other phonemes

   [t] is used to represent four other phonemes

---

any pattern can be noted pre-, inter- and/or postvocalically. From Figure 7.5, we see that H. H. does seem to demonstrate a pattern with [tʃ]: In pre- and intervocalic positions, [t] is realized; postvocalically, [tʃ] is deleted.

3. Summarize the collapse of contrasts. The purpose of this overview is to discover any substitutions that represent more than one target phoneme. Therefore, all target phonemes with the same substitution are grouped together. For H. H., [k], [s], [z], and [tʃ] are replaced by [t], for example. In addition, [d] replaced [g], [dʒ], [ð], and [ʃ]. These are summarized for H. H. on Figure 7.8.

4. Look for any *sound preferences*. This is exemplified by a sound or sound combination representing several different phonemes. Sound preferences should be checked to see if any patterns exist, for example, one phone utilized for a whole class of consonants. For H. H., [t] and [d] seem to represent sound preferences; both were employed as substitutions for

four different phonemes. The summary of H. H.'s phonemic contrasts is provided in Figure 7.8. Only consonant singletons were entered in this form, but it could also be used to look at consonant cluster productions.

Further testing may be warranted for sounds that show inconsistent contrasts. This could be easily achieved by having the client look at and name pictures or read minimal pair words.

DECISION MAKING: PRIMARILY PHONETIC EMPHASIS

It is important to analyze all existing data, possibly supplementing them with additional information, before arriving at the tentative decision that the client does show evidence of a phonetic disorder. In doing so, it must always be kept in mind that phonetic and phonemic disorders can co-occur. "It would be a mistake to adopt an either/or dichotomy" (Elbert, 1992, p. 242). The following section

Prevocalic

m ✓		n ✓						
p ✓	b ✓✓ ✓	t ✓	d ✓	tʃ [t][t]	dʒ [d] [d]	k [t][t] [t]	g [d] [t]	
f [b] [b] [b]	v ∅	θ [b]	ð	ʃ [d]	Clusters [fl]→[b] [pl]→[b] [kr]→[t] [bl]→[b] [skw]→[tw] [br]→[b] [sl]→[tw] [dr]→[d] [st]→[d]			
		s [t][t]	z [t]					
w ✓✓✓		r [w] [r]		j ✓		h ✓		
Notes:								

Intervocalic

m ✓		n ✓				ŋ		
p ✓✓	b ✓	t	d	tʃ [t]	dʒ	k [t]	g [d]	
f ✓	v ✓	θ	ð [d]	ʃ [d]	ʒ	Clusters [nd]→[n] [ng]→[n] [kj]→[t] [kl]→[d] [ns]→[nt] [sm]→[fm] [θt]→[t] [str]→[t]		
		s	z [t]					
w		r [w] [w]		j		h		
		l [w]						
Notes:								

Postvocalic

m ∅✓✓		n ∅✓✓ ∅✓				ŋ ✓		
p ✓	b ∅	t ∅∅	d ✓	tʃ ∅	dʒ	k [t]	g ∅	
f ∅	v ∅	θ ∅	ð	ʃ [s]	ʒ	Clusters [mp] ✓✓ [lz]→∅ [ndʒ]→[n]		
		s ∅	z ∅ [t] ∅					
Notes:		r		[ɚz]→[ə] scissors				
		l ∅∅∅						

FIGURE 7.5 Matrix for Recording Phones According to Pre-, Inter-, and Postvocalic Word Positions for Child H. H.

outlines the factors that will help the clinician in the process of decision making when considering a primarily phonetic emphasis.

Additional Testing and Decisions

Phonetic disorders are signalled by:

1. *Preservation of phonemic contrasts.* Substitutions of one phoneme for another suggest the collapse of phonemic contrasts. However, the client's realizations should be carefully examined to see whether any production variations might exist between the two speech

m 4✓ 1∅		n 5✓ 2∅						ŋ 1✓
p 4✓ 1∅	b 4✓ 1∅	t 1✓ 2∅	d 2✓	tʃ 3[t] 1∅	dʒ 2[d]	k 5[t]	g 2[d] 1∅	
f 1✓ 1∅ 3[b]	v 1✓ 2∅	θ 1∅ 1[b]	ð 1[d]	ʃ 2[d] 1[s]	3 not tested			
		s 2[t] 1∅	z 3[t] 2∅					
w 3✓		r 3 [w] 1 [r]		j 1✓		h 1✓		

*Prevocalic
1[pl]→[b]
1[bl]→[b]
1[br]→[b]
1[dr]→[d]
1[fl]→[b]
1[kr]→[t]

1 2[w]
3 ∅

1[skw]→[tw]
1[sl]→[tw]
1st→[d]

Clusters
*Intervocalic
1nd→[n]
1[kj]→[t]
1[ns]→[nt]
1[θt]→[t]
1[ng]→[n]
1[kl]→[d]

1[sm]→[tm]
1[str]→[t]
*Postvocalic
2[mp]✓
1[lz]→∅
1[ndʒ]→[n]

Notes *Vowel nucleus* 5 [ɚ]→[ə] 2 [ɝ]→[ɜ]

FIGURE 7.6 Overall Inventory of Phones for Child H. H.

sound realizations. Even minimal form differences, if used consistently, could indicate the preservation of phonemic contrasts. Omissions of sounds should also be carefully listened to in an attempt to determine if articulatory changes can be discovered between minimal pairs with and without the deleted sound. Several investigators have demonstrated that omitted sounds may be represented by some other articulatory gesture utilized to preserve the phonemic contrasts (Smit and Bernthal, 1983; Weismer, 1984; Weismer, Dinnsen, and Elbert, 1981). Noted changes included variations in vowel duration and a final gliding articulation of the vowel preceding the deleted sound.

What to Do?

Use pictures representing minimal pairs of the target sound and the substitution or omission. Have the client spontaneously produce each word. If a dis-

> Minimal pair words for the most frequently misarticulated sounds are contained in Chapter 8.

List all target sounds together with the substitution(s) used. By examining the Overall Inventory Matrix, determine whether the substitution is consistent (occurs every time) or inconsistent (occurs only in certain contexts). Circle the appropriate word.

Collapse of Contrasts
List all target sounds that have the **same** substitution.

Targets	Substitution

Sound Preferences
List any speech sounds which are used for a wide range of target phonemes.

FIGURE 7.7 Neutralization of Phonemic Contrasts Summary Form

tinguishable articulatory contrast is realized between the two sounds, utilize narrow transcription to document the variation. Different articulatory gestures might indicate that the client is differentiating between the two phonemes but not in a conventional manner.

2. Peripheral, motor-based problems. By definition, phonetic disorders are characterized by misarticulations, that is, aberrant speech sound form representing disruptions of the relatively peripheral articulatory process and involving inadequate motor learning (Fey, 1992). Speech sound errors within the framework of phonetic disorders are also relatively consistent, that is, inadequate motor learning of the particular sound is generalized throughout the system. Therefore, consistent inventory constraints are noted regardless of the position of the sound within the word (Elbert, 1992). In addition, phonetic disorders are not cognitive-linguistic (organizational) or perceptually based problems (Kamhi, 1992).

Organizational difficulties would be reflected in disturbed phonotactics, whereas clients with perceptually based problems may not be able to discriminate between the target sound and its inaccurate production.

List all target sounds together with the substitution(s) used. By examining the Overall Inventory Matrix, determine whether the substitution is consistent (occurs every time) or inconsistent (occurs only in certain contexts). Circle the appropriate word.

Target → Substitution		Target → Substitution	
[tʃ] → [t]	~~Consistent~~ **(Inconsistent)**	[ʃ] → [s]	~~Consistent~~ **(Inconsistent)**
[dʒ] → [d]	**(Consistent)** ~~Inconsistent~~	[r] → [w]	~~Consistent~~ **(Inconsistent)**
[k] → [t]	**(Consistent)** ~~Inconsistent~~	[l] → [w]	~~Consistent~~ **(Inconsistent)**
[g] → [d]	~~Consistent~~ **(Inconsistent)**		Consistent / Inconsistent
[f] → [b]	~~Consistent~~ **(Inconsistent)**		Consistent / Inconsistent
[θ] → [b]	~~Consistent~~ **(Inconsistent)**		Consistent / Inconsistent
[ð] → [d]	**(Consistent)** ~~Inconsistent~~		Consistent / Inconsistent
[s] → [t]	~~Consistent~~ **(Inconsistent)**		Consistent / Inconsistent
[z] → [t]	~~Consistent~~ **(Inconsistent)**		Consistent / Inconsistent
[ʃ] → [d]	~~Consistent~~ **(Inconsistent)**		Consistent / Inconsistent

Collapse of Contrasts
List all target sounds that have the **same** substitution.

Targets	Substitution
[tʃ], [k], [s], [z]	[t]
[dʒ], [g], [ð], [ʃ]	[d]
[f], [θ]	[b]
[ʃ]	[s]
[r], [l]	[w]

Consonant clusters were not listed
[tʃ], [g], [f], [θ], [l], [z]
demonstrate deletions in the postvocalic position

Note [f] is articulated accurately one time

Sound Preferences
List any speech sounds which are used for a wide range of target phonemes.

[d] and [t]

FIGURE 7.8 Neutralization of Phonemic Contrasts Summary Form: Application for Child H. H.

What to Do?

Examine the client's irregular productions relative to their occurrence pre-, inter-, or postvocalically. If the production remains consistent, occurring in every tested word and position, this would suggest a phonetic disorder. However, if positional constraints are discovered, the organization or phonotactics may not be intact, pointing to a phonemic disorder (Elbert, 1992).

Often, no pattern can be discovered, that is, the client produces the sound correctly in some words and incorrectly in others. In this case, two additional factors should be considered: (1) the phonetic context and (2) the possibility of an emerging sound. Due to the possible influence of coarticulation, specific phonetic contexts may enhance or hinder the production of the target sound. Words that contain accurate sound realizations should be examined to determine if a common phonetic context exists. Emerging sound patterns in the speech of children can also result in inconsistent realizations. Support for this possibility includes the appearance of the sound in productionally "easy" contexts (e.g., single syllables or familiar words) and its stimulability at the sound or word level. If the production is influenced by the phonetic context or the sound seems just to be emerging, this would suggest a phonetic disorder.

CLINICAL APPLICATION

Phonetic or Phonemic Difficulties

Tommy's parents requested an evaluation of his speech sound skills. They were concerned that he had some misarticulations that were not age-appropriate. The initial impression of Tommy, age 7;1, was that of an alert child who was fairly intelligible but seemed to have problems with [s], [z], [r], [θ], and [ð]. Tommy passed a hearing screening, an examination of the speech mechanism, and a language screening test. A spontaneous speech sample and an articulation test revealed the following:

1. Substitution of w/r ([r] → [w]) in all word positions. The r-coloring of central vowels was also not realized. Results were consistent in single-word tasks and spontaneous speech.
2. Substitution of θ/s and ð/z ([s, z] → [θ, ð]) in all word positions with the exception of [st] blends at the beginnings or ends of words. In these blends, [s] was accurate. Such an accurate production of [s] in blends was noted only in one-word samples, not in conversational speech.
3. Substitution of t/θ and d/ð ([θ, ð] → [t, d]) in all word positions; consistent in one-word samples and spontaneous speech.

Initial analysis. Tommy did not seem to fit the typical picture of a child with a phonemic disorder. Due to the age of the child, the clinician was not too concerned about the th-problems. However, she was concerned that Tommy's errors constituted a collapse of phonemic contrasts. Further testing was warranted.

Preservation of phonemic contrasts. Minimal pairs were used to test Tommy's productions of [w] versus [r]. The clinician noticed subtle differences in attempted [r]-productions when contrasted to his realization of [w]. For example, there was not too as much lip rounding when he tried to say a word beginning with [r] when compared to his [w] realization. Tommy was not stimulable for [r] at the sound level. When Tommy was asked to produce minimal pairs with [s] and [θ], his [s] sounded like a [θ] in certain contexts and like a dentalized [s] ([s̪]) in others. He was stimulable for [s], [z], [θ], and [ð] at the sound and word levels.

Peripheral motor-based difficulties. Errors were consistent across word positions. The accurate production of [s] in [st] blends was thought to be the effect of coarticulation. Discrimination of minimal pairs with [s] versus [θ] and [z] versus [ð] demonstrated an accuracy of over 90 percent. Discrimination of [w] versus [r] was 70 percent accurate.

Clinical decision making. The clinician decided that Tommy showed more evidence of a motor-based phonetic disorder than of a phonemic disorder. Further testing did not indicate perceptual or cognitive-linguistic-based difficulties. In certain contexts, Tommy distinguished productionally and perceptually between the target sounds and his substitutions.

Guidelines for Beginning Therapy

The gathering of data is completed and diagnostic decisions have been made. Any diagnosis should also lead directly into the selection of intervention goals and strategies. Although goals and strategies will constantly change, depending on the client and the noted difficulties, specific diagnostic information should aid in deciding where to begin with therapy.

Stimulability. Although stimulability is not an absolute predictor of which error sounds will improve in therapy and at which level therapy should begin (sound, syllable, word level), stimulability can be used as a probe to find out which sounds might be somewhat easier for the client to realize. If a client is stimulable for a particular sound, the clinician could attempt this sound in therapy for a trial period.

Correct Production of the Sound in a Specific Context. The collected data often give evidence of a typically misarticulated sound produced accurately within a specific word context. Such a word might appear on an articulation test or in the spontaneous speech sample. It was also suggested that articulation test results be supplemented with additional word lists. These probes could yield such a context as well. Norm productions of a word or words containing a usually misarticulated sound verify that under certain contextual conditions, the client is able to realize its regular articulation. These words, therefore, offer themselves as a therapeutic point of departure.

Sounds Affecting Intelligibility. Certain sounds affect intelligibility more than others. One main reason is their relatively high frequency of occurrence in conversational contexts. A chart displaying the frequency of occurrence of General American English consonants is provided in Appendix 7.2. Other sounds may affect intelligibility due to their conspicuous aberrant articulation. Therapeutically, high priority should be given to sounds that affect the intelligibility of the client the most.

Developmentally Earlier Sounds. Under comparable clinical circumstances, sounds that are acquired developmentally earlier should be considered first targets. The term *comparable clinical circumstances* means that both sounds were stimulable to the same degree and that the sounds in question seemed to have a comparable impact on the client's intelligibility.

CLINICAL APPLICATION

Decision Making: Where to Begin Therapy

The previous Clinical Application with Tommy can be used as an example to illustrate these guidelines for making decisions concerning where to begin therapy. See the table on page 179.

Given these variables, it would appear that in this case, [s] and [z] are good choices for initiating a trial probe in therapy. They were stimulable, appeared correctly in certain word contexts, and have a high frequency of occurrence in General American English. Therefore, they will have a definite impact on Tommy's speech intelligibility. In addition, [s] and [z] are typically developmentally earlier than [θ] and [ð]. However, due to the high frequency of occurrence of [r] in General American English and relative early mastery in the acquisition process, [r] should probably be targeted before [θ] and [ð].

Sound	Stimulable	Correct Word Context	Intelligibility	Development
[r]	no	no	high frequency	earlier than [s], [z], [θ], [ð]
[s], [z]	yes, sound/word	yes, st-blends	high frequency	relatively late
[θ], [ð]	yes, sound/word	no	[ð] high, [θ] low	later sound

DECISION MAKING: PRIMARILY PHONEMIC EMPHASIS

If a phonemic impairment is suspected, a thorough *phonological assessment* becomes necessary. Data for a phonological assessment can be organized in a number of ways. The following organizational scheme is one that has been described either partially or totally by several authors (e.g., Elbert and Gierut, 1986; Fey, 1992; Grunwell, 1987; Howell and Dean, 1994; Ingram, 1989b; Lowe, 1994). This organization will help the clinician in answering important assessment questions and in the planning of therapy goals. The categories found in this organizational scheme are:

1. inventory of speech sounds
2. distribution of speech sounds
3. syllable shapes and constraints
4. phonological contrasts
5. phonological error patterns

Inventory and Distribution of Speech Sounds

The inventory and distribution of speech sounds are discussed earlier in this chapter. Figures 7.1, 7.2, and 7.3 are provided to aid in organizing and analyzing these parameters.

Syllable Shapes and Constraints

The term **syllable shape** refers to the structure of the syllables within a word. Therefore, the unit of analysis is the word; that is, each word is described according to occurring vowels, designated as *V*, and consonants, *C*, within that word. Syllable shapes vary, with the productionally easiest ones being open syllables such as *eye* or *go*. Syllable shapes in General American English can be very complex, containing up to three consonants prevocalically and four postvocalically. Syllable shapes are important because clients with phonological disorders may delete syllables, use predominantly open syllables, or demonstrate specific consonant preferences in the production of syllables (Crystal, 1981; Hodson and Paden, 1991; Pollock and Schwartz, 1988).

A **syllable constraint** refers to any restriction or limitation established in the production of syllable shapes. Children acquiring speech in a normal manner use many different syllable shapes at an early age. When Stoel-Gammon (1987) analyzed the speech of thirty-two 2-year-olds, she found that thirty-one of the thirty-two children produced two different types of closed syllables while over

> More information can be found in the Syllable Structure section of Chapter 2.

half of them demonstrated CVCVC structures and word-initial clusters. Approximately half of the 2-year-olds in this investigation were also realizing word-final clusters. Therefore, even children with an emerging phonological system should demonstrate both open and closed syllable structures.

The information about syllable shapes and any possible constraints can be obtained from the articulation test and the spontaneous speech sample. Both the type and frequency of occurrence of the syllable shapes of each word should be noted. Worthwhile information is also gained by determining whether discrepancies exist between the responses on the articulation test and the conversational speech sample. Specific syllable constraints in the speech sample could in part explain a decrease in the client's intelligibility.

Table 7.2 provides the most frequent one-syllable word shapes reported by French, Carter, and Koenig (1930) in one-syllable words. Several two-syllable shapes are included; more could be added. According to Shriberg and Kent (1995), approximately 77 percent of the words spoken by adult speakers of General American English are one-syllable words and both one- and two-syllable words comprise almost 94 percent of those spoken. The main goal of our analysis is to determine whether the client has basic syllable structures and, if so, which ones. Simple open and closed syllable shapes of one- and two-syllable words should be a portion of the client's repertoire.

What to Do?

1. Analyze the client's sample to determine if one-, two-, and when appropriate, three- or more syllable words exist. Note if there is a large proportion of any single syllable type. For example, it is remarkable if the client uses primarily one-syllable words.

2. Analyze any reductions in the syllable number or syllable shapes. Reductions in the number of syllables include multisyllable words in which syllable deletions occur. For example, *telephone*, a three-syllable word, might be reduced to [tɛfoʊn]. Changes in the syllable shape are exemplified by words in which deletion of consonants has altered the original syllable shape. For example *house*, a CVC shape, might become [haʊ] a CV shape.

TABLE 7.2 Common One- and Two-Syllable Shapes

SHAPE	EXAMPLES
V	a, I
CV	go, he
CCV	grow, tree
VC	up, on
VCC	ask, oops
CVC	hop, doll
CCVC	trees, brush
CVCC	hopped, lamp
CCVCC	stopped, drink
Two-Syllable	
CVCVC	wagon, shovel
CVCCV	window, candy
CVCCVC	bathtub, jumping

CLINICAL APPLICATION

Syllable Shapes with H. H.

Analyzing the data from the Goldman-Fristoe test for H. H. demonstrated:

1. the presence of one- and two-syllable words
2. three-syllable words (*telephone, pajamas*) were reduced to two syllables—however, H. H. could produce three syllables (see Santa Claus and Christmas tree)
3. syllable shapes of one-syllable CVC words were frequently reduced to a CV structure, although in the majority of cases, the CVC structure was maintained
4. the majority of two-syllable words were reduced in shape by final consonant deletion

Based on this sample, H. H. can produce one- and two-syllable words; however, the syllable shapes were often reduced, that is, produced as open syllables in two-syllable words.

Phonological Contrasts

The organization and analysis of data for determining phonological contrasts are dealt with earlier in this chapter. See the Phonemic Contrasts: Differentiating Phonetic from Phonemic Disorders section and Figure 7.7.

Phonological Error Patterns

Phonological assessment attempts to evaluate the phonological system of each client as accurately as possible. An accurate assessment leads to both an effective diagnosis and successful subsequent therapy. Although the client's productions must be compared to the adult model, it should also be kept in mind that the client's realizations represent a system in themselves. A **system** refers to an orderly combination of parts forming a complex unity. A central goal of any phonological assessment is to understand the client's phonological system. Identifying and categorizing the error patterns are an important aspect of this understanding. Knowledge of existing patterns within the system will lead directly to important therapeutic decisions. On the other hand, a lack of this knowledge can easily result in misinterpreting patterns as inconsistencies in the client's phonological system. The totality of sound realizations of each client exemplifies a system; it is the clinician's task to discover and evaluate the system accurately.

There are a number of methods available for analyzing error patterns. While some techniques are more productionally based—analyzing the speech sound form—others attempt to analyze the client's phonemic system. Recalling that phonetic and phonemic disorders can, and often do, occur together, the following form- and function-based frameworks are offered: (1) place-manner-voice, (2) distinctive feature, (3) phonological process, and (4) assessing phonological knowledge as an application of generative phonology.

Place-Manner-Voice Analysis. The place-manner-voice analysis is a productionally based system; it depicts speech sound form. As its name implies, this analysis describes error patterns according to a rather broad phonetic feature classification system. Place, manner, and voicing characteristics of each error sound are compared to those representing the norm production features. This comparison can then be examined to determine if any patterns emerge within the sound system of the client. In this context, patterns are defined as the frequent use of specific place, manner, and voicing features. The place-manner-voice analysis is designed only to classify substitutions of one sound for another. Distortions and deletions are not accounted for by this system.

The following place-manner-voice categorization system is taken from Howell and Dean (1994):

Place of Articulation

Labial	[p], [b], [f], [v], [m], and [w]
Dental	[θ] and [ð]
Alveolar	[t], [d], [s], [z], [n], and [l]
Postalveolar	[ʃ], [ʒ], [tʃ], and [dʒ]
Palatal	[j], [r]
Velar	[k], [g], and [ŋ]
Glottal	[h]

Manner of Articulation

Stop-plosives	[p], [b], [t], [d], [k], and [g]
Fricatives	[f], [v], [θ], [ð], [s], [z], [ʃ], [ʒ], and [h]
Affricates	[tʃ] and [dʒ]

Nasals   [m], [n], and [ŋ]
Liquids   [l] and [r]
Glides   [w] and [j]

Voicing
Voiced   [b], [d], [g], [v], [ð], [z], [ʒ],
                [ʤ], [m], [n], [ŋ], [l], [r],
                [w], and [j]
Voiceless   [p], [t], [k], [f], [θ], [s], [ʃ],
                [tʃ], and [h]

Figure 7.9 provides a graph of the consonants of General American English according to this system, while Figure 7.10 presents a Place-Manner-Voicing Summary Sheet.

What to Do?

Transfer the information from the Overall Inventory of Phones Matrix (Figure 7.3) to the Place-Manner-Voicing Summary Sheet (Figure 7.10) in the following way:

1. Target sound and its substitution are written in the left-hand column.

2. Compare the substitution to the target sound noting any place, manner, and/or voicing features that were affected. The appropriate change in feature(s) should be circled. Some substitutions will be only one-feature changes; others could be changes in place, manner, *and* voicing characteristics.

3. List the specific place, manner, and/or voicing change that occurred in the column marked Specific Changes. For example, if a child substituted a [t] for [k] ([k] → [t]) "place" would be circled, and "velar → alveolar" recorded in the blank after the place feature.

4. List the number of times this particular feature change occurred. This should be marked down in the Number of Errors column.

5. List each single-sound substitution according to the prescribed directions. After all substitutions and feature changes have been listed, look for patterns of errors by using the summary at the bottom of the sheet.

Figure 7.11 is the Place-Manner-Voicing Summary Sheet filled out for H. H.

	Labial		Dental		Alveolar		Post-alveolar		Palatal		Velar		Glottal	
Stops	p	b			t	d					k	g		
Nasals		m				n						ŋ		
Fricatives	f	v	θ	ð	s	z	ʃ	ʒ					h	
Affricates							tʃ	ʤ						
Liquids						l				r				
Glides		w								j				

Shaded areas are voiced sounds.

FIGURE 7.9 Place-Manner-Voice Features of General American English Consonants

Target	→	Substitution	Circle Differences	Specific Changes	No. of Errors
————	→	————	Place Manner Voicing	———————— ———————— ————————	———— ———— ————
————	→	————	Place Manner Voicing	———————— ———————— ————————	———— ———— ————
————	→	————	Place Manner Voicing	———————— ———————— ————————	———— ———— ————
————	→	————	Place Manner Voicing	———————— ———————— ————————	———— ———— ————
————	→	————	Place Manner Voicing	———————— ———————— ————————	———— ———— ————

Summary

PLACE		MANNER		VOICING	
Change	No. of Occ.	Change	No. of Occ.	Change	No. of Occ.
————	——	————	——	————	——
————	——	————	——	————	——
————	——	————	——	————	——
————	——	————	——	————	——
————	——	————	——	————	——
————	——	————	——	————	——

Distortions ————————————————————————

Deletions ————————————————————————

FIGURE 7.10 Place-Manner-Voicing Summary Sheet   *(continued)*

FIGURE 7.10   Continued

Place-Manner-Voicing Summary Sheet (continued)

Target	→	Substitution	Circle Differences	Specific Changes	No. of Errors
————	→	————	Place Manner Voicing		
————	→	————	Place Manner Voicing		
————	→	————	Place Manner Voicing		
————	→	————	Place Manner Voicing		
————	→	————	Place Manner Voicing		
————	→	————	Place Manner Voicing		
————	→	————	Place Manner Voicing		
————	→	————	Place Manner Voicing		
————	→	————	Place Manner Voicing		

Place-Manner-Voicing Summary Sheet

Target	→	Substitution	Circle Differences	Specific Changes	No. of Errors
[t∫]	→	[t]	(Place) (Manner) Voicing	postalveolar → alveolar _3_ affricate → stop _3_	
[dʒ]	→	[d]	(Place) (Manner) Voicing	postalveolar → alveolar _2_ affricate → stop _2_	
[k]	→	[t]	(Place) Manner Voicing	velar → alveolar _5_	
[g]	→	[d]	(Place) Manner Voicing	velar → alveolar _2_	
[f]	→	[b]	Place (Manner) (Voicing)	fricative → stop _3_ voiceless → voiced _3_	

Summary

PLACE		MANNER		VOICING	
Change	No. of Occ.	Change	No. of Occ.	Change	No. of Occ.
postalveolar → alveolar	8	affricate → stop	5	voiceless → voiced	6
velar → alveolar	7	fricative → stop	12	voiced → voiceless	3
dental → labial	1	liquid → glide	5		
dental → alveolar	1				
palatal → labial	3				
alveolar → labial	2				

Distortions [r]

Deletions [m], [n], [b], [t], [t∫], [g], [f], [v], [θ], [s], [z], [l]

FIGURE 7.11 Place-Manner-Voicing Summary Sheet for Child H. H.　　　　(continued)

CLINICAL APPLICATION

Place-Manner-Voicing Analysis for H. H.

Using the summary sheet, H. H.'s place, manner, and voicing substitutions could be summarized as follows:

Place: High occurrence of alveolars being substituted for postalveolar and velar phones (postalveolar and velar → alveolar).

Manner: High occurrence of stops being substituted for fricatives (fricatives → stops).

Voicing: Errors of both voiced → voiceless and voiceless → voiced consonants.

In summary, place-manner-voice analyses are productionally based. They provide the clinician with information about specific

FIGURE 7.11   Continued

Place-Manner-Voicing Summary Sheet (continued)

Target	→	Substitution	Circle Differences	Specific Changes	No. of Errors
[θ]	→	[b]	(Place) (Manner) (Voicing)	dental → labial / fricative → stop / voiceless → voiced	1 / 1 / 1
[ð]	→	[d]	(Place) (Manner) Voicing	dental → alveolar / fricative → stop	1 / 1
[ʃ]	→	[d]	(Place) (Manner) (Voicing)	postalveolar → alveolar / fricative → stop / voiceless → voiced	2 / 2 / 2
[ʃ]	→	[s]	(Place) Manner Voicing	postalveolar → alveolar	1
[s]	→	[t]	Place (Manner) Voicing	fricative → stop	2
[z]	→	[t]	Place (Manner) (Voicing)	fricative → stop / voiced → voiceless	3 / 3
[r]	→	[w]	(Place) (Manner) Voicing	palatal → labial / liquid → glide	3 / 3
[l]	→	[w]	(Place) (Manner) Voicing	alveolar → labial / liquid → glide	2 / 2
___	→	___	Place Manner Voicing		

changes in place, manner, and voicing that occur in the speech of the client when compared to norm realizations. Although the system evaluates actual phonetic features of speech sounds, it is rather broad-based. Some important features, such as organ of articulation, and secondary features, such as lip rounding of [ʃ], are not accounted for. Only substitutions of one sound for another can be classified according to place-manner-voice parameters. Sound deletions, distortions, assimilations, and syllable structure changes are not assessed.

Distinctive Feature Analysis.   A distinctive feature analysis compares the phonetic features of the target sound with the phonetic features of its substitution. Because the distinctive feature system is binary, (+) and (−), similarities and differences between target and substitution can be clearly ascertained. One of the advantages of this analysis is that it allows for a comparison of several sound substitutions to the target phoneme. For example, if a client substitutes [t], [d], [z], and [ʃ] for the /s/ ([s] → [t], [d], [z], and [ʃ]), similarities and differences between all sound features can be compared. In addition, correctly and incorrectly realized features across several phonemes can be examined to see if patterns exist. A pattern is characterized by frequent use of one or more identical distinctive features when the target sound and the sound substitution are compared.

Although many different distinctive feature systems exist, most clinical applications use a version of the Chomsky and Halle (1968) distinctive feature system (Elbert and Gierut, 1986; Gierut, 1992; Grunwell, 1987; Lowe, 1994; McReynolds and Engmann, 1975). These distinctive features can be found in Chapter 4, Tables 4.2 and 4.3. Any other distinctive feature system could be substituted; the principles of analysis would remain the same.

What to Do?

To describe patterns of errors, the target phoneme and its substitution(s) must be analyzed to determine the distinctive features of each. Figure 7.12 depicts an example of a worksheet that can be used to identify them. Data recorded on the Matrix for Recording Overall Inventory of Phones (Figure 7.3) can easily be transferred to this worksheet.

1. List the target phoneme and the substitution at the top of one of the boxes. If there are several substitutions for one target phoneme, each substitution should be listed in a separate box.

2. List the features that differ between the target sound and the substitution in the blank spaces under Feature Differences.

Record their (+) or (–) values. These features are taken from the distinctive feature table you are using.

3. Transfer the information from the completed worksheet to the Summary Sheet for Distinctive Feature Analysis (Table 7.3). Table 7.3 provides the number of phonemes affected by specific distinctive feature changes.

A distinctive feature worksheet and summary form are completed for H. H. in Figure 7.13 and Table 7.4.

CLINICAL APPLICATION

Distinctive Feature Analysis with H. H.

For child H. H., four distinctive features impact six different phonemes:

1. – anterior is changed to + anterior
2. + high is changed to – high
3. + continuant is changed to – continuant
4. + strident is changed to – strident

In summary, distinctive feature systems attempt to capture those phonetic features that distinguish between phonemes of a language. Although these distinctive features are primarily productionally based, they represent an important aspect of a phonemic analysis. Error patterns can clearly be seen when frequently occurring distinctive features are summarized. Distinctive feature analyses cannot account for deletions, assimilations, or changes of the syllable structure.

Phonological Process Analysis. A phonological process analysis is a means of identifying substitutions, syllable structure, and assimilatory changes that occur in the speech of clients. Each error is identified and classified as one or more of the phonological processes.

Distinctive Feature Analysis Form

List all target sounds together with the substitution(s). Use the Chomsky-Halle distinctive feature system to determine which features differ between the target sound and the substitution. List these differences with their "+" and "−" values in the space under the sounds.

FIGURE 7.12 Worksheet for Distinctive Feature Analysis

Distinctive Feature Analysis Form

List all target sounds together with the substitution(s). Use the Chomsky-Halle distinctive feature system to determine which features differ between the target sound and the substitution. List these differences with their "+" and "−" values in the space under the sounds.

Row 1

Target → Substitution	
tʃ → t	
Feature Differences	
−anterior	+anterior
+high	− high
+del.rel.	−del.rel.
+strident	−strident

Target → Substitution	
dʒ → d	
Feature Differences	
−anterior	+anterior
+high	− high
+del.rel.	−del.rel.
+strident	−strident

Target → Substitution	
k → t	
Feature Differences	
−coronal	+coronal
−anterior	+anterior
+high	− high
+back	− back

Target → Substitution	
g → d	
Feature Differences	
−coronal	+coronal
−anterior	+anterior
+high	−high
+back	−back

Target → Substitution	
f → b	
Feature Differences	
+cont.	−cont.
−voice	+voice
+strident	−strident

Row 2

Target → Substitution	
θ → b	
Feature Differences	
+coronal	−coronal
+cont.	−cont.
−voice	+voice

Target → Substitution	
ð → d	
Feature Differences	
+cont.	−cont.

Target → Substitution	
ʃ → d	
Feature Differences	
−anterior	+anterior
+high	−high
+cont.	−cont.
−voice	+voice
+strident	−strident

Target → Substitution	
ʃ → s	
Feature Differences	
−anterior	+anterior
+high	−high

Target → Substitution	
s → t	
Feature Differences	
+cont.	−cont.
+strident	−strident

Row 3

Target → Substitution	
z → t	
Feature Differences	
+cont.	−cont.
+voice	−voice
+strident	−strident

Target → Substitution	
r → w	
Feature Differences	
+conson.	−conson.
+vocalic	−vocalic
+coronal	−coronal
−high	+high
−back	+back
−round	+round

Target → Substitution	
l → w	
Feature Differences	
+conson.	−conson.
+vocalic	−vocalic
+coronal	−coronal
+anterior	−anterior
+lateral	−lateral
−high	+high
−back	+back
−round	+round

Target → Substitution	
— → —	
Feature Differences	

Target → Substitution	
— → —	
Feature Differences	

FIGURE 7.13 Distinctive Feature Worksheet for Child H. H.

TABLE 7.3 Summary Sheet for Distinctive Feature Analysis Using the Chomsky-Halle Distinctive Feature System

FEATURE	FEATURE CHANGE	NO. OF PHONEMES AFFECTED	FEATURE CHANGE	NO. OF PHONEMES AFFECTED
Sonorant	+ to –	_____	– to +	_____
Consonantal	+ to –	_____	– to +	_____
Vocalic	+ to –	_____	– to +	_____
Coronal	+ to –	_____	– to +	_____
Anterior	+ to –	_____	– to +	_____
Nasal	+ to –	_____	– to +	_____
Lateral	+ to –	_____	– to +	_____
High	+ to –	_____	– to +	_____
Low	+ to –	_____	– to +	_____
Back	+ to –	_____	– to +	_____
Round	+ to –	_____	– to +	_____
Continuant	+ to –	_____	– to +	_____
Delayed Release	+ to –	_____	– to +	_____
Voiced	+ to –	_____	– to +	_____
Strident	+ to –	_____	– to +	_____
Summary:				

Patterns of error are described according to the most frequent phonological processes present and/or to those that affect a class of sounds or sound sequences. The processes utilized to identify substitutions are again primarily productionally based; however, they do account for sound and syllable deletions as well as several assimilation processes.

As with all analysis systems, various authors and their protocols delineate somewhat different processes (Bankson and Bernthal, 1990; Dean, Howell, Hill, and Waters, 1990; Hodson, 1986; Ingram, 1981; Khan and Lewis, 1986; Shriberg and Kwiatkowski,

1980). Certain processes seem to occur more frequently in the speech of children developing their phonological systems in a normal manner. Others, labelled idiosyncratic processes, occur infrequently in the normal population (Stoel-Gammon and Dunn, 1985). On most protocols, substitution processes are limited to consonants, but vowel processes have been identified as well (Pollock and Keiser, 1990; Reynolds, 1990; Stoel-Gammon and Herrington, 1990). The most frequently cited phonological processes are reviewed in Chapter 4. See the Natural Phonology section.

TABLE 7.4 Summary Sheet for Distinctive Feature Analysis: Application H. H.

FEATURE	FEATURE CHANGE	NO. OF PHONEMES AFFECTED	FEATURE CHANGE	NO. OF PHONEMES AFFECTED
Sonorant	+ to –		– to +	
Consonantal	+ to –	2	– to +	0
Vocalic	+ to –	2	– to +	0
Coronal	+ to –	3	– to +	2
Anterior	+ to –	1	– to +	6
Nasal	+ to –		– to +	
Lateral	+ to –	1	– to +	0
High	+ to –	6	– to +	2
Low	+ to –		– to +	
Back	+ to –	2	– to +	2
Round	+ to –	0	– to +	2
Continuant	+ to –	6	– to +	0
Delayed Release	+ to –	2	– to +	0
Voiced	+ to –	1	– to +	3
Strident	+ to –	6	– to +	0

Summary:

–ant. to +ant: ʧ → t, ʤ → d, k → t, g → d, ʃ → d, ʃ → s

+high to –high: ʧ → t, ʤ → d, g → d, k → t, ʃ → d, ʃ → s

+cont to –cont: f → b, θ → b, ð → d, ʃ → d, s → t, z → t

+strident to –strident: ʧ → t, ʤ → d, f → b, ʃ → d, s → t, z → t

---

CLINICAL APPLICATION

Phonological Processes Used to Identify Vowel Errors

Several common and idiosyncratic substitution processes that describe changes in consonant productions have been identified. However, children with phonological disorders may also evidence impaired vowel systems. The following processes have been used to describe vowel substitutions in children (Bauman-Waengler, 1991; Pollock and Keiser, 1990):

1. *Vowel backing:* A front vowel is replaced by a back vowel of a similar tongue height. Example: [ɪ] → [ʊ].

2. *Vowel fronting:* A back vowel is replaced by a front vowel of a similar tongue height. Example: [u] → [i].

3. *Centralization:* A front or back vowel is replaced by a central vowel. Example: [ɛ] → [ʌ].

4. *Decentralization:* A central vowel is replaced by a front or back vowel. Example: [ʌ] → [ʊ].

5. *Vowel raising:* A front vowel is replaced by a front vowel with a higher tongue position, or a back vowel is replaced by a back vowel with a higher tongue position. Example: [æ] → [ɛ].

6. *Vowel lowering:* A front vowel is replaced by a front vowel with a lower tongue position, or a back vowel is replaced by a back vowel with a lower tongue position. Example: [u] → [ʊ].

7. *Diphthongization:* A monophthong is realized as a diphthong. Example: [ɛ] → [ɛⁱ]

8. *Monophthongization (or diphthong reduction):* A diphthong is realized as a monophthong. Example: [aɪ] → [a].
9. *Complete vowel harmony:* A vowel change within a word that results in both vowels being produced the same. Example: [tɛdi] → [tɛdɛ]
10. *Tenseness harmony:* A lax vowel becomes tense when there is another tense vowel in the same word. Example: [mɛni] → [meni]
11. *Height vowel harmony:* A vowel is replaced with a vowel that is closer in tongue height to another vowel in the same word. Example: [bæskɪt] → [bɛskɪt]

There are several assessment protocols that analyze phonological processes in articulation tests or in spontaneous speech (Bankson and Bernthal, 1990; Dean, Howell, Hill, and Waters, 1990; Grunwell, 1985a; Hodson, 1986; Ingram, 1981; Khan and Lewis, 1986; Lowe, 1996; Shriberg and Kwiatkowski, 1980). All of them identify each aberrant production according to the phonological process or processes that best represent the changes that have occurred. Most protocols also summarize the phonological processes by counting the total number of specific processes. Table 7.5 represents a protocol for summarizing the established phonological processes from the articulation test and the spontaneous speech sample.

What to Do?

1. Go through the matrix for recording phones according to pre-, inter-, and postvocalic word positions (Figure 7.2) and the matrix for recording the overall inventory of phones (Figure 7.3). Identify the phonological process that best describes the change. More than one phonological process might apply to a given misarticulation. For example, if a child substitutes [d] for [s] ([s] → [d]), this needs to be identified as stopping and voicing.

TABLE 7.5 Phonological Process Analysis Summary Sheet

PROCESSES	NUMBER OF OCCURRENCES
Syllable Structure Changes	
Cluster reduction	_____
Cluster deletion	_____
Reduplication	_____
Weak syllable deletion	_____
Final consonant deletion	_____
Initial consonant deletion	_____
Other _____	_____
Substitution Processes	
Consonant cluster substitution	_____
Fronting	_____
Labialization	_____
Alveolarization	_____
Stopping	_____
Affrication	_____
Deaffrication	_____
Denasalization	_____
Gliding of liquids	_____
Gliding of fricatives	_____
Vowelization	_____
Derhotacization	_____
Voicing	_____
Devoicing	_____
Other _____	_____
_____	_____
_____	_____
Assimilation Processes	
Labial assimilation	_____
Velar assimilation	_____
Nasal assimilation	_____
Liquid assimilation	_____
Other _____	_____
_____	_____
_____	_____

2. Tally the number of times the child used each process. On the summary form, list the processes and their frequency of occurrence.

The phonological processes and their frequency of occurrence for H. H. are contained in Table 7.6. A word-by-word analysis of his phonological processes is contained in Appendix 7.1.

CLINICAL APPLICATION

Phonological Process Analysis for H. H.

H. H. demonstrates a high frequency of occurrence of the following phonological processes:

Consonant cluster reduction	Fronting
Final consonant deletion	Stopping

Assessing Productive Phonological Knowledge. Elbert and Gierut (1986) present an approach to analyzing a child's *productive*

Some protocols figure the *percentage of occurrence* for each phonological process. This percentage is derived from the total number of times the process *did* occur divided by the number of times the process *could have* occurred in the presented material. Quantitative criteria are then suggested to guide in selecting processes for intervention. For example, Hodson and Paden (1983) recommend that a pattern should be established at least 40 percent of the time before it is targeted for intervention. The Hodson protocol (Hodson, 1986), using a predetermined set of responses, provides the number of times each process could occur within the sample. However, this protocol does not account for a spontaneous speech sample. Counting the number of times each process could occur within the entire sample can be a long and difficult task. If the frequency of occurrence of each process appears necessary, it might be easier and more time-efficient to select a protocol or a computer program that provides this information.

TABLE 7.6 Summary of Phonological Processes for Child H. H.

PROCESSES	NUMBER OF OCCURRENCES
Syllable Structure Changes	
Cluster reduction	16
Cluster deletion	1
Reduplication	0
Weak syllable deletion	2
Final consonant deletion	17
Initial consonant deletion	1
Other _____	_____
Substitution Processes	
Consonant cluster substitution	9
Fronting	15
Labialization	5
Alveolarization	1
Stopping	20
Affrication	0
Deaffrication	0
Denasalization	0
Gliding of liquids	6
Gliding of fricatives	0
Vowelization	0
Derhotacization	8
Voicing	10
Devoicing	3
Other _____	_____
_____	_____
_____	_____
Assimilation Processes	
Labial assimilation	_____
Velar assimilation	_____
Nasal assimilation	_____
Liquid assimilation	_____
Other _____	_____
_____	_____
_____	_____

phonological knowledge. The authors postulate that "the way in which the child *uses* the sound system allows us to determine what the child *knows* about the sound system." (Elbert and Gierut, 1986, p. 50). This approach emphasizes first that the child's performance must be described independently of the adult norm system. It is only *after* the child's phonological knowledge is assessed that comparisons are made between the child's phonological system and the adult model. Elbert and Gierut view this approach as an application of generative phonology. As such, the analysis procedures seem to be particularly useful with children who have severe phonological disorders or complex patterns of errors. This analysis may not be appropriate for children who exhibit only one or two sound errors or for those who produce sound distortions.

The child's productive phonological knowledge is determined by (1) the breadth of the distribution of sounds and (2) the use of phonological rules. The breadth of the distribution of sounds consists of

1. the phonetic inventory,
2. the phonemic inventory, and
3. the distribution of sounds in the phonemic inventory.

The following definitions and examples are given for each:

1. Breadth of the Distribution of Sounds
   A. *Phonetic inventory:* Includes all the sounds that the child produced. Whether these sounds concur with the target sound or not is unimportant. The phonetic inventory would include sounds and sound substitutions listed on the matrix for recording the overall inventory of phones (Figure 7.3). Thus, all sounds accurately articulated and those used as substitutions would be listed.

B. *Phonemic inventory:* Lists only those sounds that are used contrastively, that is, those that signal meaning differences. One way to determine the phonemic inventory is by testing the child's production of minimal pairs. If a phonemic contrast is neutralized, that is, if the child uses the same sound for two phonemes, this should be evaluated in more depth by using additional minimal pair words in both pre- and postvocalic positions. The Neutralization of Phonemic Contrasts Summary Form (Figure 7.7) could also be used as a portion of this analysis. Those sounds that do appear on the summary form should be further tested using minimal pairs. For example, for H. H. [k], [s], [z], and [tʃ] were all realized as [t]. Minimal pairs such as *keys, Cs, Zs, cheese,* and *Ts* could be presented to see if H. H. produces differences between the pairs.

C. *Distribution of sounds in the phonemic inventory:* Includes an analysis of the distribution of sounds by (1) word position and (2) morphemes. Word position distribution examines whether sounds that contrast meaning are used by the child in *all* versus *some* word positions. This could include a comparison of the articulation test, the spontaneous speech sample, and other selected words to see if the child does produce some errors inconsistently, that is, correct only in some contexts and incorrect in others. For example, a child who says [wæmp] for *lamp* and [wʊk] for *look* but can realize [l] correctly in *yellow* and *telling* demonstrates a distribution by word position. *Distribution by morpheme* examines whether sounds are used contrastively for *all* versus *some* target morphemes. For example, H. H. substitutes [b] for [f] in *fishing, feather,* and *finger* but articulated [f] correctly in *telephone.*

The phonological rules operating in the child's system are categorized according to static and dynamic rules.

2. The Use of Phonological Rules

   A. *Static rules:* Describe the phonotactic constraints operating within the child's system. There are three types of static rules:

   (1) *Inventory constraints:* Certain sounds do not occur in the phonetic or phonemic inventories.

   (2) *Positional constraints:* Certain sounds occur only in certain word positions but not in others.

   (3) *Sequence constraints:* Certain sound combinations do not occur.

   B. *Dynamic rules:* Alter the production of sounds by changing segments in specific contexts or environments. There are two types of dynamic rules:

   (1) *Allophonic rules:* Describe phonetic variations in the production of a sound. Free variation and complementary distribution can be employed to provide evidence of whether specific phonetic variations are or are not employed to signal phonemic differences.

   a. *Free variation:* Refers to sounds that co-occur in the same position for the same word. Although these sounds have the potential to signal a difference in meaning, in this phonological system they do not. Therefore, for this particular system, they are not meaning-differentiating phonemes. For example, a child sometimes produces [tɑ] and sometimes [kɑ] for *car*. Although the production differences between [t] and [k] are linguistically relevant, they do not signal phonemic differences in the child's system. [t] and [k] are in free variation. Free variations are random, that is, unpredictable in terms of specific contextual factors.

   b. *Complementary distribution:* Refers to those sounds that occur in mutually exclusive contexts. These variations are context-conditioned and their occurrence is predictable. Here again, phonetic differences are not signalling a difference in meaning; the phonetic difference is not phonemically relevant. For example, a child realizes all word-initial stops as voiced and all word-final stops as voiceless. Thus, *pin* and *bin* are produced as [bɪn], while *rip* and *rib* were realized as [rɪp]. Variations like these are context-conditioned and predictable. Although [p] and [b] can both be produced, they never occurred in the same context; they were mutually exclusive. In this example, [p] and [b] would stand in complementary distribution. The child does not use [p] and [b] to signal phonemic differences.

   (2) *Neutralization rules:* Refers to the collapse of a phonemic contrast between sounds in certain contexts or environments. According to Elbert and Gierut (1986), three conditions must be met before the neutralization rule is operating:

   a. The presence of the phonemic contrast must be evidenced somewhere in the child's system. The underlying assumption is that the phonemic contrast must somehow be there before it can be neutralized.

   b. This phonemic contrast must be missing in other environments.

   c. There must be evidence of morphophonemic alternations. Such alternations are produced when a specific sound in a specific morpheme is changed in a new morphemic environment. For example, the child says [aʲs] for *ice*, however, when saying *icy*, [s] changes to [t] and the word becomes [aʲti].

Dynamic rules may be optional or obligatory. *Optional rules* are those that are applied only in some cases or to some morphemes. Obligatory rules, on the other hand, are those that always apply to all morphemes when the particular rule conditions are met. Box 7.1 provides additional references that expand on the concepts of free variation and complementary distribution. The reader is referred to these sources for additional examples.

Based on information gained from the breadth of distribution of sounds, the use of phonological rules, and the nature of the child's lexical representations, Elbert and Gierut postulate six different levels of productive phonological knowledge. Type 1 knowledge represents the most productive knowledge and Type 6 the least:

Box 7.1_____

Determining Phonological Rules: Selected References

Dinnsen, D. A. (1984). Methods and empirical issues in analyzing functional misarticulations. In M. Elbert, D. A. Dinnsen, & G. Weismer (Eds.), *Phonological theory and the misarticulating child*, ASHA Monograph No. 22. Rockville, MD: ASHA.

Elbert, M., & Gierut, J. (1986). *Handbook of clinical phonology: Approaches to assessment and treatment.* Boston: College-Hill Press.

Grunwell, P. (1987). *Clinical phonology* (2nd ed.). Baltimore: Williams and Wilkins.

Hyman, L. (1975). *Phonology: Theory and analysis.* New York: Holt, Rinehart, and Winston.

Type 1: Adultlike lexical representation for all target morphemes in all word positions. No phonological rules are noted. Type 1 knowledge is signalled by norm production of sounds. Elbert and Gierut (1986) note that children generally have Type 1 knowledge of nasals and glides.

Type 2: Adultlike lexical representation for all target morphemes in all word positions; however, obligatory or optional dynamic phonological rules may be functioning as well. For the most part, the child's production of these sounds is comparable to the target, but some rule-governed irregular productions do occur.

Type 3: Adultlike lexical representation in all word positions but only for some morphemes. This type of knowledge can be described by "fossilized forms," that is, forms that were produced incorrectly at an early age and are now resistive to change. Fossilized productions of names and pets' names are commonly observed.

Type 4: Adultlike lexical representation in some word positions for all target morphemes. Type 4 knowledge is signalled by positional constraints. Irregular sound realizations are noted but only in certain word positions.

Type 5: Adultlike lexical representation in some word positions for some target morphemes. Type 5 knowledge is signalled by those representations that were noted in both Type 3 and Type 4 levels. Thus, positional constraints and fossilized forms are both operating on a sound.

Type 6: Nonadultlike lexical representation in all word positions of all target morphemes. These sounds reflect inventory constraints; they are always produced in an aberrant manner relative to the target sound.

Figure 7.14 is a schematic drawing of the decision-making process that occurs for each of these six types of productive phonological knowledge.

MEASURES OF INTELLIGIBILITY AND SEVERITY

Measures of severity and intelligibility can be especially helpful in documenting the neces-

sity for or progress in therapy. Measures of severity and intelligibility can be selected that meet the specific needs of the assessment and the age and the speech status of the particular client.

Measures of Intelligibility

Intelligibility refers to a judgment made by a clinician based on how much of an utterance can be understood. Measurements of the degree of speech intelligibility are based on a subjective, perceptual judgment that is generally related to the percentage of words that are

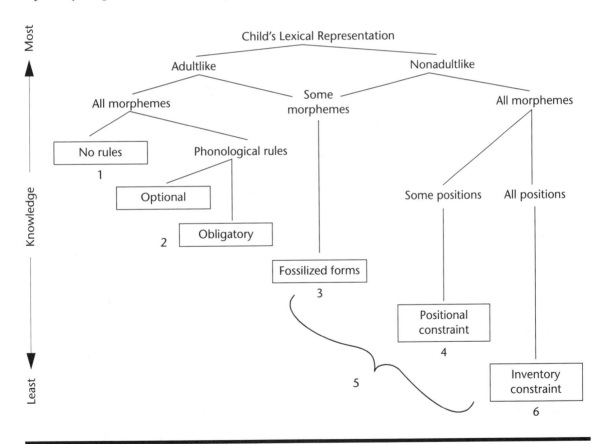

FIGURE 7.14 Decision Tree for Ranking Child's Phonological Knowledge on a Continuum

Source: From *Handbook of Clinical Phonology: Approaches to Assessment and Treatment* (p. 62), by M. Elbert and J. Gierut, 1986, Austin, TX: PRO-ED, Inc. Copyright 1986 PRO-ED, Inc. Reprinted with permission.

understood by the listener. Factors influencing speech sound intelligibility include the number, type, and consistency of speech sound errors (Bankson and Bernthal, 1998b). Clearly, the number of errors is related to the overall intelligibility. However, just adding up the errors does not yield an adequate index of intelligibility. For example, Shriberg and Kwiatkowski (1982a, 1982b) reported a low correlation between the percentage of consonants correct and the intelligibility of a speech sample.

The intelligibility of an utterance is influenced by several factors. Connolly (1986) lists the following:

1. loss of phonemic contrasts
2. loss of contrasts in specific linguistic contexts
3. the number of meaning distinctions that are lost due to the lack of phonemic contrasts
4. the difference between the target and its realization
5. the consistency of the target-realization relationship
6. the frequency of abnormality in the client's speech
7. the extent to which the listener is familiar with the client's speech
8. the communicative context in which the message occurs

Although intelligibility remains essentially a subjective evaluation, many authors have attempted to quantify it and to apply their results to a wide array of children and adults with communication disorders (e.g., Boothroyd, 1988; Bross, 1992; Hodson and Paden, 1981; Kent, Miolo, and Bloedel, 1994; Leinonen-Davis, 1988; Ling, 1976; Monsen, 1981; Shriberg and Kwiatkowski, 1982a; Webb and Duckett, 1990; Weiss, 1982; Wilcox, Schooling, and Morris, 1991; Yorkston and Beukelman, 1981). A summary of intelligibility measures is outlined in Box 7.2.

Measures of Severity

Articulatory competency can also be measured by different severity classifications. Severity measures are attempts to quantify the degree of involvement. Shriberg and Kwiatkowski (1982a, 1982b) developed a metric for measuring the severity of involvement in children with phonological disorders. They suggest calculating the *percentage of consonants correct* (PCC). Based on research, this type of calculation was found to correlate most closely to listener's perceptions of severity. Quantitative estimates of severity using the PCC give the clinician an objective measure to establish the relative priority of those who might need therapy, for example. The PCC calculations can be translated into the following severity divisions:

>90%	mild
65–85%	mild-moderate
50–65%	moderate-severe
<50%	severe

Box 7.3 provides the procedure for determining the percentage of consonants correct.

SUMMARY

The goal of this chapter was to show how the data gathered in the appraisal section of our assessment could be utilized for several different types of analyses. The first portion of this

---

Shriberg, Austin, Lewis, McSweeny, and Wilson (1997) have expanded the original concept of Percentage of Consonants Correct (PCC) to other measures that examine the percentage of vowels correct (PVC) and a matrix that weights distortion errors, the Articulation Competence Index (ACI), to mention just two of the ten total indexes. A conversational speech sample is the basis for all calculations. For information on the various metric values, see Shriberg et al. (1997).

Box 7.2

Measures of Intelligibility

In spite of the fact that there is not a general procedure for measuring intelligibility, the percentage of words understood in a speech sample is a common way to calculate intelligibility (Gordon-Brannan, 1994). Intelligibility can be categorized according to several indices. The following is based on the frequency of occurrence of misarticulated sounds (Fudala and Reynolds, 1994):

Level 6: Sound errors are occasionally noticed in continuous speech.
Level 5: Speech is intelligible, although noticeably in error.
Level 4: Speech is intelligible with careful listening.
Level 3: Speech intelligibility is difficult.
Level 2: Speech is usually unintelligible.
Level 1: Speech is unintelligible.

Kent, Miolo, and Bloedel (1994) summarized a number of procedures that have been used, or could be used, to assess intelligibility. The following are selected for the purpose at hand.

Procedures that emphasize phonetic contrast analysis:

CID Word Speech Intelligibility Evaluation (Word SPINE), for children and adolescents with severe and profound hearing impairments, Monsen, 1981.
CID Picture Speech Intelligibility Evaluation (Picture SPINE), for children and adolescents with severe and profound hearing impairments, Monsen, Moog, and Geers, 1988.
Ling's Phonologic and Phonetic Level Speech Evaluation (PPLSE), for hearing-impaired individuals, Ling, 1976.

Children's Speech Intelligibility Test (CSIT), for children of any age, especially for very young children or children with cognitive or motor limitations, Kent, Miolo, and Bloedel, 1994.

Procedures that emphasize phonological process analysis:

Assessment of Phonological Processes–Revised (APP–R), for children with object-naming competence, Hodson and Paden, 1983.
Functional Loss (FLOSS), for children with limited phonological systems, Leinonen-Davis, 1988.
The RULES Phonological Evaluation, for children with phonological disorders, Webb and Duckett, 1990.
Vihman-Greenlee Phonological Advance Measure, for children, especially those with phonological disorders, Vihman and Greenlee, 1987.

Procedures that emphasize word-level intelligibility:

Assessment of Intelligibility of Dysarthric Speech, for adults and older children, Yorkston and Beukelman, 1981.
Preschool–Speech Intelligibility Measure (P–SIM), for preschool children, but could be used with older children, Wilcox, Schooling, and Morris, 1991.
Weiss Intelligibility Test (WIT), for children and adolescents, Weiss, 1982.

---

chapter demonstrated how to organize the data collected from the appraisal portion outlined in Chapter 6. A preliminary analysis included forms and procedures to determine the distribution of speech sounds. These procedures were exemplified using a case

study of the child H. H. The next step in the diagnostic process examined the data to determine if a neutralization of phonemic contrasts existed. Based on the definitions of phonetic-articulatory versus phonemic-phonological impairments, the possibility of

Box 7.3_____

Determining the Percentage of Consonants Correct (PCC)

What is measured?	A five- to ten-minute conversational sample is tape-recorded and analyzed.
What to score?	Only consonants are scored using this metric. The examiner is required to make correct versus incorrect judgments on individual consonant productions. The following sound changes are considered incorrect:

1. deletion of a target consonant
2. substitution of a target consonant, including the substitution of a glottal stop or a cognate
3. partial voicing of a prevocalic consonant
4. any distortions
5. addition of a sound to a correct or incorrect target sound
6. initial [h] deletion and final n/ŋ substitutions in stressed syllables only. For example [ɪt] for *hit* and [rɪn] for *ring* would be incorrect. However, in unstressed syllables—for example, saying [fɪʃən] for *fishing*—would be considered correct. Acceptable allophonic variations are considered correct. For example, the intervocalic allophonic variation of [t] in *water* [wɑɾɚ] is considered correct.

What not to score?	Do not score utterances that are unintelligible or consonants in the second or successive repetitions of a syllable. For example, if the child says [bə beɪbi], score only the first [b]. Also, do not score target consonants in the third or successive repetitions of adjacent words unless the articulation changes. For example, if the child says [trit], [trit], [trit], only the consonants in the first two words are counted. However, if the child changes the articulation saying [trit], [twit], [trit], then the consonants in all three utterances are counted.
Calculation:	The percentage of consonants correct is calculated in the following manner:

$$\frac{\text{Number of correct consonants}}{\text{Number of correct plus incorrect consonants}} \times 100$$

_____

differentiating characteristics of these two disorders was discussed. The following section of this chapter outlined further testing that might be necessary for children presenting a phonetic disorder.

The remaining portion of this chapter outlined the procedures for a comprehensive phonological assessment. These included the inventory and distribution of speech sounds, analysis of the syllable shapes and con-straints, phonological contrasts, and analyzing phonological error patterns. There are several different ways to analyze the patterns of errors in a phonological assessment. The following means were exemplified: place-manner-voicing, distinctive feature, phonological process, and the assessment of productive phonological knowledge. Each of these analyses offers differing results. For each one, sample forms and procedures were supplied as well as a continued implementation of each analysis using the case study of H. H. Finally, measures of severity and intelligibility were described. These measures can be used to document the need for, and progress in, therapy as well as serve as a basis for clinical research.

APPENDIX 7.1

1. Transcription of H. H. According to Pre-, Inter-, and Postvocalic Positions

Target Word	Child's Production	Position	Description
1. house	[haʊ]	postvocalic	[s] deletion
2. telephone	[tɛfoʊ]	[unstressed syllable deletion—not counted] postvocalic	[n] deletion
3. cup	[tʌp]	prevocalic	[k] → [t]
4. gun	[dʌn]	prevocalic	[g] → [d]
5. knife	[naɪ]	postvocalic	[f] deletion
6. window	[wɪnoʊ]	intervocalic	[nd] → [n]
7. wagon	[wædən]	intervocalic	[g] → [d]
wheel	[wi]	postvocalic	[l] deletion
8. chicken	[tɪtə]	prevocalic intervocalic postvocalic	[tʃ] → [t] [k] → [t] [n] deletion
9. zipper	[tɪpə]	prevocalic vowel nucleus	[z] → [t] [ɚ] → [ə]
10. scissors	[tɪtə]	prevocalic intervocalic nucleus + postvocalic	[s] → [t] [z] → [t] [ɚz] → [ə]
11. duck	[dʌt]	postvocalic	[k] → [t]
yellow	[jɛwoʊ]	intervocalic	[l] → [w]
12. vacuum	[ætu]	prevocalic intervocalic postvocalic	[v] deletion [kj] → [t] [m] deletion
13. matches	[mætət]	intervocalic postvocalic	[tʃ] → [t] [z] → [t]
14. lamp	[wæmp]	prevocalic	[l] → [w]
15. shovel	[dʌvə]	prevocalic postvocalic	[ʃ] → [d] [l] deletion

Target Word	Child's Production	Position	Description
16. car	[tɑə]	prevocalic vowel nucleus	[k] → [t] [ɚ] → [ə]*
17. rabbit	[wæbɪ]	prevocalic postvocalic	[r] → [w] [t] deletion
18. fishing	[bɪdɪn]	prevocalic intervocalic postvocalic	[f] → [b] [ʃ] → [d] [ŋ] → [n], this is considered a variation in regular pronunciation and not an error, not counted
19. church	[tɜ]	prevocalic vowel nucleus postvocalic	[tʃ] → [t] [ɝ] → [ɜ] [tʃ] deletion
20. feather	[bɛdə]	prevocalic intervocalic vowel nucleus	[f] → [b] [ð] → [d] [ɚ] → [ə]
21. pencils this	[pɛntə] child would not say	intervocalic postvocalic	[ns] → [nt] [lz] deletion
22. carrot	[tɛwə]	prevocalic intervocalic postvocalic	[k] → [t] [r] → [w] [t] deletion
orange	[oʊwɪn]	intervocalic postvocalic	[r] → [w] [ndʒ]→ [n]
23. bathtub	[bætʌ]	intervocalic postvocalic	[θt] → [t] [b] deletion
bath	[bæ]	postvocalic	[θ] deletion
24. thumb finger	[bʌm] [bɪnə]	prevocalic prevocalic intervocalic vowel nucleus	[θ] → [b] [f] → [b] [ŋg] → [n] [ɚ] → [ə]
ring	[ɹɪŋ]	prevocalic	[r] → [ɹ]
25. jump	[dʌmp]	prevocalic	[dʒ] → [d]
26. pajamas	[dæmi]	[unstressed syllable deletion—not counted] prevocalic [dʒ] → [d] [i] in end noted as a diminutive, final consonant deletion not counted

---

*[ɑɚ] is considered to be a centering diphthong, therefore, it is the nucleus of the syllable. If you transcribed the utterance [kɑr], then this would be considered postvocalic [r] → [ə].

Target Word	Child's Production	Position	Description
27. plane	[beɪn]	prevocalic	[pl] → [b]
blue	[bu]	prevocalic	[bl] → [b]
28. brush	[bʌs]	prevocalic	[br] → [b]
		postvocalic	[ʃ] → [s]
29. drum	[dʌm]	prevocalic	[dr] → [d]
30. flag	[bæ]	prevocalic	[fl] → [b]
		postvocalic	[g] deletion
31. Santa Claus	[tænə dɑ]	prevocalic	[s] → [t]
		intervocalic	[nt] → [n], considered a normal assimilation, counted as correct
		intervocalic	[kl] → [d]
		postvocalic	[z] deletion
32. Christmas tree	[tɪtmə ti]	prevocalic	[kr] → [t]
		intervocalic	[sm] → [tm]
		intervocalic	[str] → [t]
33. squirrel	[tw3ə]	prevocalic	[skw] → [tw]
		vowel nucleus	[ɝ] → [3]
		postvocalic	[l] deletion
34. sleeping	[twipɪn]	prevocalic	[sl] → [tw]
		postvocalic	[ŋ] → [n] this is considered a variation in regular pronunciation and not an error, not counted
bed	[bɛd]		
35. stove	[doʊ]	prevocalic	[st] → [d]
		postvocalic	[v] deletion

2. Phonological Processes for H. H.

Target Word	Child's Production	Position	Description
1. house	[haʊ]	postvocalic	final consonant deletion
2. telephone	[tɛfoʊ]		weak syllable deletion
		postvocalic	final consonant deletion
3. cup	[tʌp]	prevocalic	velar fronting
4. gun	[dʌn]	prevocalic	velar fronting

Target Word	Child's Production	Position	Description
5. knife	[nɑˑ]	postvocalic	final consonant deletion
6. window	[wɪnoᶷ]	intervocalic	cluster reduction
7. wagon	[wædən]	intervocalic	velar fronting
wheel	[wi]	postvocalic	final consonant deletion
8. chicken	[tɪtə]	prevocalic	stopping
		intervocalic	velar fronting
		postvocalic	final consonant deletion
9. zipper	[tɪpə]	prevocalic	stopping + devoicing
		vowel nucleus	derhotacization
10. scissors	[tɪtə]	prevocalic	stopping
		intervocalic	stopping + devoicing
		nucleus	derhotacization
		postvocalic	final consonant deletion
11. duck	[dʌt]	postvocalic	velar fronting
yellow	[jɛwoᶷ]	intervocalic	gliding
12. vacuum	[ætu]	prevocalic	initial consonant deletion
		intervocalic	cluster reduction + cluster substitution (velar fronting)
		postvocalic	final consonant deletion
13. matches	[mætət]	intervocalic	stopping
		postvocalic	stopping + devoicing
14. lamp	[wæmp]	prevocalic	gliding
15. shovel	[dʌvə]	prevocalic	stopping + fronting + voicing
		postvocalic	final consonant deletion
16. car	[tɑə]	prevocalic	velar fronting
		nucleus	derhotacization*
17. rabbit	[wæbɪ]	prevocalic	gliding
		postvocalic	final consonant deletion
18. fishing	[bɪdɪn]	prevocalic	stopping + labialization + voicing
		intervocalic	stopping + fronting + voicing
		postvocalic	not counted, normal variation
19. church	[tɝ]	prevocalic	stopping
		nucleus	derhotacization
		postvocalic	final consonant deletion

*If this word was transcribed as [kɑr], this would be vowelization.

Target Word	Child's Production	Position	Description
20. feather	[bɛdə]	prevocalic intervocalic nucleus	stopping + labialization + voicing alveolarization + stopping derhotacization
21. pencils	[pɛntə]	intervocalic postvocalic	cluster substitution (stopping) cluster deletion
22. carrot	[tɛwə]	prevocalic intervocalic postvocalic	velar fronting gliding final consonant deletion
orange	[oᵘwɪn]	intervocalic postvocalic	gliding cluster reduction
23. bathtub	[bætʌ]	intervocalic postvocalic	cluster reduction final consonant deletion
bath	[bæ]	postvocalic	final consonant deletion
24. thumb	[bʌm]	prevocalic	stopping + labialization + voicing
finger	[bɪnə]	prevocalic intervocalic nucleus	stopping + labialization + voicing cluster reduction + velar fronting derhotacization
ring	[ɹɪŋ]	prevocalic	derhotacization
25. jump	[dʌmp]	prevocalic	stopping
26. pajamas	[dæmi]	 prevocalic postvocalic	weak syllable deletion stopping diminutive—use of [i]
27. plane	[beˈn]	prevocalic	cluster reduction + voicing
blue	[bu]	prevocalic	cluster reduction
28. brush	[bʌs]	prevocalic postvocalic	cluster reduction palatal fronting
29. drum	[dʌm]	prevocalic	cluster reduction
30. flag	[bæ]	prevocalic postvocalic	cluster reduction, cluster substitution (stopping + labialization + voicing) final consonant deletion

31. Santa Claus	[tænə dɑ]	prevocalic
		intervocalic
		
		intervocalic
		
		postvocalic
			stopping
			[nt] → [n] considered normal assimila-
			  tion, not counted
			cluster reduction, cluster substitution
			  (velar fronting + voicing)
			final consonant deletion

Target Word	Child's Production	Position	Description
32. Christmas tree	[tɪtmə ti]	prevocalic	cluster reduction, cluster substitution (velar fronting)
		intervocalic	[sm] → [t] cluster reduction, cluster substitution (stopping)
		intervocalic	[str] → [t] cluster reduction
33. squirrel	[twɝə]	prevocalic	cluster reduction, cluster substitution (velar fronting)
		nucleus	derhotacization
		postvocalic	final consonant deletion
34. sleeping	[twipɪn]	prevocalic	cluster substitution (stopping, gliding)
		postvocalic	not counted, normal variation
bed	[bɛd]		
35. stove	[doᵘ]	prevocalic	cluster reduction, cluster substitution (voicing)
		postvocalic	final consonant deletion

3. Spontaneous Speech Sample for H. H.

Looking at pictures:

[dæ ə pɪtə əv ə tɑ]
That a picture of a dog.

[hi ə bɪ dɑ]
He a big dog.

[hi baᵘ ən hæ ə tɑwə]
He brown and has a collar.

[oᵘ dæ ɪt ə tɪti]
Oh, that is a kitty.

[wi hæf ə tɪti]
We have a kitty.

[wi dɑt aᵘ tɪti ə wa:ŋ taˈm]
We got our kitty a long time.

Conversation with Mom:

[tæn wi do tu mədanoᵘ]
Can we go to McDonald?

[aˈ wʌ ə tibɝdə]
I want a cheeseburger.

[aˈ wʌ fɛnfaˈθ]
I want french fries.

[wɛ ɪt bɪwi]
Where is Billy?

[hi tʌm tu mədanə wɪt ʌt]
He come to McDonald with us?

[xxxxx mɑˈ haᵘ]
xxxx My house.

[mɑmi lɛ do]
Mommy let go

[lɛ do naᵘ]
Let go now.

Talking about summer vacation:

[wi doᵘf tu dæmɑt]
We drove to Grandma.

[si wɪf ɪn oᵘ +haᴵo]
She live in Ohio.

[si hæt ə fɑm]
She has a farm.

[si hæt wɑtə taᵘt]
She has lot'a cows.

[taᵘt ju noᵘ mu taᵘ]
Cows, you know, moo cow.

[deᴵ it ə ho wɑt]
They eat a whole lot.

APPENDIX 7.2

Proportional Occurrence of Consonant Phonemes in First-Grade, Third-Grade, and Fifth-Grade Children's Speech[1]

	Percent of All Consonants					
	1st Grade		3rd Grade		5th Grade	
RANK	CONSONANT	PERCENT	CONSONANT	PERCENT	CONSONANT	PERCENT
1	n	13.63	n	13.46	n	12.59
2	r	8.20	r	8.73	r	9.01
3	t	7.91	t	7.77	t	7.69
4	m	7.49	s	7.48	s	7.31
5	s	6.94	d	6.53	d	6.81
6	d	6.31	m	6.30	m	5.43
7	w	5.57	w	5.22	l	5.33
8	l	4.96	l	5.05	w	5.05
9	k	4.96	ʔ[2]	4.92	k	4.82
10	z	4.58	k	4.76	z	4.62
11	ʔ[2]	4.49	ð	4.58	ð	4.52
12	ð	4.42	z	4.28	ʔ	3.65
13	h	3.37	b	3.13	h	3.04
14	b	3.18	h	3.07	b	2.94
15	g	2.90	g	2.52	g	2.56
16	f	2.21	p	2.34	j	2.53
17	p	2.12	f	2.18	p	2.49
18	v	1.64	j	1.88	f	2.30
19	j	1.41	v	1.58	v	2.12
20	ŋ	1.05	ŋ	1.19	ŋ	1.38
21	θ	1.03	θ	.96	ʃ	1.33

(continued)

APPENDIX 7.2   Continued

	Percent of All Consonants					
	1st Grade		3rd Grade		5th Grade	
RANK	**CONSONANT**	**PERCENT**	**CONSONANT**	**PERCENT**	**CONSONANT**	**PERCENT**
22	ʃ	.84	ʃ	.94	θ	1.04
23	ʤ	.53	ʧ	.57	ʧ	.74
24	ʧ	.51	ʤ	.57	ʤ	.69
25	ʒ	0	ʒ	0	ʒ	0

Source: From *Clinical Phonetics* (2nd ed.) (p. 352), by L. D. Shriberg and R. D. Kent, 1995, Boston: Allyn & Bacon. Copyright © 1995 by Allyn & Bacon. Reprinted by permission.
1. These data are adapted from Carterette and Jones (1974).
2. /ʔ/ is included as a "phoneme" of English in the original data.

THERAPY FOR PHONETIC ERRORS

This chapter describes techniques that can be used to treat phonetic errors in the speech of children and adults. As previously defined, phonetic errors are motor production problems. This chapter emphasizes a *phonetic approach,* which has also been referred to in the literature as a *traditional* or *motor approach* (e.g., Bankson and Bernthal, 1998c; Creaghead, Newman, and Secord, 1989; Lowe, 1994; Van Riper, 1978; Weiss, Gordon, and Lillywhite, 1987). Using this approach, the client is directed to position the articulators in such a way that a specific speech sound within normal limits results. Therapy progresses from one error sound to the next. In addition, several of the treatment protocols cited in the literature also include tasks used to improve auditory discrimination skills (e.g., Van Riper and Emerick, 1984; Weiner, 1979; Winitz, 1975, 1989).

The goal of this chapter is to provide a solid information base for clinicians to use in their efforts to help their clients achieve a norm production of specific speech sounds. This foundation entails an understanding of how the sound is normally produced and knowledge of the client's misarticulation. In a continuing attempt to unite phonetic and phonological treatment principles, the linguistic function (exemplified by sound frequency, phonotactics, and examples of minimal pairs) will be provided for several of the sounds.

The sounds chosen for inclusion in this chapter represent the most frequently misarticulated sounds noted by McDonald (1964). Where applicable, the voiced or voiceless cognates are also treated. For each individual sound, not all possible misarticulations are addressed. Rather, only the most frequent misarticulations referenced in the research or as a result of personal clinical experience are included. Therefore, for some sounds, [s] for example, most of the misarticulations treated are distortions. For other sounds, such as [l], the majority of the errors are sound substitutions.

DECISION MAKING: WHEN TO USE A PHONETIC APPROACH

Historically, phonetic approaches were first described in Europe around the turn of the century (Gutzmann, 1895; Kussmaul, 1885). Their first documentation within the United States is attributed to Scripture (1902), Ward (1923), and Scripture and Jackson (1927). Through the years, many authors have added to and modified these beginnings, including Mosher (1929), Nemoy (1954), Nemoy and Davis (1937), West, Kennedy, and Carr (1937), Van Riper (1939a, 1939b), Young and Hawk (1955), Mysak (1959), West and Ansberry (1968), and Winitz (1969), to mention just a few. Van Riper's "Speech Correction" (1939b) is often cited as the text that popularized these techniques that have been used by clinicians for decades.

Any contemporary view of treatment needs to stress what is current, what is new. Thus, due to their noncontemporary roots, one might hesitate to take traditional-motor approaches seriously. In addition, after so much emphasis has been placed on analyzing the phonemic systems of our clients, the question arises: Should a traditional phonetic approach still be used? The answer to this question is yes. There is definitely a place for these methods within our contemporary understanding of phonetic-phonological disorders and their remediation.

Phonetic Errors

In **phonetic** or **traditional-motor approaches,** each error sound is treated individually, one after the other. This treatment principle stands in contrast to a **multiple-sound approach,** which attempts to theoretically influence several error sounds simultaneously. Traditional-motor approaches should not be automatically used with all clients who exhibit a single-sound error. A client with a

single-sound error who has problems with the *function* of the sound within the language system, that is, with the underlying system that governs the use of this particular sound, is probably demonstrating a phonemic disorder. Omissions and substitutions of an isolated speech sound can be phonemic disorders. In such cases, other therapy options may be more suitable. The question is never how many sounds are involved but rather whether the errors, single or multiple, are phonetic or phonemic in nature. If they are phonetically based, the best treatment option may be a traditional-motor, phonetic approach.

Decision Making: A Phonetic Approach with Phonemic Disorders?

As previously discussed, a phonetic approach will probably be chosen if the client demonstrates a phonetic disorder. This does not necessarily mean that it is unsuitable for clients with phonemic disorders. Certain portions of these techniques may prove helpful when working with children who demonstrate phonemic disorders. The following guidelines are presented to aid in the decision-making process of when to initiate a phonetic approach with children exhibiting phonemic-phonological disorders.

Phonological approaches emphasize the function of sounds within a specific language system. Consequently, the internalization of

---

A simplistic solution defines phonetic and phonemic problems according to the number of error sounds observed: If only one or possibly a couple of sounds are in error, we have a phonetic problem; multiple sound errors are phonemic (Paul, 1995). However, the assumption that single-sound errors must be motoric, phonetic in nature while multiple-sound errors reflect conceptual, phonemic problems has been refuted (Locke, Bleile, Fey, and Folkins, 1996).

phonological rules and contrasts are the main goals of phonological therapies. If, however, the sound is not in the child's repertoire, and remains elusive in spite of phonological treatment attempts, the phonetic approach could be implemented to establish its norm articulation. This does not mean that a clinician needs to go through all steps of the phonetic approach but that certain ideas and procedures of the phonetic approach can prove useful. Thus, one of the treatment goals would be to help the child produce the appropriate phonetic features of the speech sound. This in turn could facilitate the primary goal, that is, increasing the child's ability to understand and utilize the phonological rules and contrasts with that particular sound.

Bankson and Bernthal (1998c) report that the traditional-motor or phonetic approach "can also be incorporated into treatment programs for clients reflecting linguistic or pattern-based errors, especially if the patterns reflect motor constraints (e.g., prevocalic voicing or certain cluster simplifications)" (p. 333). Based on these authors' recommendation, if motor constraints can be identified in the patterns of clients with phonemic disorders, the traditional, phonetic approach constitutes a viable option.

THERAPY SEQUENCE

This section outlines possibilities for sequencing therapy when working with phonetic disorders. These sequences have been described by numerous authors (e.g., Secord, 1989; Van Riper, 1978; Van Riper and Emerick, 1984; Van Riper and Irwin, 1958; Waengler and Bauman-Waengler, 1984; Winitz, 1975) and have been utilized by clinicians for decades. Although the following sequencing is presented, clinicians will find that certain stages will be necessary for some clients while for others they might prove unnecessary. The

specific client's needs and capabilities will cause changes in the sequencing of every therapy program.

Each of the treatment phases assumes that the client enters that particular stage with minimal competency and moves to the next stage when a certain level of accuracy has been achieved. The necessary level of accuracy before preceding to the next stage of treatment is usually relatively high. Paul (1995) notes that correct usage is typically set at 80 percent to 90 percent in structured intervention contexts. Therefore, during structured activities within a therapy setting, 80 percent to 90 percent accuracy would be needed before proceeding to the next stage. However, is this high accuracy necessary in spontaneous speech before a client is dismissed from therapy? As dismissal criteria, Lee, Koenigsknecht, and Mulhern (1975) have suggested a much lower level of accuracy for spontaneous, natural contexts. They argue that termination criteria in spontaneous contexts should be set at 50 percent accuracy. It appears that once children use targeted behaviors in spontaneous speech the majority of the time, it is probable that progress will continue toward more consistent usage. These percentages appear reasonable but, again, may vary according to the individual clinician's expectations and client's capabilities.

General Overview of Therapy Progression

Sensory-Perceptual Training/Ear Training. In this phase of therapy, the client develops the ability to discriminate between the target sound and other sounds, including the irregular production that he or she uses. During sensory-perceptual training, the client is not asked to attempt a production of the target sound but only to judge its distinctness from other sounds. The stages of this phase are those outlined by Van Riper and Emerick (1984).

Identification. The clinician describes and demonstrates knowledge of the sight, sound, and feel of the target sound. For young children, the target sound is often given a name, such as naming [s] the hissing-snake sound. For older children and adults, models and diagrams along with more complex articulatory descriptions can be employed. The goal is recognition and discrimination of the sound in *isolation* when contrasted to other similar and dissimilar sounds. Winitz (1975) adds that discrimination contrasts should at first address speech sounds that are productionally and, therefore, acoustically very different; only later should the client be asked to discriminate between the target sound and the error production. For example, if the client substitutes [θ] for [s], phonetically very different sounds should be presented at first—[s] versus [m], for example. Only at the end of the training period should [s] versus [θ] be introduced. Winitz (1975) believes that phonemic contrasts arranged in a hierarchical order from dissimilar to similar are more efficient than just contrasting the error production to the target sound.

Isolation. Next, the target sound is produced by the clinician in a variety of contexts which vary in word position (initially, medially, and finally) and context complexity (words, phrases, and sentences). The client must indicate when the target sound is heard. The goal of this phase is recognition of the target sound in words and identification of the position of the target sound within that word.

Stimulation. In this phase, variations of the target sound are presented in large quantities; that is, the client is bombarded with them. Variations might include louder or softer and slower or faster presentations of words containing the target sound. In addition, longer or shorter durations of the target sound within words could be presented. The client should also be able to identify the target sound when various speakers (with a tape recorder or in a group setting) say words, sentences, and finally paragraphs that contain it. The goal of this phase is continued identification of the target sound as context and speaker change.

Discrimination. Here, norm and error productions of the target sound are presented by the clinician. The error productions should mirror those of the client. These specific misarticulations are presented by the clinician in contexts of varying complexity, from words to sentences to tongue twisters with several of the misarticulations within one utterance. Van Riper and Emerick (1984) label this error detection. The second part of this sensory perceptual training phase is error correction. Here, the client is asked to explain why the sound is in error and, possibly, what needs to be done to correct it. For example, the clinician says [θoᵘp] for the word *soap*. The client must identify the error and explain that the tongue was peeking between the teeth, which is wrong for *soap*. For children, the error correction phase must be preceded by careful preparation so that they are capable of making these types of observations. The final goal of this stage is to emphasize the client's ongoing self-monitoring skills. Now clients must recognize the error production every time it occurs in their speech. For this self-monitoring phase, Winitz (1975) suggests that when the client misarticulates, the clinician should wait a few seconds and then imitate the client's production. This should be followed by the clinician correctly repeating the word several times.

Whether sensory-perceptual training is necessary for every client remains a controversial issue (see, for example, Briere, 1966; Dickson, 1962; Monnin, 1984; Sonderman, 1971; Williams and McReynolds, 1975). At least two factors should be considered before implementing these procedures: the age of the client and whether specific auditory discrimination difficulties are noted for the individual client. Age becomes a factor as many of the tasks used to achieve the goals of the training are metalinguistic skills. Metalinguistic skills require the child to think and talk about language. Identifying the position of a sound in a word is a metalinguistic skill, for example. The child must first understand the concept that a "word" is made up of individual "sounds" and their relative relationship to one another. The ability to segment words into sounds develops during the early school-age years (Fox and Routh, 1975; Liberman, Shankweiler, Fischer, and Carter, 1974). Therefore, for younger children, certain aspects of sensory-perceptual training may not be appropriate. Second, clinicians should

| Auditory perceptual testing was discussed in Chapter 6 and guidelines and assessment protocols were provided. |

carefully evaluate the specific auditory perceptual skills of their clients. The term *specific perceptual skills* refers to clients' abilities to differentiate between their error production and the target sound. If testing reveals no difficulties with specific discrimination tasks, sensory-perceptual training does not seem warranted.

In the previous discussion, sensory-perceptual training is seen as a phase before production training which, depending on the client's capabilities, may or may not be implemented. However, sensory-perceptual training in the form of self-monitoring remains a necessity during the next phases of therapy. Clinicians will constantly need to help their clients develop discrimination of "correct" versus "incorrect" productions. This type of self-monitoring is not an optional portion of therapy. However, clinical decision making should address the question of whether the aforementioned stages of sensory-perceptual training are necessary prior to work on the actual production of the target sound.

Production of the Sound in Isolation. The goal of this phase of therapy is to elicit a norm production of the target sound alone, not in combination with other sounds. An isolated production can easily be achieved with fricatives, glides, and liquids, for example, sounds which can be prolonged. For stop-plosives, young children might find it easier to articulate the target sound together with a central vowel, [kʌ] for example, or with a noticeable aspiration: [kʰ].

There are several possibilities for eliciting the target sound. Beginning clinicians often have the idea that this will be a task that can be achieved in a very short time. This is indeed often the case. However, if norm or near-norm articulation is not obtained within a reasonable time frame (five to ten minutes), persisting with the procedure will probably cause frustration to both the client and the clinician. In this case, either the technique should be changed or other preexercises should be initiated to prepare the client for the norm articulation. The following possibilities are offered for eliciting the target sound in isolation:

Auditory Stimulation/Imitation. In this procedure, the clinician provides examples of the target sound and the client is asked to imitate the sound. A similar procedure is implemented for stimulability testing (see Chapter 6). Many authors (e.g., Irwin, 1965; Milisen, 1954; Powers, 1971; Van Riper, 1978; Weiss et al., 1987) have suggested that this method be used first to elicit a new sound. The client is instructed to "watch me and do exactly what I do." If this works, it is perhaps the easiest and quickest way to achieve the target sound. Unfortunately, though, it does not always succeed.

Phonetic Placement Method. In the **phonetic placement method**, the clinician instructs the client how to position the articulators in order to produce a norm production. The phonetic production features of the target sound and the error production are analyzed to determine which articulatory changes need to be initiated so that an accurate production results. In the next section of this chapter, these methods will be described in detail for the most common misarticulations.

Sound Modification Method. The **sound modification method** is based on deriving the target sound from a phonetically similar sound that the client can accurately produce. The phonetically similar correctly articulated sound is used as a starting point. Specific adjustments to the articulators are then suggested, which should result in the target sound. The following section of this chapter offers sound modification methods for the most common misarticulations.

Once the target sound has been produced acceptably in isolation, the next task is to stabilize it. This is typically achieved by having the client repeat it immediately. At first, this will probably need to be carried out in front of a mirror with careful monitoring and feedback by the clinician. When the production is more stable, the client should articulate the sound a number of times successively, with a softer or louder voice, for example, and when possible, with different durations. This does not need to develop into a tedious drill for client and clinician but can easily be achieved in activities that are fun and motivating. For example, the clinician could hide colored cards or favorite objects around the room. Every time the client finds the object, the target sound could be repeated. The clinician constantly provides feedback as to the acceptabil-

ity of the productions, also asking the client to attempt judgments of the accuracy of his/her own productions.

Is an Isolated Production Necessary? Using Facilitating Contexts. Some clients can produce the target sound quite accurately in some word contexts but not in others. The coarticulatory context conditions seem to aid the client's production of a target sound. Supporting contexts have been labelled facilitating contexts (McDonald, 1964). Van Riper (1978) introduced the term *key words* for those words in which the target sound was correctly produced.

Facilitating contexts or *key words* are often found in the analysis of the client's articulation test or a conversational speech sample. Additional materials examining facilitating contexts include McDonald's (1964) deep testing and Secord's (1981a) probes of articulatory consistency. Van Riper (1978) describes how these key words can be used to simplify the production of the target sound in isolation. For example, the target sound is isolated by prolonging the sound within the word or by syllabifying the word. In one case, results of an evaluation demonstrated a d/g substitution. However, the word *finger* was found with a correct production of [g]. The facilitating context of a postdorsal-velar nasal [ŋ] aided the client in producing a postdorsal-velar stop. To take advantage of this situation for the purpose of producing an isolated [g], the client first says "fin-ger," separating the word between [ŋ] and [g]. The "ger" is then reduced to [g].

Facilitating contexts can also be used to begin therapy at the word level. For example, if a small core of words is found with an acceptable production of the target sound, these words can be employed to stabilize the production. As Van Riper (1978) pointed out, key words can be used as a model for the client. Acoustic and articulatory differences are then pointed out between the articulation of these key words and aberrant target sound productions in other words. When the client can feel and hear the target sound, a transition is attempted to other words. For this transition, it is important that the clinician understand the facilitating context(s) in which the sound occurs. For example, is the target sound always preceded or followed by certain vowels or consonants? Are the key words one- or two-syllable words? Does the target sound occur in a stressed or unstressed syllable? If the clinician can predict the facilitating context, words can be added with similar coarticulatory conditions.

CLINICAL APPLICATION

Using Facilitating Contexts

Using the example of *finger,* an analysis suggests that the abutting [ŋ] had a facilitating effect on a norm [g] production; both organ and place of articulation are the same for both sounds. Additional words satisfying this coarticulatory context condition include *singer, linger, hunger,* and *longer.* After these words are accurately articulated, a logical sequence might be to proceed to [ŋ] + [k]: *monkey, stinky, thinker.*

Facilitative contexts can be very effective in therapy. If appropriate words can be found, it is relatively easy to isolate the sound in question: an excellent start for the isolation phase of production. If, in a given situation, the use of meaningful words is especially important, facilitative contexts can also be employed for work at the word level. As always, the final clinical choice will depend on the circumstances and capabilities of the individual client.

Nonsense Syllables. The goal of this therapy phase is to maintain accuracy of the production of the target consonant when it is embedded in varying vowel contexts. The therapeutic efficacy of this phase can be greatly increased by ordering the nonsense syllables from those that are easiest for the client to produce to those that are more difficult. The typical sequencing is target sound + vowel (CV), vowel + target sound (VC), and vowel + target sound + vowel (CVC). However, this sequence may change based on the difficulty the individual client demonstrates with each type of nonsense syllable. Vowels can be arranged in a hierarchical order from those that provide favorable coarticulatory conditions to those that do not. Suitable vowel sequences will be suggested for each of the misarticulations discussed in the following section. However, articulatory ease and production accuracy of the individual client will ultimately determine the sequencing of vowels.

Many clinicians skip the nonsense syllable phase of treatment and move directly to the target sound produced in words. One reasoning is that words are more meaningful and interesting to the client than drillwork with nonsense syllables. Work with nonsense syllables does not need to be a tedious exercise. Coming up with motivating and enjoyable activities that incorporate nonsense syllables requires only clinical imagination. In addition, while words are more meaningful to children than nonsense syllables, the word material should always be carefully evaluated. Some of the small "articulation cards" with black and white line drawings depicting words, for example, are not easily recognizable to either the clinician or the client. Such material stretches the concept of meaningfulness. Finally, and probably most important, some clients need work with nonsense syllables before they can produce words with any acceptable level of accuracy. If the client produces under 50 percent accuracy in two to three practice sessions, the word level is probably still too difficult. The clinician could then work with nonsense sylla-bles or utilize consonant-vowel words such as *see, sow,* and *saw* until the production has sta-bilized. In addition, working with nonsense syllables eliminates the interference of the "old" error with the "new" production of the target sound which is inherent in meaningful word material. Years of practice with the "old" aberrant articulation of the target sound will often override the "new" articulation, espe-cially in familiar words. For example, a child may be quite able to produce the nonsense syllable [ki] accurately in the context of other nonsense syllables. However, when attempt-ing the word *key,* the child might suddenly re-vert back to the "old" substitution and produce [ti].

Words. The goal of this therapy phase is to maintain productional accuracy of the target sound within the context of words. A large variation exists within this category from one-syllable CV structures to multisyllabic words in which the target sound appears sev-eral times, often in consonant clusters. Orga-nizing words from relatively easy to more difficult to produce will prove helpful. This should be done in a systematic manner using the articulatory complexity of the word as a guideline. Several factors affect the articula-tory complexity of words. These include the length of the word, the position of the sound within the word, the syllable structure, the syllable stress, coarticulation factors, and the client's familiarity with the word.

The Length of the Word. Typically, the fewer the number of syllables, the easier the word is to produce. This would indicate that one-syl-lable words should be attempted before two- and three-syllable words (Secord, 1989).

The Position of the Sound within the Word. A sound in the initial position of a word or syl-lable appears to be the easiest. Word- and syl-lable-final sounds are typically more difficult. Thus, target sounds should generally be placed at the beginning of a word before at-tempts are made to realize the target sound at the end of a word (Secord, 1989).

The Syllable Structure. Open syllables (CV) are generally easier than closed syllables (CVC). Considering ease of production, the syllable structure may on occasion have precedence over the length of the word. Two syllable words with a reduplicated CVCV structure, such as *Daddy* or *teddy,* may be easier than CVC words such as *bed* or *mad* (Bankson and Bernthal, 1998c).

The Syllable Stress. A target sound is easier to produce in a stressed syllable than in an un-stressed one. Therefore, when choosing two-syllable words, the target sound should first appear in the stressed syllable (McDonald, 1964).

Coarticulation Factors. Certain words may be easier to articulate than others due to the in-fluence of coarticulation. This relates not only to preceding and following vowels but also to the neighboring consonants within the word. Knowledge of the vowel and consonant artic-ulations will aid in developing a list of words ordered from relatively easy to produce to more difficult (Winitz, 1975). However, the fi-nal decision as to ease and difficulty of pro-duction will be with our client when these words are implemented. Clinicians may find that certain words will be "too difficult," that is, the target sound is consistently misarticu-lated within that word. These words should then be attempted at a later time when the regular articulation of the target sound is more stabilized.

Coarticulatory factors also include the number of times the target sound appears in a word and whether it appears as a singleton or as a portion of a consonant cluster. Words that contain the target sound only once are normally easier to articulate than those that might have the target sound more than once. Thus, *cape* is easier than *cake*. Also, words that contain the target sound as a singleton will typically be easier than if the target sound is a portion of a consonant cluster. Thus, *sale* is productionally easier than *snail*.

Familiarity. Familiar words are usually articulated more accurately than unfamiliar words (Secord, 1989). Therefore, clinicians should begin with words that the client knows well or those that are more frequent in the speech of the particular group the client represents. With some clients, however, familiar words may also prove to be more difficult. The impact of years of practice misarticulating a familiar word in a multitude of settings may prove hard to overcome. These words may then need to be targeted later when the production and self-monitoring skills of the client have improved.

Structured Contexts—Phrases and Sentences.
The goal of this therapy phase is to maintain accuracy of production of the target sound as words are placed into short phrases and sentences. However, at this point, phrases and sentences should not yet be spontaneous but rather structured and elicited. If spontaneous sentences are used, it is possible that the client will choose words containing combinations with the target sound that are still too difficult. This presupposes that clinicians will begin work at this phase while still continuing the work at the word level. This is a logical supposition because clinicians will typically select a core set of words that can be accurately produced and then put these words into short phrases and sentences.

A *carrier phrase* with a target word at the end is one of the easiest ways to elicit a short phrase. At the beginning, the carrier phrase should probably not contain any other words with the target sound. Another relatively simple way to elicit an utterance is to embed one target word within the carrier phrase, which can be modified to create some degree of spontaneity. For example, if a child is working on [s], the carrier phrase could be "I see a _____." The clinician could have objects or pictures prepared (at first without any s-sounds) which the client identifies to complete the phrase.

During this therapy phase, the clinician moves from highly structured to less structured tasks. At the same time, the clinician might begin to implement target words with more syllables and consonant clusters.

Spontaneous Speech.
The goal of this phase is to maintain accuracy of production when the target sound appears spontaneously in conversation. This goal is first addressed within the therapy setting; however, the client needs to transfer this production accuracy to more and more situations outside therapy. This transfer of behavior to conversational speech in various settings is often referred to as *carryover*.

Both within and outside the therapy setting, this therapy phase should proceed in a systematic manner. One way of accomplishing this is to vary the length of conversation time. Clinicians could start with five minutes of conversation, increasing the time interval as the client's accuracy increases. Initially, before the conversation begins, the client should be aware that the clinician is "listening for our sound." Later, the time interval can be extended and specific contexts that trigger the production of the target sound in many different words included. For example, pictures are available containing words with the target sound which could serve as the basis for conversation. Also, certain topics might lend themselves to the production of specific sounds. For example, a topic that includes racing, race cars, and race car drivers would probably trigger [r] in a variety of contexts.

After a relatively high level of accuracy is achieved within the therapy setting, the next decisive step is correct production of the sound outside, in the real world. Parents and teachers can serve as valuable assistants during this phase of therapy. When working outside the therapy setting, the amount of time implemented and the specific tasks should be discussed with the assisting helper. This phase can become overwhelming to both the helper and the client if both suddenly think that the sound needs to be produced accurately all the time in every outside setting.

CLINICAL APPLICATION

Structuring a Home Program

When structuring a home program, the clinician needs to make sure that the speech assistant (caregiver, teacher, relative, etc.) is informed of several variables:

1. When? Which portion of the day should be set aside for the program?
2. How long? How many minutes should be spent on this program?
3. How often? How many times per day should this program be implemented? Should it be a daily occurrence?
4. What should be done? In detail, what should the assistant do? Does the assistant have written instructions as well as words, phrases, and topics that should be used in the home program?
5. How should accuracy be judged? How should the assistant determine which productions are acceptable and which not?
6. What should be done if a production is considered unacceptable? How should the assistant react to an aberrant production?
7. How should the assistant motivate and reward the client? What type of reward system should be implemented so that the client stays motivated and continues to work within the home program?

One question that the clinician needs to ask is: How can I be sure that the assistant understands what is to be done? This is an important question. If the assistant does not really understand in detail what has to be accomplished, this can often lead to frustration for both the client and the assistant. (The author had a caregiver assistant who, rather than implement two five-minute sessions during the day, thought that one thirty-minute session twice a week would be better. After two long sessions, the child refused to work at home.) Bringing the assistant into therapy can partially solve this problem. The assistant can see and hear which productions are considered accurate and which are not acceptable. After a period of observation, have the assistant take an active role in the therapy session. Helpful advice can then be given to the assistant to guide in making decisions about correct and incorrect productions as well as implementation of activities.

Katie, who was in second grade, was working on [s] in structured conversation. Katie's mother expressed her willingness to work at home with her.

1. When? After discussing this with the mother, a quiet one-on-one time after dinner was considered the best way to begin.
2. How long? Ten minutes was a good time frame to begin with.
3. How often? Every weekday.
4. What should be done? Written instructions were put into a small spiral notebook which the mother could transport in her purse between therapy and home. The clinician described in some detail what the topic of the conversation should be. These topics had been practiced in therapy and Katie was able to reach a fairly high degree of success with them.
5. How should accuracy be judged? After participating in two therapy sessions, the mother knew what to listen for. Reminders were also written into the notebook. Katie originally had a θ/s substitution. The mother was aware that [s] should have a clear, sharp quality and not sound like [θ].
6. What should be done if a production was considered unacceptable? It was decided that a small stop sign that was constructed in therapy would be used to signal any unacceptable [s] productions. The mother would simply hold up the sign when she heard [θ]. Katie knew that when the sign went up, she should repeat the whole sentence and try to monitor her [s] production.

7. How should the assistant motivate and reward the client? It was decided that if Katie participated for the ten minutes of therapy, she could play on the computer, uninterrupted by her two brothers, for fifteen minutes. Also, at the end of each week of therapy, Katie could pick out one of the videos that the family would watch on the weekend.

Even when an assistant is employed, the clinician should also monitor the client's level of accuracy in situations outside the immediate therapy setting. This can be accomplished in a variety of ways. For example, tape recordings can be brought from home, the clinician and child could go to buy an ice cream, or go window shopping at a toy store. The clinician could also drop by the child's classroom or call on the telephone to check on the accuracy of sound production outside the therapy setting.

Dismissal and Reevaluation Criteria. The last phase of therapy examines dismissal and reevaluation criteria. Fifty percent accuracy during natural spontaneous speech was mentioned earlier as criterion for dismissal. This relatively low percentage was suggested under the assumption that the client's competency will continue to increase on its own. Such a supposition needs to be checked by some type of reevaluation process. A reevaluation can be as simple as stopping by the child's classroom and listening to conversation, or it can be more structured, involving administration of an articulation test and obtaining a conversational speech sample. Whichever means is employed, *reevaluation* is a portion of our clinical responsibility. It is the only way to ensure that therapy was indeed successful, that the client has continued to generalize across situations. The ultimate therapeutic goal is norm production within all natural, conversational

settings. A reevaluation is a way of documenting this.

INDIVIDUAL SOUND ERRORS

This section will not revisit the multitude of traditional-motor approaches that have been suggested throughout the years but focus on those based on the phonetic features of the target sound in relationship to the error production. Knowledge of the correct phonetic placement and the existing differences between the norm production and the misarticulation will be instrumental in facilitating these techniques. Other traditional-motor approaches that may not be quite as "phonetically" oriented are referenced in numerous sources. For example, a compilation of phonetic placement, moto-kinesthetic, and sound approximation techniques can be found in Secord's *Eliciting Sounds* (Secord, 1981b).

This section will contain both phonetic placement and sound modification techniques for the following: s-sounds ([s] and [z]), sh-sounds ([ʃ] and [ʒ]), k-g sounds, l-sounds, r-sounds (including [r] and the central vowels with r-coloring, [ɝ] and [ɚ]), th-sounds ([θ] and [ð]), voicing problems (e.g., [p] for [b] substitution), f-v sounds, affricates ([tʃ] and [dʒ]), and consonant clusters. The discussion is seen as a reference. It contains a considerable amount of detail that will become necessary when a clinician is actually working with a client and encountering difficulties achieving an accurate production. The proposed methods also allow the clinician several possibilities for establishing a norm realization for each of the previously noted sounds.

MISARTICULATIONS OF [s] AND [z]

One of the most common speech sound errors is the aberrant production of [s] (McDonald, 1964; Weiss, 1980). Most children at some point in their development have difficulty with [s] realizations. Since [s] and [z] are counted among the latest developing speech sounds, they may pose difficulties into the first school year for some children. It is also a frequent deviation heard in the speech of adults. Whether at the grocery store or on television, one can often hear adults with irregular [s] articulations.

The phonetic production characteristics of [s] and [z] consist of several related physiological factors that make their articulation somewhat complicated. First, [s] and [z] are both fricatives. All fricatives are physiologically complex because a rather narrow opening between place and organ of articulation must be maintained over a longer period of time. In fact, the fricatives are also the longest sounds in duration (Bauman and Waengler, 1977; Lehiste, 1970). Throughout this time frame, production requirements necessitate not only a narrow opening between the organ and place of articulation but also maintenance of the right amount of expiratory air flow. There is a precise balance between the articulatory effort required to create the narrow opening and the expiratory air pressure.

If this balance is off even to a small degree, it becomes perceptually noticeable. In addition, aberrant productions can easily cross phonemic boundaries. Thus, if the tongue is too far forward, [s] might sound like [θ]. The same relationship exists between [z] and [ð]. In addition, the voiceless [s] occurs very frequently in General American English. In summary: [s] and [z] are physiologically difficult, perceptually sensitive, and produced in practically every utterance.

Phonetic Description

Norm productions of [s] and [z] are articulated in essentially two different ways: as an apico-alveolar or as a predorsal-alveolar fricative (Carrell and Tiffany, 1960). These differences are delineated in Table 8.1. The apico-alveolar variation is produced with the tongue tip up, while the predorsal-alveolar [s] is realized with the tongue tip down behind the lower incisors. Sagittal grooving of the tongue, which directs the airstream toward the opening between organ and place of articulation, is essential for both types of productions. In order to achieve this, the lateral edges of the tongue are

TABLE 8.1 Production Differences: Apico-Alveolar versus Predorsal-Alveolar [s] and [z]

	PHONETIC DESCRIPTION	
	Apico-alveolar fricative	*Predorsal-alveolar fricative*
	[s] voiceless [z] voiced	[s] voiceless [z] voiced
Notable Differences	Tongue tip up behind upper incisors	Tongue tip down behind lower incisors
Organ of Articulation	Apex (tip of tongue)	Predorsal (front portion of tongue)
Place of Articulation	Alveolar ridge	Alveolar ridge
Productional Notes	Narrow opening between tongue tip and alveolar ridge	Tongue arches towards alveolar ridge, narrow opening between predorsal section of tongue and alveolar ridge
	Sagittal grooving of tongue Lateral edges of tongue elevated	Sagittal grooving of tongue Lateral edges of tongue elevated

elevated and touch the first molars to avoid lateral air escape. Although the apico-alveolar articulation is probably the most common, many speakers produce predorsal-alveolar [s] and [z]. Each type of s-production has its therapeutic advantages and disadvantages, which will be discussed in a later section.

Linguistic Function

Frequency of Occurrence. [s] ranks among the top five sounds in frequency of occurrence. While not as frequent as [s], [z] ranks eleventh within the twenty-four consonants of General American English. The most frequent word-initial clusters include [st], [str], and [sp], while frequently encountered word-final clusters are [st], [ns], [nz], [ks], [ts], [rz], and [nts] (Dewey, 1923; French, Carter, and Koenig, 1930; Roberts, 1965).

Phonotactics. Both [s] and [z] can occur initiating and terminating a syllable. However, in spontaneous speech, the frequency of occurrence of [s] and [z] in initial, medial, and final word-positions is not comparable. In the speech of first-, second-, and third-grade children, half of the [s]-sounds occurred initiating a word; the other half were divided fairly equally between medial and final positions. On the other hand, over 90 percent of the [z] sounds were found in word-final position (Mader, 1954).

Tables 8.2 and 8.3 provide the more frequent consonant clusters with [s] and [z]. Word examples are also given. All consonant clusters are based on the lists provided by Blockcolsky, Frazer, and Frazer (1987).

Morphophonemic Function. Word-final clusters ending in [s] or [z] can be used, for example, to signal 1) plurality, as in boo<u>ks</u>, goa<u>ts</u>, ne<u>sts</u>; 2) third person singular, as in he ju<u>mps</u>, she bui<u>lds</u>; and 3) possessives, as in Mo<u>m's</u>, Da<u>d's</u>. Within phrases, contractible auxiliaries and copulas with the verb *to be* also

TABLE 8.2 Consonant Clusters with [s]

WORD-INITIATING		WORD-TERMINATING			
[sf]	sphere (a very infrequent cluster)	[fs]	coughs, roofs		
[sk]	school, skate	[sk]	mask, desk	[ks]	blocks, books
[sl]	sled, sleep	[ls]	false, pulse		
[sm]	small, smile				
[sn]	snow, snack	[ns]	dance, bounce		
[sp]	speed, spin	[sp]	wasp, crisp	[ps]	mops, tips
[st]	stop, stove	[st]	ghost, fast	[ts]	kites, cats
[sw]	sweet, sweater				
[skr]	scratch	[rs]*	horse, nurse		
[skw]	square	[lts]	melts, belts		
[spl]	splash	[mps]	lamps, jumps		
[spr]	spring, spray	[nts]	ants, presents		
[str]	street, string	[rst]*	first, worst	[rts]*	hearts, skirts
		[sks]	desks, masks		
		[sts]	nests, tastes		

*Consonant clusters with [r]. If these are considered centering diphthongs, these examples do not really represent consonant clusters. However, because they are included in most consonant cluster lists, they have been included in this one as well.

TABLE 8.3 Consonant Clusters with [z]

Word- or syllable-initiating clusters with [z] do not exist in General American English.

WORD-TERMINATING

[bz]	ribs, tubs	[vz]	knives, waves
[dz]	adds, toads	[zd]	closed, sneezed
[gz]	bags, bugs	[ldz]	builds, folds
[lz]	bells, shells	[lvz]	wolves, elves
[mz]	teams, games	[rdz]*	birds, cards
[nz]	cans, rains	[rlz]*	girls, curls
[ŋz]	wings, rings	[rvz]*	curves, dwarves
[rz]*	bears, ears		
[ðz]	bathes, breathes		

*Consonant clusters with [r]. If these are considered centering diphthongs, these examples do not really represent consonant clusters. However, because they are included in most consonant cluster lists, they have been included in this one as well.

demonstrate consonant clusters with [s] and [z]. Examples include "the man's happy" and "the cat's eating."

Minimal Pairs.   Minimal pairs are often used to test the perceptual accuracy of the error production versus the norm production of clients. Several authors (e.g., Grunwell, 1987; Locke, 1980c; Winitz, 1984) have devised protocols to test these types of auditory perceptual skills. In addition, minimal pair contrast therapy, which will be discussed in Chapter 9, employs pairs of words that differ by only a single phoneme. Sounds which are frequently contrasted to [s] and [z] include [θ] and [ð], [ʃ] and [ʒ], and [t] and [d]. Tables 8.4 and 8.5 contain a few examples of minimal pair words and sentences incorporating sound oppositions with [s] and [z]. Sound oppositions contrasting [s] and [z] to [ʃ] and [ʒ] are contained in the next section on [ʃ] and [ʒ] misarticulations.

TABLE 8.4 Minimal Pair Words and Sentences Contrasting [s] and [z] to [θ] and [ð]

[s] VERSUS [θ]		[z] VERSUS [ð]		[s] VERSUS [θ]		[z] VERSUS [ð]	
sank	thank	Zen	then	bass	bath	breeze	breathe
sick	thick			Bess	Beth	close	clothe
sink	think			face	faith	seize	seethe
sing	thing			mass	math	she's	sheathe
saw	thaw			miss	myth	Sue's	soothe
sigh	thigh			moss	moth	tease	teethe
sin	thin			mouse	mouth		
song	thong			pass	path		
sought	thought						
sum	thumb						

He was *sicker* after dinner.
He was *thicker* after dinner.

He had to *saw* the pipes.
He had to *thaw* the pipes.

The captain was *sinking*.
The captain was *thinking*.

Something was wrong with his *sum*.
Something was wrong with his *thumb*.

Did he *breeze* close by her?
Did he *breathe* close by her?

They walked by the *closing* store.
They walked by the *clothing* store.

There's a strange-looking *moss* on the tree.
There's a strange-looking *moth* on the tree.

The boy had a big *mouse*.
The boy had a big *mouth*.

TABLE 8.5   Minimal Pair Words and Sentences Contrasting [s] and [z] to [t] and [d]

[s] VERSUS [t]		[s] VERSUS [t]		[z] VERSUS [d]		[z] VERSUS [d]	
sell	tell	ace	ate	Z	D	as	add
cent	tent	base	bait	zing	ding	bees	bead
sack	tack	brass	brat	zip	dip	buzz	bud
sag	tag	case	Kate	zoo	do	cries	cried
sail	tail	kiss	kit	zoom	doom	dries	dried
sank	tank	hiss	hit	zipper	dipper	knees	need
sea	tea	lice	light			rose	rode
seam	team	mice	might			size	side
sew	toe	nice	night			toes	towed
sip	tip	peace	Pete			ways	wade
sock	talk	rice	write			trays	trade

He wanted to *sell* his story.
He wanted to *tell* his story.

He looked at the big *zipper*.
He looked at the big *dipper*.

The *seam* was split.
The *team* was split.

The airplane *zipped* through the clouds.
The airplance *dipped* through the clouds.

He thought it was *nice*.
He thought it was *night*.

It wasn't the right *size*.
It wasn't the right *side*.

She gave him a large *kiss*.
She gave him a large *kit*.

The *bees* can't be lost.
The *bead* can't be lost.

Initial Remarks

Several important variables must first be considered when confronted with a child or adult displaying an [s] problem. First, the disorder may be the result of a hearing loss, specifically a high-frequency hearing loss. Acoustically, both [s] and [z] have high-frequency components (6,000 to 11,000 Hz). Because all sound productions are monitored auditorily, even a moderate loss in these frequency areas might impair intensity relationships between formant regions and, therefore, lead to a distorted production. This makes a hearing evaluation prior to our conventional diagnostic testing indispensable. If a high-frequency hearing loss is present, our diagnostic evaluation and the subsequent therapy planning need to be organized quite differently.

Second, certain minor structural changes may affect [s] as well. This might include missing teeth in a school-age child or new dentures in an adult. Although circumstances like these may not cause [s] problems per se, an individual's inability to compensate for such structural deviations can result in unusual production characteristics.

Third, such diagnoses as "tongue thrust" or "tongue thrust swallow" also need to be considered. The term **tongue thrust** refers to excessive anterior tongue movement during swallowing and a more anterior tongue position during rest (Christensen and Hanson, 1981). Hanson (1988) suggests that a more appropriate term would be *oral muscle pattern disorders*; this would avoid the misconception that clients forcefully push their tongues forward. Controversy continues to surround these disorders and their impact on articulation, especially the articulation of [s] and [z]. Not everyone with a tongue thrust does develop [s] problems. On the other hand, there is a higher incidence of children with s-distortions who do demonstrate an oral muscle pattern disorder (Fletcher, Casteel, and Bradley, 1961; Hanson, 1988). Although an interdisciplinary approach is strongly urged, it is within the scope of practice of speech-language pathologists to diagnose and treat oral muscle pattern disorders (ASHA, 1991). Prior to ASHA's 1991 position statement, an ad hoc committee report (ASHA, 1989) suggested, as do several clinicians (Hanson, 1988, 1994; Hanson and Barrett, 1988; Hilton, 1984), that treatment, often called oral myofunctional therapy, may facilitate the correction of [s] difficulties. Knowledge of the diagnostic and treatment procedures of oral muscle pattern disorders will at times be necessary to complement work with [s] and [z] misarticulations. Box 8.1 contains literature citations that refer to the topic of tongue thrust.

Finally, the auditory discrimination abilities of the client need to be carefully evaluated. One portion of a clinician's assessment battery should include specific auditory perceptual testing (see Chapter 6). If the client demonstrates auditory discrimination problems between norm productions of [s] and [z] and the client's specific error realization, auditory discrimination training should probably be implemented.

Types of Misarticulation

As with all treatment plans, a solid diagnostic foundation needs to be established before treating misarticulations of [s] and [z]. It is important to find out exactly what the client does articulatorily during the sound realization, that is, how the client produces the error sound. Although the term *distortion* is often used to label abnormal sound changes, this seldom provides enough diagnostic information. The following guidelines are presented to help distinguish between different [s] and [z] "distortions":

Box 8.1_____

Examples of Recent Tongue Thrust Literature

Bigenzahn, W., Fischman, L., & Mayrhofer-Krammel, U. (1992). Myofunctional therapy in patients with orofacial dysfunctions affecting speech. *Folia Phoniatrica, 44*(5), 235–242.

Christensen, M., & Hanson, M. (1981). An investigation of the efficacy of oral myofunctional therapy as a precursor to articulation therapy for pre-first grade children. *Journal of Speech and Hearing Disorders, 46*, 160–167.

Hale, S. T., Kellum, G. D., Richardson, J. F., Messer, S. C., Gross, A. M., & Sisakun, S. (1992). Oral motor control, posturing, and myofunctional variables in 8-year-olds. *Journal of Speech and Hearing Research, 35*, 1203–1208

Hannuksela, A., & Vaananen, A. (1987). Predisposing factors for malocclusion in 7-year-old children with special reference to atopic diseases. *American Journal of Orthodontal-Dentofacial Orthopedics, 92*, 299–303.

Hanson, M. L. (1994). Oral myofunctional disorders and articulatory patterns. In J. Bernthal & N. Bankson (Eds.), *Child phonology: Characteristics, assessment, and intervention with special populations* (pp. 29–53). New York: Thieme Medical Publishers.

Hanson, M. L., & Barrett, R. H. (1988). *Fundamentals of orofacial myology.* Springfield, IL: Charles C. Thomas.

Lindner, A., & Modeer, T. (1989). Relation between sucking habits and dental characteristics in preschool children with unilateral crossbite. *Scandinavian Journal of Dental Research, 97*, 278–283.

Subtelny, J. D., Mestre, J. C., & Subtelny, J. (1964). Comparative study of normal and defective articulation of /s/ as related to malocclusion and deglutition. *Journal of Speech and Hearing Disorders, 29*, 269–285.

---

1. *Interdental [s] problems.* This is a frequent form of distortion. As the name interdental implies, the tongue is actually placed between the upper and lower incisors during this /s/ realization. The visibility of the tongue tip between the teeth is a diagnostic indicator for this aberrant production. Interdental [s] and [z] productions sound very much like [θ] and [ð].

Phonetic transcription of the error: If the misarticulation does cross phonemic boundaries, [θ] or [ð] are transcribed.

2. *Addental [s] problems.* This is probably the most frequently encountered s-distortion. Although *addental* actually means "at the teeth," the tongue tip may be positioned either touching or too closely approaching the posterior surface of the upper incisors. In both cases, the tongue is too far forward for norm [s] and [z] productions. Auditorily, /s/ and /z/ may again sound like /θ/ and /ð/ realizations. This is, however, not always the case. If the tongue tip is not touching but merely too closely approaching the upper incisors, the [s] may simply lose its sharp, clear tone and sound "dull" or "flat." Although the auditory impression is helpful, it can be misleading. More accuracy is afforded if the clinician can peek into the client's mouth, possibly by tilting the head back during the [s] realization. The forward positioning together with the flattened edges of the tongue might then become visible. The flattened edges of the tongue would indicate the absence of the sagittal groove necessary for regular [s] and [z] realizations.

Phonetic transcription of the error: [s̩] or [z̩]

3. *Lateral [s] problems.* As the name suggests, this [s] misarticulation is characterized by a lateral airflow during /s/ realizations. The tip of the tongue is in direct contact with the alveolar ridge (or may even be located more anteriorly, that is, in contact with the upper incisors). In addition, there is no sagittal grooving. The lateral edges of the tongue are flattened, not touching the upper molars as they should be. Under these conditions, the air can freely flow laterally into the cheeks. This lateral escape of air can occur on both sides (bilaterally) or on one side only (unilaterally). If unilateral, one of the tongue's lateral edges is in a normal position for [s] articula-

tion. Auditorily, lateral lisps are very noticeable. There is an unusual, openly conspicuous "slurping" noise component associated with lateral [s] and [z] production.

Phonetic transcription of the error: [s̝] or [z̝]

4. *Palatal [s] problems.* This faulty [s] articulation is characterized by a more palatal placement of organ and place of articulation than is normally the case. Therefore, predorsal or even mediodorsal portions of the tongue become the organ of articulation. The place of articulation is no longer the alveolar ridge but palatal areas. Palatal [s] lacks a sharp, clear friction noise; it approaches [ʃ]-quality. Their closest qualitative approximation is to a whispered (voiceless) [j] sound. One can achieve this effect by moving the tongue slightly posteriorly during a regular [s] production.

Phonetic transcription of the error: [s̠] or [z̠]

5. *Strident [s] problems.* Unlike all the previously noted [s]-sound deviations, the strident is named not for its phonetic production features but for the auditory impression it creates. This [s] sounds "strident" which, by definition, amounts to a shrill, irritating quality. Strident [s] articulations often have a whistlelike component. This whistle is achieved by an imbalance between air pressure and the opening through which the air

One can use the so-called tapping method to determine the exact location of airflow during lateral [s] productions. For this method, the fingertips are used to apply intermittent pressure lightly at different points along each side of the cheek. One executes this moving horizontally from the back to the front of the cheek at the level where upper and lower teeth approximate one another. By placing pressure on the portion of the cheek where the faulty air escape occurs, the lateral airflow will be momentarily interrupted. If the air escape is one-sided, we will hear a sudden cessation of the lateral airflow only when we are tapping at the specific point on the respective side. If it is bilateral, we should hear it on both sides.

must flow. In general, there are many ways to whistle: some do it through their fingers while others pucker their lips to form various degrees of small openings, for example. The same is true for strident [s] formations: There are many ways to produce this effect. The whistling component can be caused by too much air pressure through an adequate opening or adequate air pressure through a very narrow opening. This narrowed opening may be caused by too deep of a groove across the tongue tip. Sometimes, during a phase of therapy, a clinician may well discover with alarm that the client's [s] sounds suddenly strident. This is usually not due to inadequate tongue placement but rather to an increased overall effort. The child is consciously trying to produce a correct [s] and, in effect, overdoes it with either too much air pressure or an overtensed narrow opening. Luckily, as the child continues to practice, the intermittent stridency normally disappears.

Stridency may also be caused by a lack of airstream concentration across the front teeth due to certain dental anomalies, such as the separation of the upper incisors or an irregular dental position (Luchsinger and Arnold, 1965). For some adults, stridency may result when new dentures are worn. As the alignment of new dentures is always somehow different from the original set of teeth, certain motoric modifications need to be made. Until this compensation becomes routine, articulatory efforts may result in a strident [s] and/or [z].

Phonetic transcription of the error: [s̪] or [z̪]

6. *t/s substitution.* This misarticulation is marked by the substitution of [t] for [s], as in [tʌn] for *sun*; it involves a change in the manner of articulation from a fricative to a stop. According to phonological processes, the term *stopping* is the label used for t/s substitutions. This type of substitution is often seen in the speech of very young normally developing children. However, for some children, it

persists. Because this misarticulation represents the substitution of one phoneme for another, clients with a t/s substitution should be evaluated for a phonemic disorder.

Phonetic transcription of the error: [t] or [d]

7. *Nasal s-problems.* These deviations are characterized by nasality during the production of [s] and [z]. Nasal [s] and [z] problems may be organic or functional in nature. Organic ones result from physical anomalies or neuromotor disorders that affect the structure or function of the velum. Examples include the speech characteristics of individuals with cleft palate or specific dysarthrias. Functional problems are marked by the absence of any known physical anomalies or neuromotor problems. Noted etiologies for functional nasal deviations include articulatory dyspraxia and the imitation of faulty sound patterns, for example, the imitation of a parent with a cleft palate. Also considered functional is the maintenance of learned patterns that originally had an organic cause (Luchsinger and Arnold, 1965; Stern, 1927).

Distinguishing functional from organic velopharyngeal competency is the work of a team of professionals. Although an in-depth account of these procedures is not within the scope of this chapter, a few guidelines will be given. First, there is a higher degree of probability that a functional problem exists if the nasality is restricted to [s] and [z]. Organic problems will usually have an effect on *all* speech sounds, particularly those consonants that require a high degree of intraoral occlusion and the buildup of air pressure (stops, fricatives, affricates). Second, most of the functional nasal distortions demonstrate air escape through the nose only. Simultaneous oral and nasal airflow during [s] articulation is not as frequent (Arnold 1943,

> For a discussion of nasality due to organic problems and its impact on articulation, see the Cleft Palate section of Chapter 10.

1954). Nasal airflow and its influence on [s] productions can be verified by pinching the nostrils closed. The nasal resonance will immediately disappear during the occlusion of the nasal passageway and be audible again if the nostrils are released. Third, functional nasal productions are usually accompanied by a normal tongue placement for [s] and [z].

Phonetic transcription of the error: [s̃] or [z̃]

CLINICAL APPLICATION

A Strident Problem

Josh was a bright child who was doing well in first grade. His teacher was satisfied with the skills that he was acquiring in reading and writing. However, several children had recently started to tease Josh about his conspicuous [s] production. Josh was aware of his irregular pronunciation and was beginning to withdraw from speaking situations and become aggressive when he was teased. The teacher referred Josh to the speech-language pathologist.

Assessment revealed that Josh's only speech-language problem appeared to be this [s], which was articulated with a clear and shrill whistle in all contexts. The clinician began to analyze the phonetic characteristics this child was demonstrating. Organ, place, manner, and voicing were appropriate. However, it appeared that the more Josh tried to say the sound correctly, the louder the whistle-like component became. Using her phonetic skills, the clinician remembered that there must be a precise balance between the air pressure and the narrow opening between organ and place of articulation for [s] productions. If there is an imbalance between air pressure and the opening through which the air must flow, a whistling component could result. This whistling component, often referred to as a "strident s," can be caused by too much air pressure through a slightly narrowed opening or normal air pressure through a very narrow opening. Thinking about Josh's efforts when attempting to articulate this sound correctly, the clinician was confident that she had found the phonetic reason for Josh's problem. After explanations, some exercises, and some experimenting with openings and air pressure, Josh could say [s] sounds without a whistle.

Therapeutic Suggestions

Two approaches seem viable when working with a child or adult displaying an isolated [s] misarticulation: the phonetic placement method (Scripture and Jackson, 1927) and the sound modification method (Van Riper, 1978). Simply stated, phonetic placement amounts to describing the organ, place, and manner of production of the sound in question to the client. Systematic work toward realizing that goal is then implemented in an attempt to change the aberrant production characteristics. Naturally, with children, this needs to be accomplished in an age-appropriate manner. A mirror might be used as visual feedback, while the clinician serves as an auditory feedback system. Although this approach is widely used, it is often not easy to describe what exactly needs to be done with the tongue and the airflow, for example, in a manner that the child can easily understand and follow. The sound modification method, on the other hand, uses another sound or sounds that the child can produce in a regular manner as a point of departure for achieving the target sound (Secord, 1981b). Therefore, [t], which the child can produce, might be used to achieve [s], which the child misarticulates. The sound modification method is easier to apply if the speech sound chosen as a starting point has certain phonetic similarities to the misarticulated sound. This way, a bridge is built between the similar sound that can be correctly articulated by the child and the target sound that is in error. Both methods will be discussed for problems encountered with [s] and [z].

Phonetic Placement

Decision Making: Apico- or Predorsal Placement. Although most people realize apico-alveolar [s] and [z], a predorsal articulation is not without merit. For the apico-alveolar [s], the tongue tip is hovering, so to speak, near the alveolar ridge. This precarious position must be precisely maintained over the entire duration of the sound. In contrast, for the predorsal [s], the tongue tip is resting behind the lower incisors. This provides an easily identifiable spot for the tongue tip, which does not waver or fluctuate; it is something definite to "hold on to." For this reason, the predorsal [s] is noted as being a more stable production (Kramer, 1939; Krech, 1969; Waengler and Bauman-Waengler, 1984). Such relative stability is often especially important for children whose motor capabilities are not yet fully developed. In addition, a large percentage of [s] and [z] misarticulations are interdental or addental in nature; that is, the tongue tip is elevated but too far forward. To now move the tongue tip down for the predorsal-alveolar version provides a solution that is quite different from the child's previous attempts. The natural tendency to return to the previous incorrect [s] is diminished. It is often easier for a child to accomplish a different, new production task than to attempt minor adjustments of a previous one. The final decision of apico-alveolar or predorsal-alveolar [s] will depend on the client's motor abilities or restrictions and on the type and degree of [s] misarticulation.

Phonetic Placement: Apico-Alveolar [s]. For interdental or addental [s] misarticulations, the tongue tip must be moved back. The client, after instruction, glides the tongue posteriorly from the interdental or addental [s] position to the alveolar ridge. This necessitates visual aid, such as an articulation mirror, and reliable auditory feedback in the form of the therapist noting the exact time during this procedure when [s] is perceived as being appropriate. In addition, the lateral edges of the tongue need to be elevated. This can be aided by implementing specific tongue exercises (see Box 8.2) prior to the phonetic placement.

One could practice slightly "rolling the tongue," for example, prior to this manipulation so that the client becomes aware of the necessary elevation of the lateral edges.

For some children, the phonetic placement technique may be too demanding. They seem unable to manipulate the tongue while simultaneously trying to produce a sound. In these cases, it could be less frustrating to have the tongue tip pushed back passively during the production of the "old" [s] articulation. This can be accomplished by using a tongue depressor, which is placed between the upper and lower teeth and gently pushing the tongue tip back until the appropriate position is reached. The client should be instructed to focus attention on how the new tongue position feels and which changes had to be made to achieve this regular production. In addition, the clinician must serve as a reliable feedback system until the child can correctly discriminate, both auditorily and motorically, between the "new" and the "old" sound.

For lateral [s] realizations, the edge(s) of the tongue is not elevated and the tongue tip is in direct contact with the alveolar ridge. Therefore, the client must learn (1) to raise the lateral edges and (2) to direct the airstream over the tip of the tongue, thus releasing the previous contact. To heighten awareness of raising the lateral edges, one could start with tongue rolling exercises. To demonstrate contact versus no contact of the tongue tip with the alveolar ridge, one could use a rather forceful [t] sound (contact) with excessive aspiration (no contact). During the release phase, the client should be directed to notice the airflow over the front edges of the tongue. To develop the necessary central airflow, Secord (1981b) suggests that the client blow through a straw which has been placed along the sagittal groove of the tongue. A smaller cylindrical object (such as a small bamboo stick) can also be used to aid central airflow

Box 8.2

Tongue and Lip Exercises

Tongue and lip exercises can often be utilized with beneficial results. They are employed not to strengthen the articulators or increase their coordination per se but rather to heighten the child's awareness of tongue and lip movements. Van Riper (1963) states that "they can be said to be useful in teaching the student to manipulate his articulatory apparatus in many new and unaccustomed ways" (p. 267). Many clinicians question or flatly deny the therapeutic benefit of these exercises. A decision to use tongue and lip exercises will, therefore, be based on the clinician's philosophy and the needs of the individual client. If used, these exercises should be practiced for a limited time only and should always be specifically selected to reflect the problem at hand. The following are examples of tongue and lip exercises.

TONGUE EXERCISES

1. Stick the tongue out flat and wide.
2. Stick the tongue out narrow and long.
3. Stick the tongue out slightly with its tip up then down.
4. Tongue out as far as possible, then tongue tip up and down.
5. Tongue out as far as possible, move the tongue in and out.
6. Tongue out, then move to the left, center, right, center.
7. Tongue out, then move to the far right then far left.
8. Tongue out, then move to the right, the left; next up, then down.
9. Push the tongue tip against the cheeks, bulging out the cheeks to look like you have a golf ball in your mouth.
10. Move tongue slowly on the outside of the mouth around the red of the lips, first clockwise, then counterclockwise.
11. Move tongue slowly on the inside of the mouth from right to left passing by the closed lips. (This can be combined with # 9.)
12. Move tongue slowly on the inside of the lips in a clockwise, then counterclockwise direction.
13. Let the tongue "wash" the outside of the teeth from incisors to molars.
14. Let the tongue "wash" the inside of the teeth from incisors to molars.
15. Tap the tongue against the palate.
16. Move the tongue along the palate from behind the upper incisors posteriorly to the soft palate.
17. Move the tongue around the palate in circles, first clockwise then counterclockwise.
18. Let the tongue tip push against the inside of the lower incisors.
19. Roll the tongue.
20. Hold the tongue roll while you stick the tongue out.

LIP EXERCISES

1. Pucker lips, then relax; repeat.
2. Spread the lips, then relax; repeat.
3. Round the lips in a wide O, relax; repeat.
4. Use combinations of 1, 2, and 3. Round to spread, round to pucker, pucker to spread.
5. Use combinations of 1, 2, and 3 with articulation: *o* to *i, o* to *u, u* to *i.*
6. "Bite" the lips. First the upper and then the lower lips are "sucked into" the slightly open rows of teeth. Relax by bringing the teeth together in a neutral position.
7. "Rub" both lips together. First right and left, then forward and backward.
8. Make a "crooked" mouth, first to the right and then to the left.

while simultaneously creating more of a medial grooving of the tongue. The stick is placed sagitally on the tongue. During [s] attempts, the clinician pushes slightly down-

ward on the stick. This should help create more of a grooving effect while also hindering the contact of the tongue with the alveolar ridge.

The palatal [s]-production is characterized by a tongue position placed too posteriorly. Therefore, the client must slowly glide the tongue forward, being careful to maintain the grooving of the tongue. Tongue exercises such as numbers 15 and 16 could prove helpful prior to this manipulation.

A lack of balance between expiratory airflow and the degree of opening necessary for the production causes a strident [s]. Thus, the client needs to experiment with reducing the air pressure during the production and/or slightly increasing the opening between the organ and place of articulation. Air pressure can be reduced by having the client say the sound softly. Increasing the opening can be accomplished by a slight lowering of the tongue, possibly by lowering the mandible slightly. Table 8.6 provides an overview of necessary articulatory adjustments for the various error productions of [s].

Phonetic Placement: Predorsal-Alveolar [s]. With the predorsal-alveolar [s], the client must understand that the tip of the tongue must always stay behind the lower teeth. With visual or tactile aids (the specific portion of the tongue and the alveolar ridge can be touched while looking in a mirror), the client should be directed so that the front or blade portion of the tongue approximates the alveolar ridge. The lateral edges are again elevated.

Particularly for lateral misarticulations, the predorsal [s] has advantages over the apico-alveolar type. Moving the tongue tip down behind the lower incisors eliminates the problem of the contact between the tongue tip and the alveolar ridge, which not only characterizes this misarticulation but is often the reason for the relaxed lateral edges. Palatal [s] misarticulations with their characteristic posterior positioning of both organ and place of articulation may also benefit from the placement of the tongue behind the lower incisors. By choosing the predorsal-alveolar production, the whole tongue is more anteriorly situated.

Sound Modification Methods. Sound modification methods are based on the concept of utilizing a similar, appropriately articulated sound to aid in the production of the misarticulated sound. A similar sound refers to one that is comparable in some of its phonetic production features. This method is easiest to implement when several direct phonetic similarities exist between the sound to be modified and the target sound. However, some successful techniques have evolved out of very limited articulatory similarities.

TABLE 8.6 Overview of Error Productions and the Necessary Articulatory Adjustments for an Apico-Alveolar [s]

ERROR PRODUCTION	ARTICULATORY ADJUSTMENTS
Interdental	Tongue tip must be moved posteriorly. Lateral edges of the tongue may require elevation.
Addental	Tongue tip must be moved posteriorly. Lateral edges of the tongue may require elevation.
Lateral	Tongue tip contact with the alveolar ridge must be released. Raise the lateral edges of the tongue. Direct airflow over the tip of the tongue.
Palatal	Tongue tip must be moved anteriorly.
Strident	Reduce air pressure or increase the opening between the organ and place of articulation.

1. *[t]-[s] Method.*
   a. Begin with a series of rapid [t] repetitions, which typically produce intermittent [s]-like fricatives. This effect is increased if the child is asked to produce [t] with lots of air pressure. Have the child listen for the sound in between the [t] repetitions; then ask the child to try to prolong this intermittent [s].
   b. Begin with a [t] production in which the stop phase is prolonged, building up air pressure behind the occlusion. The client is then instructed to release the [t] very slowly. The result should approximate [s].

2. *[ʃ]-[s] Method.* Three steps are necessary to change [ʃ] to a normal [s] production:
   a. Eliminate the lip rounding associated with the production of [ʃ]. Have the client smile while saying [ʃ].
   b. Move the friction that occurs between organ and place of articulation more anteriorly. Have the client move the tongue slightly forward.
   c. Increase the sagittal grooving of the tongue. Have the client raise the lateral edges of the tongue toward the upper molars.

3. *[f]-[s] Method.* This method assumes that the tongue tip for [f] is already situated behind the lower incisors; therefore, a predorsal [s] is the goal.
   a. Pull the middle of the lower lip away from contact with the upper incisors during the production of [f].
   b. Raise the front portion of the tongue slightly as the upper and lower incisors come closer together.

For this modification, the client must be aware that a friction sound should be maintained during the entire attempt.

4. *[i]-[s] Method.* Phonetic similarities between [i] and [s] consist of the lip spreading and the high, anterior tongue placement for both sounds. For [i], the tongue tip is typically in a lowered position while the anterior portion of the body of the tongue is elevated toward the palate (Shriberg and Kent, 1995). Thus, this modification will normally result in a predorsal (tongue tip down) [s].
   a. Instruct the client to bring the teeth slightly closer together during the [i] production.
   b. Elevate the front portion of the tongue until a friction-type sound is heard.
   c. Raise the lateral edges of the tongue toward the upper molars.

Functional Nasal [s] and [z] Problems. Therapy for functional nasal [s] and [z] problems does not fit readily into the categorizations of phonetic placement or sound modification methods. The reason for the aberrant nasal [s] is not a deviant tongue placement but rather the inadequate velopharyngeal closure leading to nasal emission. Specific consonants can be used as a bridge to promote sufficient velar closure.

1. *[t]-[s].* If [t] can be produced without hypernasality, instruct the client to hold the stop phase of the [t], building up pressure during the occlusion. [t] is then *slowly* released, producing [s]. Complete velopharyngeal closure is normally necessary when producing [t]. By increasing the air pressure, the occlusion is strengthened due to the higher degree of production effort. This heightened effort may

---

The [i] could easily be modified to a voiced [z] if a decision has been made to initiate work with that sound. In addition, the [i]-[z] method has the advantage of maintaining voicing throughout the modification, which is not the case with the [i]-[s] method. See the later section on Where to Begin: [s] or [z].

promote more velopharyngeal closure for the following [s] approximation as well. Visual and auditory feedback should also be implemented to increase the client's awareness of nasal emission versus no nasal emission.

2. *[f]-[s].* Requisites for this method are an [f] production without hypernasality and the correct tongue placement for [s]. During [f], the client removes the labiodental contact (similar to the previously noted [f]-[s] method), gliding the tongue to an [s] approximation. Important here is that the client should continue to think about the [f] noise and keep that noise going. This method is based on the assumption that adequate velopharyngeal closure for [f] will now extend to [s]. Again, visual and auditory feedback should be implemented.

Where to Begin: [s] or [z]?   When attempting to achieve an isolated sound production, most clinicians automatically begin with voiceless [s]. The reasoning seems to be that the fricative, while complicated enough for the client, should not be further burdened with the addition of voicing. However, beginning with [z] could be advantageous under certain conditions.

First, voiced consonants normally are produced with less air pressure than the voiceless ones. An increased air pressure can at times be counterproductive to establishing norm articulations. Especially with an apico (tongue tip up) [s], this increased air pressure could lead to the client "losing" the precariously new approximation between organ and place of articulation.

A second factor that supports a choice of [z] is the ability of the voicing component to mask minor productional differences. Listeners seem to be more critical of even slight deviations of the voiceless [s]. The same artic-

ulatory features used for the production of [z] are not as noticeable. Naturally, we do not want the client to acquire an [s] that is somehow not acceptable.

The following scenario can serve as an example. We have begun work on [s]; however, even with our best efforts and those of the child, the production is still slightly off target. We have tried several times to correct for the minor mispositionings, but the articulation is still not quite accurate. We are becoming somewhat frustrated; the child, we feel, is already frustrated. This could be a good time to attempt a voiced [z]. If the articulatory variation is minor enough, the voicing should provide us with an acceptable sound. While giving the child (finally) success, it also allows practice time for the new sound. This practice with [z] is often all the child needs to perfect the [s] articulation.

A third consideration in favor of [z] is a coarticulatory consideration. If the voiceless [s] is placed in a consonant-vowel (or vowel-consonant) context, the client must change the voicing halfway through the utterance. This sudden change in voicing could strain an already difficult articulatory-motor task. By utilizing [z], voicing can be maintained throughout the production. To attain [s] once [z] is acceptable is relatively easy. If the child whispers [z], [s] will result. The next task is to put the isolated sound production into specific contexts.

Coarticulatory Conditions

The phonetic context in which a target sound is placed can have a considerable impact on the production of that sound. There are certain contexts that can support the production features of the target sound and others that might undermine them. Phonetic contexts that support the production of a target sound can be used effectively by clinicians in certain phases of therapy. On the other hand, ignoring coarticulatory contexts may lead to endangering a "new" sound production that is still relatively unstable. Facilitative coarticulatory conditions rely on knowledge of, and comparison between, phonetic features.

If the newly acquired [s] is practiced in syllables or words, the vowels that precede or follow it should be considered. Recall that [s] is articulated with the tongue in a relatively anterior position and with some degree of lip spreading; [i] seems phonetically comparable. Both [s] and [i] require unrounding of the lips while the anterior portion of the tongue is elevated toward the palate. This is not the case with [u]. This vowel is produced with the back of the tongue elevated and requires lip rounding. The coarticulatory effects of the lip rounding on [s] can be demonstrated by saying the word *Sue.* The lip rounding for [u] is already present as one begins to say the initial [s]. This lip rounding and the additional posterior tongue placement could actually work against a newly acquired [s] articulation.

Examining phonetic comparability, it would seem that the front vowels are better suited for our initial context work with [s]. The front vowels [i], [ɪ], [eᴵ], [ɛ], and [æ] support the relatively forward tongue placement and the lack of lip rounding. The back vowels have specific features that lack support for [s] and [z]. First, a more posterior tongue placement is associated with all back vowels. In addition, the degree of lip rounding increases from [ɔ] to [oᵁ] and from [ʊ] to [u]. The [ɑ] is considered to be an unrounded vowel. Thus, if lip rounding presents a problem for [s], the low back vowel [ɑ] should demonstrate more favorable coarticulatory conditions than the mid- and high-back vowels.

The phonetic context should be kept in mind when moving through every stage of therapy. By contrasting the phonetic features of the target sound and the surrounding consonants and vowels, a hierarchy of contexts can be established that move step-by-step from more to less supportive coarticulatory conditions. Not every client will need such small steps. However, for those who do, this hierarchy will prove invaluable. On the other hand, some clients may demonstrate phonetic contexts that may be more facilitating for them than those previously mentioned. The clinician should then use those specific contexts. The suggested sequence should not be seen as part of a "therapy cookbook" approach to be followed with every client but as one possibility that incorporates phonetic comparability.

Word Examples. The following one-syllable words are ordered from relatively easy to more difficult coarticulatory conditions:

[s] Words	[z] Words
see - seap - seam - seat - seed - seen	zee - zeal - Zeke
sip - sit - sin - sing	zip - zing - zipped - zinc
say - same - save - sail	Zane
set - said - sell	Zeb - Zed - Zen
sap - Sam - sat - sash - sang	zap - zag - zapped - zagged
sum - sun - suck - sung	
sob - sod - sock - song	czar
sow - soap - sewed - soak soot	zone - zoned
Sue - soup - suit - soon	zoo - zoom - zoomed

CLINICAL APPLICATION

Analyzing Coarticulatory Conditions

When analyzing words according to coarticulatory conditions, several factors should be kept in mind:

1. *The vowel following or preceding the target sound.* Consider the comparability of production features of certain vowels relative to the target sound. Some vowels will have production features that are phonetically similar to the target

sound, while others will be clearly different. For example, the lip rounding of the high-back vowels and the lip spreading of [s] are dissimilar articulatory conditions.

2. *The syllable structure of the word.* Consider the articulatory gesture as a whole. A word that contains a consonant followed by a vowel (CV) is a less complex articulatory unit than one with a CVC structure. CVCC words are relatively more complex than either CV or CVC structures.

3. *The phonetic features of the surrounding consonants.* Consider the movement of the articulators for the production. Organ, place, manner, and voicing of the target sound can be compared to the other consonants within the word. Again, production similarities may be used to create favorable coarticulatory conditions. For example, the organ, place, and voicing of [s] and [t] are phonetically the same. This is not the case for [s] and [k].

   Other consonants may provide supportive coarticulatory conditions based on the absence of specific production features. For example, the tongue is not directly involved in the articulation of the bilabials and [h]. Within an articulatory unit, if [s] precedes or follows a sound that does not require tongue movement, then the coarticulatory effects on [s] are minimal. The tongue movement for [s] is not influenced by any preceding or following articulatory necessities. Therefore, [m], [p], [b], and [h] can provide supportive coarticulatory conditions for those consonants in which the tongue is the active organ of articulation.

4. *The misarticulation of the client.* Consider the type of misarticulation the client demonstrates. The client is accustomed to this motor pattern; it has been practiced for a longer period of time. The new motor task, the norm articulation of the target sound, is relatively new. If the new motor task is put into a phonetic environment similar to the misarticulation, the newly established articulation could be jeopardized. For example, a child's misarticulation of [s] involves a tongue position that is too anterior, an addental or interdental [s] problem. If this [s] is in a word together with [θ], this could trigger the original misarticulation. Or, if the child has a lateral [s], it is probably not a good idea to practice words that contain [l] initially, a lateral sound that might trigger the lateral [s] misarticulation.

MISARTICULATIONS OF [ʃ] AND [ʒ]

In the following section, typical norm and aberrant productions of [ʃ] and [ʒ] are described. Specific phonetic placement and sound modification methods are then addressed. Because [s] and [ʃ] show many similarities in error productions as well as in the diagnostic procedures that would be implemented, the reader is referred back to the section on [s] misarticulations at several points.

Phonetic Description

Phonetically, [s] and [ʃ] are closely related. However, the sagittal groove is considerably wider for [ʃ] than it is for [s] (Fletcher and Newman, 1991). Therefore, the tongue is somewhat flatter for [ʃ] than for [s]. This is one reason why the friction noise for [ʃ] is not as "sharp" as that for [s]. In addition, the place of articulation is not the alveolar ridge, as with the [s]; it is located slightly posterior to it, at the anterior portion of the palate, the postalveolar or prepalatal area. Finally, [ʃ] has lip rounding rather than the lip spreading common for [s] productions. Putting this all together, the phonetic description of [ʃ] is a voiceless coronal-postalveolar or coronal-prepalatal fricative with lip rounding. The voiced counterpart of [ʃ] is [ʒ].

Linguistic Function

Frequency of Occurrence. The voiceless [ʃ] is an infrequent sound ranking twentieth out of the twenty-four General American English consonants. The voiced [ʒ] is the most infrequent sound in General American English, occurring only in words of foreign origin, such as *beige* or *rouge* (Dewey, 1923; French, Carter, and Koenig, 1930; Roberts, 1965).

Phonotactics. Both [ʃ] and [ʒ] can occur initiating and terminating a syllable. There are very few consonant clusters with [ʃ] and [ʒ].

TABLE 8.7 Consonant Clusters with [ʃ] and [ʒ]

WORD-INITIATING [ʃ]	WORD-TERMINATING [ʃ]	WORD-TERMINATING [ʒ]
[ʃr] shrimp, shrub	[rʃ] marsh, harsh [ʃt] washed, wished	[ʒd] rouged, massaged

Table 8.7 provides the more frequent consonant clusters. Word examples are also given.

Morphophonemic Function. Word-final clusters that end in [ʃ] or [ʒ] can be used to signal past tense in regular verbs that end in these sounds, for example, *splashed* and *massaged*.

Minimal Pairs. Frequent sounds that are substituted for [ʃ] and [ʒ] include [s] and [z] and [t] and [d]. Examples of minimal word pairs and sentences are contained in Tables 8.8 and 8.9.

Initial Remarks

Preliminary considerations are similar to those presented for [s]. Thus, hearing acuity, minor structural or functional deviations, and the auditory discrimination abilities of the client need to be assessed before beginning work on the isolated articulation of [ʃ] and [ʒ].

Types of Misarticulation

The most common forms of [ʃ] and [ʒ] misarticulations fall into these categories:

TABLE 8.8 Minimal Pair Words and Sentences Contrasting [ʃ] and [ʒ] to [s] and [z]

[ʃ] VERSUS [s]		[ʒ] VERSUS [z]	[ʃ] VERSUS [s]		[ʒ] VERSUS [z]	
shack	sack	no words found	bash	bass	beige	base
shag	sag		clash	class		
shame	same		gash	gas		
shave	save		leash	lease		
she	see		mesh	mess		
shed	said		plush	plus		
sheep	seep					
sheet	seat					
shell	cell					
shine	sign					
ship	sip					
shock	sock					
shoe	Sue					
shoot	suit					
show	sew					
shy	sigh					
What a *shine*! What a *sign*!			It was a big *bash*. It was a big *bass*.			
The *shell* was very small. The *cell* was very small.			He broke the *leash*. He broke the *lease*.			
It was a large *shock*. It was a large *sock*.			The *clash* was over. The *class* was over.			

TABLE 8.9 Minimal Pair Words and Sentences Contrasting [ʃ] and [ʒ] to [t] and [d]

[ʃ] VERSUS [t]		[ʒ] VERSUS [d]	[ʃ] VERSUS [t]		[ʒ] VERSUS [d]	
shack	tack	no words found	bash	bat	rouge	rude
shag	tag		cash	cat	beige	bade
shake	take		fish	fit		
shape	tape		flash	flat		
sharp	tarp		hash	hat		
she	tea		mash	mat		
shed	Ted		rash	rat		
shell	tell		rush	rut		
ship	tip		wish	wit		
shop	top					
shoe	two					
shoot	toot					

He found a large *shack* in the woods.
He found a large *tack* in the woods.

The *ship* was broken.
The *tip* was broken.

He tried to *shake* it.
He tried to *take* it.

It was a long *shape*.
It was a long *tape*.

She had a funny *wish*.
She had a funny *wit*.

He couldn't find his *cash*.
He couldn't find his *cat*.

What a *fish* he had.
What a *fit* he had.

It was a large *flash*.
It was a large *flat*.

1. *Lateral [ʃ] problems.* Lateral [ʃ] misarticulations demonstrate lateral airflow. This is triggered by (1) a firm contact of the frontal portions of the tongue with the prepalatal area and (2) a lowering of the lateral edges of the tongue. The resulting [ʃ] is auditorily highly conspicuous; there is a noticeable noise component to the sound. Lateral [ʃ] errors can be bilateral or unilateral. Means of verifying laterality have been discussed in the section on [s] problems.

Phonetic transcription of the error: [ʃ] or [ʒ]

2. *Addental [ʃ] problems.* For these misarticulations, the tongue placement is too far forward with the tongue approximating the alveolar ridge rather than the prepalatal area. Reduced medial grooving of the tongue may also be present. If a child demonstrates an addental [s] production, the likelihood exists that [ʃ] may also be addental.

Phonetic transcription of the error: [ʃ] or [ʒ]

3. *Palatal [ʃ] problems.* These productions are characterized by a more posterior tongue articulation: Organ and place of articulation are too far back. There is a shift from coronal-postalveolar or prepalatal to predorsal-medio-palatal (or possibly even mediodorsal-medio-palatal) tongue placement. Because of this, these misarticulations are often perceptually similar to a voiceless [j].

Phonetic transcription of the error: [ç], a voiceless palatal fricative or [ʝ], a voiced palatal fricative

4. *Nasal [ʃ] problems.* These productions are characterized by nasality during the production of [ʃ] and [ʒ]. Comparable to the nasal [s]

problems, the nasality can be functional or organic in nature. The previous discussion for functional nasal [s] problems applies to nasalized [ʃ] as well.

Phonetic transcription of the error: [ʃ̃] or [ʒ̃]

5. *Unrounded [ʃ] productions.* Frequently, children produce [ʃ] with acceptable positioning of organ and place of articulation but without the necessary lip rounding. These productions remain auditorily conspicuous; the sound is "off." Upon noticing the lips of the client during [ʃ], it will become clear that there is no (or not enough) lip rounding.

Phonetic transcription of the error: [ʃ] or [ʒ]

Therapeutic Suggestions

Phonetic Placement. Although most [ʃ] and [ʒ] realizations are produced with the tongue tip up, approximating the area directly behind the alveolar ridge, [ʃ] can also be produced with the tongue tip down behind the lower incisors. As with the tongue tip down [s], the tongue arches upward with the front portion of the tongue approximating the postalveolar or prepalatal area. The following descriptions are given for both tongue tip up (coronal-postalveolar or prepalatal) and tongue tip down (predorsal-prepalatal) [ʃ] and [ʒ].

Phonetic Placement: Coronal-Postalveolar or Prepalatal Placement. For lateral [ʃ], the contact between organ and place of articulation needs to be released. In addition, the lateral edges of the tongue should be elevated, creating a medial groove of the tongue. Techniques suggested for lateral [s] problems can also be used here. However, differences between the production of the [s] and [ʃ] should be kept in mind: for [ʃ], the placement of the tip of the tongue is approximating an area slightly behind the highest point of the alveolar ridge. In addition, there is not as much medial sagittal grooving of the tongue and lip rounding is required.

If the client is demonstrating an addental [ʃ]-production, the tongue tip needs to be slightly retracted. This can be achieved by having the client prolong the addental [ʃ] and then glide the tongue slowly back. The clinician will need to monitor and identify when the change results in an acceptable [ʃ]. Another way to achieve this goal is to push the tongue back with a tongue depressor. Its flat portion is placed interdentally and a gentle attempt is made to displace the blade of the tongue posteriorly.

The tongue placement for palatal [ʃ] is too far back. Thus, during the prolongation of [ʃ], the client should be directed to glide the tongue forward. Medial grooving of the tongue as well as lip rounding should be maintained.

[ʃ] problems resulting from not enough lip rounding require only the addition of lip protrusion during this production. By placing both hands on the cheeks, the client can push the lips forward during the [ʃ] attempts. This manipulation paired with visual and auditory feedback should give the client initial success in achieving a [ʃ] with lip rounding.

Phonetic Placement: Predorsal-Prepalatal Placement. First, the tip of the tongue is placed down touching the inside of the lower incisors. Second, the front portion of the tongue has to arch upward, creating a narrow opening between the predorsal portion of the tongue and the area directly behind the alveolar ridge. A slight medial groove is also necessary; therefore, the lateral edges of the tongue have to come into contact with the upper molars. If these conditions are met, only lip protrusion has to be added in order to realize an acceptable [ʃ].

Sound Modification Methods

1. *[s]-[ʃ] Method.* Because [s] and [ʃ] sounds are phonetically similar, clients who have difficulty with [ʃ] often demonstrate [s] problems as well. If that is the case, this method cannot be used. If [s] is intact, though, the [s]-[ʃ] method would certainly be a good choice. Only lip rounding and a slight retraction of the tongue are initially required. Fortunately, both requirements are often fulfilled simultaneously. If the lips are clearly protruded, the tongue tip has a tendency to retract a bit (Goguillot, 1889; Weinert, 1974). If this natural retraction is still not enough, the client should be instructed to glide the tongue back slightly. If the [ʃ] is still auditorily somewhat off, slight adjustments may need to be made.

2. *[t]-[ʃ] Method.* The main phonetic dissimilarity between [t] and [ʃ] pertains to the manner of articulation: stop versus sibilant fricative. Organ and place of articulation are close enough to be usable.

    a. Begin with a prolonged [t] production (prolonging the implosion phase) with lip protrusion.

    b. Maintaining the lip protrusion, instruct the client to slowly release the [t] while gliding the tongue back slightly.

3. *[tʃ]-[ʃ] Method.* The goal of this method is to isolate the friction portion of the affricate. This can be done in the following manner:

    a. Begin with a very slow production of [tʃ], making sure that lip protrusion is realized.

    b. Instruct the client to lengthen the final fricative portion of the affricate.

Functional Nasal [ʃ] Problems. Each of the following methods must first be evaluated to see if adequate velopharyngeal closure, that is, no hypernasal resonance is noted for the sounds coupled with [ʃ].

1. *[t]-[ʃ].* This is similar to the technique described in functional nasal [s] problems. The addition of lip rounding will be necessary for [ʃ] realizations.

2. *[tʃ]-[ʃ].* First, a forceful [tʃ] is produced, one with an increased buildup of air pressure behind the point of closure. The [t] portion is then slowly released. The client should be instructed that this release should be only minimal. Our goal is a slightly narrower opening between organ and place of articulation than is normally the case with [ʃ] productions. This narrow opening with its increased air pressure should help support the velopharyngeal closure necessary for [ʃ].

Coarticulatory Conditions

When describing context conditions that support regular [ʃ] productions, two questions must be considered: First, is the problem based on difficulties with the tongue placement or is it primarily due to not enough lip rounding? The answer will play a role in the selection of coarticulatory conditions.

If the problem is a result of faulty tongue placement, that is, if addental, palatal, or lateral [ʃ] realizations result, the sequence of supportive vowel coarticulations follows those described for [s]. Thus, the front vowels [i], [ɪ], [eⁱ], [ɛ], and [æ], particularly the high-front vowels [i] and [ɪ], support the relatively high anterior position of the tongue during regular [ʃ] productions.

If the [ʃ] misarticulation is primarily due to a lack of lip rounding, a different coarticulatory sequence is proposed. Now the natural lip rounding of the back vowels would support the articulatory necessities for [ʃ]. The high-back vowels [u] and [ʊ] with the most lip rounding would be especially helpful, followed by [oᵘ] and [ɔ]. Even the central vowels [ɝ] and [ɚ], which are produced with some degree of lip rounding, could support the lip protrusion necessary for [ʃ]. The unrounded features of the low-back vowel [ɑ] and the front vowels would initially not be indicated.

Word Examples. The following one-syllable words are ordered from relatively easy to more difficult coarticulatory conditions:

[ʃ] Words

Primary Problem: Tongue Placement	Primary Problem: Lip Rounding
she - sheep - sheet - she'd - shield	shoe - shoot
ship - shin - shipped - shift	should - shook
shape - shame - shade - shave - shake	show - showed - shown - shore
shed - chef - shell - shelf	sure - shirt
shack - shag - shaft	shot - shawl - shock - shocked - shop
shut - shove	shack - shag - shaft
shop - shot - shawl - shock - shocked	shed - shell - chef - shelf
show - showed - shown - shore	shade - shave - shake - shape - shame
should - shook	shin - shift - ship - shipped
shoe - shoot	she - sheet - she'd - shield - sheep

MISARTICULATIONS OF [k] AND [g]

Many children go through a phase of substituting [t] for [k] and [d] for [g]. For example, Preisser, Hodson, and Paden (1988) reported that this is the most common deviation involving the [k] and [g] sounds in children from 18 to 29 months of age. Some children seem to "get stuck" in this usually short transient period. In spite of a normal progression in other aspects of their speech/language development, they might retain the t/k (d/g) substitution into their preschool or even school years. This poses obvious dangers because the child's enormous increase in vocabulary during this time necessitates the understanding and observation of the phoneme oppositions /t/ versus /k/ and /d/ versus /g/. Many minimal pairs exemplify these contrasts in General American English—*tea* versus *key,* for instance.

Phonetic Description

[k] and [g] are voiceless or voiced postdorsal-velar stops: The back of the tongue is raised, creating a complete blockage of the expiratory airflow at the anterior portion of the velum. A buildup of air pressure occurs until the tongue suddenly moves away from the velum, releasing the air into the oral cavity. Typically, [k] is produced with higher pressure and more tension than [g]. That makes [k] in most cases aspirated and [g] unaspirated. However, the [k] is not usually aspirated in certain context conditions—in word-medial position and as a component of a consonant cluster, for example.

Linguistic Function

Frequency of Occurrence. [k] and [g] occur fairly frequently in General American English. Out of twenty-four consonants, [k] is ranked within the top ten most frequent consonants, while [g] ranks approximately fifteenth (Carterette and Jones, 1974; Mader, 1954; Mines, Hanson, and Shoup, 1978). Frequent word-initiating consonant clusters include [gr], [kw], [kl], and [kr]. Frequent word-final clusters with these sounds are [ks] and [kt] (Dewey, 1923; French, Carter, and Koenig, 1930).

Phonotactics. Both [k] and [g] can occur initiating and terminating a syllable. Most [g] sounds occur initiating words, while [k] sounds are fairly equally distributed across initial, medial, and final word positions (Mader, 1954). Tables 8.10 and 8.11 list the more frequent [k] and [g] consonant clusters with word examples.

Morphophonemic Function. Word-final clusters that end in [ks] or [gz] can be used to signal plurality, as in boo<u>ks</u>, le<u>gs</u>, or do<u>gs</u>. In number and tense marking, [k] occurs with [t]

TABLE 8.10   Consonant Clusters with [k]

WORD-INITIATING		WORD-TERMINATING	
[kl]	clown, clean	[kl]	uncle, tickle
[kr]	cry, crumb	[ks]	box, six
[sk]	school, sky	[kt]	backed, looked
[skr]	scream, scrape	[lk]	milk, silk, elk
[skw]	squeak, squirt	[rk]	dark, work
		[rkt]	worked, parked
		[sk]	ask, desk
		[sks]	asks, disks

TABLE 8.11   Consonant Clusters with [g]

WORD-INITIATING		WORD-TERMINATING	
[gl]	glad, glue	[gz]	pigs, bugs
[gr]	grape, grouch	[gd]	wagged, flagged
[gw]	Gwen, very infrequent		

or [s] to produce words such as p<u>ick</u>ed and p<u>ick</u>s. The [g] preceding either [d] or [z] can also mark number and tense in verbs such as lo<u>gg</u>ed or wa<u>gs</u>. Within phrases, contractible auxiliaries and copulas with the verb *to be* also demonstrate clusters with [k] and [g]. Examples include "the du<u>ck's</u> waddling" and "the do<u>g's</u> barking."

Minimal Pairs.   The most common substitution for [k] and [g] are [t] and [d]. Table 8.12 provides examples of minimal pairs and sentences contrasting these sounds.

Initial Remarks

Due to the fact that [k] and [g] misarticulations are often substitutions of one speech sound for another, it is especially important that the client be evaluated for a phonemic disorder.

TABLE 8.12   Minimal Pair Words and Sentences Contrasting [k] and [g] to [t] and [d]

[k] VERSUS [t]		[k] VERSUS [t]		[g] VERSUS [d]		[g] VERSUS [d]	
cake	take	ache	ate	gate	date	bag	bad
cop	top	back	bat	gown	down	beg	bed
cape	tape	bake	bait	go	doe	bug	bud
cub	tub	beak	beat	got	dot	leg	led
key	tea	bike	bite	gull	dull	sag	sad
kite	tight	knock	knot				
cool	tool	lake	late				
car	tar	like	light				
corn	torn	neck	net				

They didn't like the cold *coast*.	The *cub* was small.	They had a *bake* sale.
They didn't like the cold *toast*.	The *tub* was small.	They had a *bait* sale.
The teacher *caught* the boy.	The *gate* was fixed.	He twisted his *neck*.
The teacher *taught* the boy.	The *date* was fixed.	He twisted his *net*.
He was stuck in the *car*.	There is a scratch on her *back*.	He *likes* it.
He was stuck in the *tar*.	There is a scratch on her *bat*.	He *lights* it.
Hand me the *key*.	The *lock* was big.	Her big brother made her *beg*.
Hand me the *tea*.	The *lot* was big.	Her big brother made her *bed*.

Types of Misarticulation

1. *[t] and [d] substitutions.* These are the most common aberrant productions noted for [k] and [g]: [t] replaces the voiceless [k], while [d] is substituted for the voiced [g]. Thus, the manner of articulation is maintained but the point of contact between organ and place of articulation is moved anteriorly: a coronal-alveolar replaces a postdorsal-velar articulation.

Phonetic transcription of the error: [t] or [d]

2. *Substitution of a postdorsal-velar fricative.* Here the manner of articulation is affected: A narrow opening between organ and place of articulation replaces the complete contact necessary for a stop-plosive production. Thus, the back of the tongue is not raised sufficiently to form the necessary closure. Organ and place of articulation remain the same.

Phonetic transcription of the error: [x], a voiceless postdorsal-velar fricative and [ɣ], a voiced postdorsal-velar fricative.

3. *Substitution of a postdorsal-uvular stop.* The client produces a stop-plosive but the place of articulation is too far back in the mouth. The result is a [k] or [g] that sounds "guttural."

Phonetic transcription of the error: [q], for voiceless and [ɢ], for voiced postdorsal-uvular stops.

Therapeutic Suggestions

Phonetic Placement. In cases of [t] for [k] substitutions, it is necessary to prevent the tip of the tongue and/or its neighboring frontal portions from reaching the alveolar ridge. Therefore, the tip of the tongue must remain down, behind the lower incisors. Visibility offered by a relatively wide opening of the mouth and subsequent observation in an articulation mirror during all phases of the activity can be helpful. This placement may be preceded by tongue exercises that emphasize identifying the front versus the back portions of the tongue, hard palate, and velar areas.

Some clinicians have suggested that the child cough or gargle in an attempt to demonstrate the area of the mouth and tongue involved in the articulation.

Another application is to place the client's little finger sagittally holding down the front half of the tongue while the client produces the "old k-sound." Under this condition, the tip of the tongue is prevented from making contact with the alveolar ridge. If enough of the tongue body is held down (not just the tongue tip but the entire length of the client's little finger should be positioned on the tongue), and the client continues to make a stop-plosive sound, [k] should result.

A similar procedure uses a tongue depressor placed flat and transversely into the child's mouth, the edge of the tongue depressor pushing at the corners of the mouth. The anterior portions of the tongue rest under the tongue depressor. This method is again an attempt to hinder the elevation of the front part of the tongue. With this part of the tongue secure under the tongue depressor, a [t] for [k] substitution is difficult to attain.

If the client produces a *postdorsal-velar fricative* instead of the regular stop production, the manner of articulation must be changed. The client should be instructed about the necessary elevation of the back of the tongue and the explosive release of the obstructed airstream. [t] could be used initially to illustrate the buildup of air pressure and the quick release. During a rather forceful [t] production, the client should note the feeling of the air pressure followed by the burst of air. The emphasis should be on the close contact between organ and place of articulation. The client then tries to duplicate this feeling when producing [k].

For a postdorsal-uvular substitution, the place of articulation must be more anteriorly placed in the oral cavity. Nemoy and Davis

(1937) suggest that the client repeat in a rapid sequence [i]-[k], [i]-[k], [i]-[k], trying to keep the tongue in the [i] position while saying the [k] sound. The pairing of the front vowel [i] with the postdorsal-uvular substitution has a tendency to create a more forward positioning of the tongue.

Sound Modification Methods

1. *[ŋ]-[g] Method.* These two speech sounds are phonetically very similar: Organ and place of articulation are directly comparable; however, [ŋ] is a nasal while [g] is a stop. The easiest way to use this modification method is to have the client:

a. Prolong [ŋ] sound while holding the nostrils closed.

b. Release the buildup of air pressure into the oral cavity; [g] should result. If [k] is the goal, have the child whisper [ŋ] with the same procedure but with an increase in air pressure.

2. *[u]-[k] Method.* This method is based on using the high-back vowel [u] to facilitate the tongue positioning for [k]. Have the client:

a. Prolong [u] and then elevate the back of the tongue.

b. Suggest that the client try to "stop" the sound by blocking it with the back portion of the tongue. The goal is to obtain complete closure between the posterior portion of the tongue and the soft palate.

c. Release the sound. If the tongue positioning for [u] is maintained, an acceptable [k] or [g] should result.

Coarticulatory Conditions

[k] and [g] also demonstrate context-dependent modifications during their productions. In the context of back vowels such as [u] or [ɑ], the articulation is made further back in the mouth. In the context of front vowels,

such as in the word *key,* the point of contact is more frontally located (Shriberg and Kent, 1995). These modifications can be used to structure coarticulatory conditions that support specific production goals.

If the goal is to move the organ and place of articulation posteriorly, for example, when a [t] for [k] substitution is realized, combining [k] with the back vowels [u], [ʊ], [oᵘ], [ɔ], and [ɑ] will be advantageous. During the production of back vowels, the posterior portion of the tongue is elevated, supporting the placement necessary for [k]. The front vowels do not provide this coarticulatory support. In fact, the high front vowels pose an additional danger in this respect. Due to the influence of the high frontal tongue placement for these vowels, the client might be tempted to revert back to the [t] substitution. With a t/k substitution, the phonetically supportive vowel sequence follows the order high-back, mid-back, low-back, central, low-front, mid-front, high-front.

If the goal is a more anterior tongue position, as in the substitution of a postdorsal-uvular stop for [k] and [g], the opposite vowel sequence would be indicated. In this case, the front vowels would aid a more anterior placement with the sequence high-front, mid-front, low-front, central, low-back, mid-back, followed by high-back vowels.

It seems advisable to let [g] follow [k] in the sequencing of therapy; the lesser degree of overall muscular effort together with the voicing component make [g] usually more difficult to achieve. According to personal clinical experience, a coarticulatory condition that seems to support [g] articulation is not a vowel context but an abutting consonant. Often in the context of [ŋ], as in the word *finger,* clients have produced a standard [g] that was not evidenced in other g-words. Verification of this observation will come from the particular client. It is always worth a trial period to search for individually based starting points.

Word Examples. The following one-syllable words are ordered from relatively easy to more difficult coarticulatory conditions for a child with a t/k substitution.

[k] Words	*[g] Words*
coo - coop - cool - cooed*-cooled*	goof - goose - goofs
could*	good* - goods*
cope - comb - cove - coal - coach - coat*	go - goal - goes - ghost* - gold*
cop - cob - cough - call - caught* - cart*	gong - gob - gone - gauze - got*
cup - cub - come - cuff - cut*	gum - gull - Gus - gush - gulp
curb - curve - curl - Kurt*	girl
cap - cab - can - car - calf - cash - cat*	gang - gap - gab - gas - gash
Ken - kept* - Kent*	guess - get* - guest*
Kay - cape - came - cane - cave - cage	gay - game - gave - gain - gate*
king - Kim - kiss - kit* - kid*	give - gill - gift* - guilt*
key - keep - keen - keel	geese

Words marked with an asterisk (*) are those containing [t] and [d]. These words will probably need to be evaluated to determine if the coarticulatory influence of [t] and [d] will have an impact on the newly acquired [k] and [g].

MISARTICULATIONS OF [l]

Problems with [l] productions are common in the speech of 3- and 4-year-old children (Prather, Hedrick, and Kern, 1975; Sander, 1972; Vihman and Greenlee, 1987). By age 4;6 to 5, normally developing children demonstrate a decrease in [l] misarticulations (Haelsig and Madison, 1986). Aberrant articulations include substitutions of [w] and [j] for [l]. Due to the relatively high frequency of oc-currence of [l] in General American English, misarticulations are also fairly conspicuous errors.

Phonetic Description

[l] sounds are phonetically described as voiced apico-alveolar laterals. During most [l] realizations, the tip of the tongue, the most frontal part of the corona, touches the alveolar ridge. The neighboring coronal areas are relaxed, allowing air to escape laterally. Whereas some articulatory modifications do occur—for example, typical changes take place when [l] is in word-initial versus word-final positions—the main feature for [l], that is, a laterally free passage for the expiratory airway, remains constant.

Common descriptions of [l] realizations state that the free lateral passage exists on both sides, that is, bilaterally. However, Faircloth and Faircloth (1973) confirm that during spontaneous speech and under certain articulatory conditions, [l] can be realized unilaterally. Heffner (1975) describes the unilateral production as a common [l] realization. Because very little air actually escapes through the lateral openings, a unilaterally free passage will usually result in a perfectly acceptable auditory [l] impression. Quite in contrast to the escape of air during lateral [s] misarticulations, the lateral airflow during [l] realizations is so minimal, its pressure so low, that our tapping method (see the section concerning lateral [s]-misarticulations on p. 225) will not suffice to detect it.

There are two [l] varieties in English, the so-called "light" (or "clear") and the "dark" [l]. Different authors have categorized the production features of the two types in various ways. Some distinguished between them using the location of the tongue tip (Wise, 1958), while others have discussed the qualitative differences (Heffner, 1975). The "light"

[l] has an [ɪ] quality that results from a convex shape of the tongue, especially its frontal portion near the palatal or prepalatal area (Heffner, 1975). The "dark" [l] has an [ʊ] or [o] quality that is caused by the elevation of the tongue's posterior portion (Shriberg and Kent, 1995). This high-back elevation produces a concave upper surface of the tongue behind the alveolar occlusion. Light l-sounds are transcribed [l], while dark l-sounds are symbolized [ɫ].

Although both [l] varieties represent one single phoneme in English, /l/, their usage is nevertheless regulated: Light [l] is typically realized in the initial word position when /l/ precedes a vowel or follows an initial consonant—for example, in the words *like, leap, play,* and *sleep.* Dark [ɫ] is found in word-final positions, as syllabics, and when it precedes a consonant (Heffner, 1975). Examples include the words *full, bottle,* and *told.* Occasional lack of tongue tip contact has also been noted in [l] following a vowel in word-final position (Giles, 1971). This becomes important to clinicians when evaluating children. If the tongue tip contact is not established, for example in the word *wheel,* the final [l] might assume an [o] or [ʊ] quality. Shriberg and Kent (1995) note that "caution should be observed in evaluating the child's proficiency for /l/ articulation. It is prudent to test /l/ production in more than one context or syllabic position before ascribing the /o/-like sound to an articulatory error" (p. 71).

Linguistic Function

Frequency of Occurrence. [l] is a frequent sound in General American English, ranked eighth in children's speech and fifth in adult's speech (Carterette and Jones, 1974; Mines, Hanson, and Shoup, 1978). Frequent word-initial clusters include [pl], [kl], and [bl], and [ld] and [lz] are commonly occurring word-

TABLE 8.13 Consonant Clusters with [l]

WORD-INITIATING		WORD-TERMINATING	
[bl]	black, blue	[lb]	bulb
[fl]	flower, flake	[ld]	mild, gold
[gl]	glue, glad	[lf]	Ralph, golf
[kl]	clean, clown	[lk]	milk, elk
[pl]	play, plane	[lm]	film, elm
[sl]	sled, slide	[lp]	help, gulp
[spl]	splash, splinter	[ls]	false, pulse
		[lt]	belt, salt
		[lθ]	health, filth
		[lv]	shelve, twelve
		[lz]	bells, dolls
		[ldz]	folds, worlds
		[lts]	belts, adults
		[lvd]	solved, shelved
		[lvz]	shelves, wolves

final clusters (Dewey, 1923; French, Carter, and Koenig, 1930; Roberts, 1965).

Phonotactics. [l] is realized in all word positions although, as previously noted, allophonic variations exist that are in part dependent on the sound's position within the word. According to Mader (1954), [l] occurs more frequently in medial and final word positions than when initiating a word. Table 8.13 lists the most frequent consonant clusters with [l].

Morphophonemic Function. The consonant cluster [lz] is used to signal plurality (do<u>lls</u>, ha<u>lls</u>), possessive (Ji<u>ll's</u>, Bi<u>ll's</u>), third person singular (he sai<u>ls</u>, she ro<u>lls</u>), and contractible auxiliaries and copulas (The ba<u>ll's</u> rolling. The do<u>ll's</u> little.). The consonant cluster [ld] signals past tense, as in sai<u>led</u> or ro<u>lled</u>.

Minimal Pairs. Common substitutions for [l] are [r], [w], and [j]. Table 8.14 contains minimal pair words and sentences exemplifying these substitutions.

Initial Remarks

Distortions and substitutions are common [l] errors. Typical substitutions include w/l, j/l, and r/l. Because these substitutions are phonemically relevant, it is important to establish whether they represent phonemic difficulties. This information should be the basis for any therapeutic decision. Also, knowledge of the articulatory features of the misarticulated [l] needs to be secured. This should include probes into contexts that would promote light and dark [l] realizations. Because their articulation is different, one type may be closer to norm production than the other.

Types of Misarticulation

1. *w/l substitution.* In word-initial position, this production is marked by the substitution of [w] for [l], as in [wæmp] for *lamp*. Because of the elevation of the back of the tongue for dark /l/ in word-final position, the substitution often has a back vowel quality, as in [teɪboʊ] for *table*.

Phonetic transcription of the error: Initiating a word or syllable: [w]; terminating a word or syllable: typically a mid-back vowel.

2. *j/l substitution.* In this substitution, a [j]-like sound replaces [l], thus, [jæmp] for *lamp*. [j] substitutions are usually heard only in word- or syllable-initial position, as in [hɛjoʊ] for *hello*. If this is a phonetically based problem, the client probably realizes that somewhat different [l] articulations are used in word-initial versus word-final position; that is, the client "understands" the contextual rules governing the allophonic [l] variations. In addition, [j] does not exist in word-final position in General American English; it always precedes a vowel. Clients with a phonetic disorder will not violate this phonotactic constraint. Therefore, in word-final position, the client will try to modify [l] accordingly. The result may again resemble a back vowel.

TABLE 8.14 Minimal Pair Words and Sentences Contrasting [l] to [r], [w], and [j]

[l] VERSUS [r]		[l] VERSUS [ɚ]		[l] VERSUS [w]		[l] VERSUS [j]	
lace	race	bowl	boar	lag	wag	lung	young
lane	rain	Dale	dare	life	wife	loose	use
led	red	feel	fear	lake	wake	lard	yard
lick	Rick	male	mare	leave	weave	Lou	you
long	wrong	mole	more	leap	weep	less	yes
lie	rye	owl	our	leak	weak	let	yet
light	right	tile	tire	light	white		
lead	read			let	wet		
lock	rock						

She knew it was the *long* way home.
She knew it was the *wrong* way home.

He stumbled on the *lock.*
He stumbled on the *rock.*

What a *deal!*
What a *dear!*

The *tile* needed to be replaced.
The *tire* needed to be replaced.

He didn't want to *leave.*
He didn't want to *weave.*

Lou cannot come to the party.
You cannot come to the party.

It was a *light* coat.
It was a *white* coat.

The *lung* fish swam in the aquarium.
The *young* fish swam in the aquarium.

Phonetic transcription of the error: Initiating a word or syllable: [j]; terminating a word or syllable: typically a mid-back vowel.

3. *r/l substitution.* In this substitution, a sound resembling [r] replaces [l], as in [ræmp] for *lamp*. [r] substitutions are typically heard in word- or syllable-initial positions only. While [r] realizations show a considerable amount of variability in their articulatory features, [r] never has coronal contact with the alveolar ridge as [l] does.

Phonetic transcription of the error: Initiating a word or syllable: [r]; terminating a word or syllable: typically a back or central vowel.

4. *l-distortion.* A common [l] distortion is created by too small an opening for lateral air escape. Lateral openings that are too small, when combined with increased air pressure, can often cause an undue friction noise during [l] productions.

Phonetic transcription of the error: [ɮ], a voiced lateral fricative

Therapeutic Suggestions

Phonetic Placement.   For norm productions of [l], the apex and coronal edges of the tongue are in direct contact with the alveolar ridge. The lateral edges of the tongue are not elevated but rather relaxed, allowing free passage of the air to the right and left of the contact at the alveolar ridge. Visibility of the articulatory events is often very helpful when establishing the placement of an isolated sound. Because visibility for most [l] productions is limited, a wide open-mouth posture can enhance it. Under this condition, the tip of the tongue should touch the alveolar ridge in such a way that a good portion of the tongue's underside becomes visible.

For w/l substitutions, the client must first realize that the lip protrusion of [w] is not present on [l]. Lip exercises numbers 1 through 5 (Box 8.2) or observation of the lips during production of [u]-[i] might help the client understand that there is no lip rounding during [l] productions. Next, tongue contact with the alveolar ridge needs to be established. The edges of the tongue should be relaxed; for example, the client could be instructed to make a "flat tongue" and then to raise the tip of the flattened tongue to the alveolar ridge. If the posterior elevation of the tongue for [w] is carried over to the [l], the client's initial realization might resemble the dark l-sound. While this [ɫ] may sound somewhat "off" in word- or syllable-initial positions, the quality should become auditorily more acceptable if it is preceded by a vowel.

If a j/l substitution is used, the client must be instructed that the tongue tip needs to touch the alveolar ridge. Because the placement of the dorsum of the tongue is fairly similar for [j] and [l], this may be the only articulatory adjustment necessary. If the resulting [l] approximation has a frictionlike component, the lateral edges of the tongue will need to be lowered to allow more airflow.

The primary consideration for r/l substitutions is contact of the tip of the tongue with the alveolar ridge. In addition, if the client is using a bunched [r], the dorsum of the tongue needs to be more forward. This more forward placement could be established by using the following [i]-[l] sound modification method.

For l-distortions caused by limited lateral airflow, the main goal is lowering the lateral edges. The edges of the tongue need to be relaxed and somewhat flattened. With a mirror and a wide-open mouth posture, the client should first practice a flattened tongue versus a rolled tongue. When this has been achieved, the tongue tip should be placed on the alveolar ridge, again trying to distinguish between a flattened versus a rolled tongue posture.

A passive method of lowering the lateral edges of the tongue is as follows: Place a narrow ribbon (approximately 1/2 inch wide) flat crosswise over the front of the tongue so that the ends hang down on each side to at least the bottom of the client's chin. Next, have the client place the tip of the tongue firmly against the alveolar ridge. During the client's attempts to produce [l], both ends of the ribbon are pulled down gently. If everything is introduced and executed properly, this will bring the rims of the tongue down, allowing lateral air flow (Gutzmann, 1912; Waengler and Bauman-Waengler, 1985).

Sound Modification Methods

1. *[d]-[l] Method.* Organ and place of articulation for these two sounds are very similar; the manner of articulation, though, is different.

    a. Use the previously mentioned method of pulling the lateral edge of the tongue down during [d] production. A second possibility:

    b. During the stop phase of [d], the client should release the air without losing the tongue tip-alveolar contact.

2. *[n]-[l] Method.* Again, only the manner of articulation distinguishes these two sounds: nasal versus lateral.

    a. Utilize the same procedure as described for the [d]-[l] method, but the client's nostrils need to be pinched closed during the [n] production.

    By employing the nasal [n], an additional factor is introduced—the change from nasal to oral resonance. This needs to be considered before implementing this modification method.

3. *[i]-[l] Method.* This method is based on similarities between the [i] and the light [l] productions.

    a. Prolong [i] ([ɪ] can also be used) while moving the tongue tip to the alveolar ridge. Although production similarities exist between [i] or [ɪ] and the light [l], this method does not offer much visual feedback for the client if an articulation mirror is being used. If visibility is important, the [ɑ] -[l] method might be a better choice.

4. *[ɑ]-[l] Method.*

    a. Prolong [ɑ] with a wide-open mouth posture.

    b. Elevate the tongue tip to the alveolar ridge. Not only is visibility good with this open mouth posture, it also helps to lower the lateral edges.

Coarticulatory Conditions

Favorable coarticulatory conditions, specifically the sequence of vowels that support regular [l] articulations, will depend on the goal to be achieved. If visibility is important, low vowels might be our choice. This allows the client a means of visual control which can be continued until [l] is somewhat stabilized. A desirable sequence of context exercises might begin with the low-back vowel [ɑ], continuing with the low-front vowel [æ]. Mid-front vowels [ɛ] and [eⁱ] and mid-back vowels [ɔ] and [oᵁ] would still offer some visibility if produced with a relatively open mouth posture. Because of the possible coarticulatory influence of the lip rounding, if the client demonstrates a w/l substitution, the mid- and high-back vowels will probably be the last in our sequence.

In the case of [l] distortions based on too small an opening for lateral air escape, the back vowels will probably be our choice. The slightly concave shape of the tongue supports the relaxing of the lateral edges. Here, the dark [l] in word-final position may be easier for our client to achieve.

If the later goal is production of both light *and* dark /l/, two coarticulatory conditions need to be considered; first, the position of /l/ within the word, second, the tendency for certain vowels to promote light versus dark [l] sounds. Back vowels, especially high-back vowels, coarticulatorily support the dark [l], while front vowels, especially high-front vowels, aid the production of light [l]. Depending on our momentary goal, light [l] or dark [ɫ], the sequence of vowels will have to vary. For the coarticulatory support of light [l] articulations, the sequence could be [l] + : high-front, mid-front, low-front, central, low-back, mid-back, and high-back vowels. The opposite sequence is suggested preceding dark [ɫ] realizations: high-back, mid-back, low-back, central, low-front, mid-front, and high-front vowels.

Several supportive coarticulatory possibilities have been suggested. Based on our momentary goal, different vowel sequences were considered. However, the order of supporting coarticulatory circumstances for the new sound achievement must be determined by whatever is easiest for our client to attain.

Word Examples. The following one-syllable words are ordered from relatively easy to more difficult coarticulatory conditions for a child with an [l] problem. Word examples are given for both light and dark /l/.

Words with Light l-sounds	Words with Dark l-sounds
Lee - leap - leaf - leave - leak - leash	pool - tool - fool - cool - school - spool
limb - lip - lid - lit - lick - live	wool* - bull - pull - full
lay - lame - late - laid - lake - lace	bowl - pole - foal - goal - coal
led - let - leg - ledge - left - lend	all - hall - ball - mall - doll - fall - call
lamb - lad - laugh - lag - lamp	hull - dull - gull - skull pal
lug - luck - love - lump - lunch	bell - tell - fell - sale - shell
law - lot - loss - log - long - lock	mail - bale - pail - Dale - nail - sale - jail
low - load - loan - loaf - loaves	ill - hill - will* - Bill - pill - fill - gill
look - looked	eel - heel - meal - deal - kneel - feel
Lou - loom - loop - loon - loot - Luke	

*If the child had a w/l substitution, these words would need to be evaluated to see whether the initial [w] might negatively impact [l] articulations.

MISARTICULATIONS OF [r] AND THE CENTRAL VOWELS WITH R-COLORING

The misarticulations in this section include those occurring with the consonantal r-sound, as in *rabbit* or *red* and/or the central vowels with r-coloring, [ɝ] and [ɚ] as in *bird* or *father*. If children have difficulty producing "r-qualities," they typically demonstrate problems with both consonantal [r] and central vowels with r-coloring (Shriberg, 1975; 1980).

Consonantal [r] develops relatively late; it is frequently still in error during the preschool years (Irwin and Wong, 1983, Kenney and Prather, 1986; Olmsted, 1971). Irwin and Wong (1983) reported that, even at age 6, only 82 percent of all [r] realizations were correct in spontaneous speech.

The central vowels with r-coloring appear to be among the last, if not the last, vowels to be mastered. Data from the Irwin and Wong (1983) study using spontaneous speech demonstrated that the central vowels with r-coloring were the last vowels to reach a fairly high percentage of norm realization. At age 3, children attained accuracy with both of these vowels only 70 percent of the time, while at age 4, accuracy levels with [ɚ] were still below 90 percent.

Although it is expected that r-sounds (both consonantal and central vowels with r-coloring) are "mastered" by school-age, there are children who persist in their difficulties with them. Typical problems include substitutions of consonantal [r] in word- or syllable-initial positions and derhotacization or vowelization of the central vowels with r-coloring.

Phonetic Description

Consonantal [r]. There are many forms of [r] articulations in General American English. In fact, /r/ might well be the most variable consonant of our language. In different contexts, the same speaker may use various tongue and lip positions when producing this sound. The different types of [r] productions are usually placed into two broad categories, the bunched and the retroflexed [r] (Shriberg and Kent, 1995).

The bunched [r] is phonetically classified as a voiced mediodorsal-mediopalatal rhotic. For this production, the corpus of the tongue is elevated toward the palate while the tongue tip points downward. The voiced expiratory air escapes sagittally through this fairly wide passage. The sides of the tongue touch the bicuspids and molars. This tongue position may vary with the vowel context and lip rounding may be present.

The retroflexed [r] is phonetically classified as a voiced apico-prepalatal rhotic. The tip of the tongue points to the alveolar ridge or its neighboring prepalatal areas. Because the lateral edges of the tongue are raised, preventing lateral air escape, the voiced expiratory air is again channelled sagittally out of the oral cavity. During this action, the dorsum of the tongue is somewhat depressed. This makes the elevation of the tip of the tongue appear even more pronounced. Often, the tip of the tongue might even be slightly bent backwards or curled up. Such an articulatory position gave these [r] realizations their characteristic name: retroflexed.

Although /r/ is extremely variable in its production features, it is therapeutically helpful to recognize some frequent allophonic variations that occur in General American English. After [θ], the [r] can be produced as a trill. The term **trill** depicts the sound produced by the vibratory action of an organ of articulation tapping rapidly against a place of articulation, in this case the tongue tip against the alveolar ridge. After [t], [r] may have a fricativelike quality. This is caused by the preceding [t], which in its release phase creates a closer approximation between organ and place of articulation than is normally the case. Also, following

The [r] is classified as a rhotic sound. But such a term refers actually just to the seventeenth letter of the Greek alphabet, rho, and says nothing about production features. Together with [l], [r] is also often referred to as a liquid. This term does not designate the phonetic features of [r] productions either. To emphasize the production features, some authors have included [r] (along with [w], [j], and [l]) in the manner of articulation known as approximants (Abercrombie, 1967; International Phonetic Alphabet, 1993; Ladefoged, 1993). Such a label indicates that an organ of articulation approaches a place of articulation, keeping a large enough distance from it so that a friction noise does not result.

voiceless consonants, such as in the words *try, cry,* and *fry,* [r] may be partially devoiced.

Central Vowels with R-Coloring. [ɝ] and [ɚ] have been called rhotic or rhotacized vowels and retroflexed vowels. The term *r-colored* or *rhotacized vowels* describes their perceptual quality: They appear to contain r-features. The second term, *retroflexed,* refers to a possible tongue position during their production. Because these vowels are by no means always produced with a retroflexed tongue articulation, this label is somewhat imprecise.

The central vowel [ɝ] occurs in stressed syllables of words and is usually produced with some degree of lip rounding. [ɚ] is the unstressed counterpart of [ɝ]. Both vowels show similar articulations, although lip rounding may be lacking when producing [ɚ]. Based on the results of palatography, Fletcher (1992) noted that tongue actions for the rhotic vowels are similar to those for the rhotic consonants. The r-like vowels can be produced in two ways. First, the tongue might be curled upward and backward in a retroflexed position. Second, the tip might be dropped down, the body of the tongue bunched and moved posteriorly in the mouth. These articulations are comparable to the "retroflexed" and "bunched" consonantal [r] productions previously discussed.

Linguistic Function

Frequency of Occurrence. Both consonantal [r] and the central vowels with r-coloring are frequent sounds in General American English. According to Carterette and Jones (1974), they are the second most frequently occurring sound category. There are many consonant clusters with [r], which are also prevalent. These include [pr], [tr], [fr], and [gr] word-initially and [rd], [rt], [rn], and [rz] word-finally (Dewey, 1923; French, Carter and Koenig, 1930; Roberts, 1965).

Phonotactics. While the consonantal [r] occurs initiating syllables or in specific clusters, the central vowels with r-coloring function as syllable nuclei. Many of the noted word-final [r] clusters, such as [rn] and [rt], contain [ɝ] (e.g., *turn, hurt*) or can be transcribed as centering diphthongs preceding a consonant (e.g., *barn, farm*); they are therefore technically not consonant clusters. However, because they are included on many consonant cluster lists, they will also be included in Table 8.15 for the purpose at hand.

Minimal Pairs. The most frequent substitutions for [r] include [w], [j], and [l]. Table 8.16 contains examples of minimal pair words and sentences with these phonemic oppositions.

Initial Remarks

Because several misarticulations of the consonantal [r] include substitutions of one phoneme for another, it is important that the phonemic system of the client be evaluated. Dialectal variations should also be examined. Dialects that characteristically lose r-coloring on central vowels include Southern, South Midland, eastern New England, and African

American or Black English Vernacular (Flexner, 1987; Iglesias and Anderson, 1995; Williams and Wolfram, 1977).

TABLE 8.15 Consonant Clusters with [r]

WORD-INITIATING		WORD-TERMINATING	
[br]	bread, broom	[rb]	Herb, curb
[dr]	dream, drink	[rd]	bird, card
[fr]	frog, friend	[rg]	iceberg, Pittsburgh
[gr]	grass, grouch	[rk]	fork, Mark
[kr]	Craig, cry	[rl]	Karl, girl
[pr]	prune, prince	[rm]	arm, worm
[ʃr]	shrimp, shrub	[rn]	barn, learn
[tr]	train, truck	[rp]	burp, chirp
		[rs]	nurse, horse
[skr]	scream, scratch	[rʃ]	harsh, kirsch
[spr]	spring, sprite	[rt]	dirt, short
[str]	straw, strong	[rv]	serve, starve
		[rz]	doors, ears
		[rdʒ]	large, George
		[rkt]	worked, parked
		[rlz]	girls, Charles
		[rst]	first, pierced
		[rts]	shirts, sports
		[rtʃ]	March, birch

CLINICAL APPLICATION

Dialect and R-Problems

The dialect of the family should always be considered when evaluating younger clients. For example, in the Midwest, a diagnostic situation presented itself in which the client demonstrated a lack of r-coloring on all rhotic vowels. The clinician was first convinced that the child had "r-problems" until she met the mother and father. Both parents, who had lived most of their lives in Boston, spoke in a similar manner. Derhotacization was a characteristic of their eastern New England dialect.

TABLE 8.16 Minimal Pair Words and Sentences Contrasting [r] with [l], [w], and [j]

[r] VERSUS [l]		[r] VERSUS [l]		[r] VERSUS [w]		[r] VERSUS [j]	
race	lace	boar	bowl	rag	wag	rung	young
rain	lane	dare	Dale	rail	whale	ram	yam
red	led	fear	feel	rake	wake	rank	yank
Rick	lick	mare	male	rate	wait	rot	yacht
wrong	long	more	mole	red	wed	rear	year
rye	lie	our	owl	ray	way	roar	your
right	light	tire	tile	right	white		
read	lead			rent	went		
rock	lock			ring	wing		
				ripe	wipe		
				ride	wide		
				raced	waste		
				rest	west		
				round	wound		
				rake	wake		
				run	won		

It was a long *rain.*
It was a long *lane.*

She won the *race* at the county fair.
She won the *lace* at the county fair.

He walked to the *right.*
He walked to the *light.*

He *feels* the earthquake.
He *fears* the earthquake.

Across the field ran a large *mare.*
Across the field ran a large *male.*

The *ring* was broken.
The *wing* was broken.

The athletes always *run.*
The athletes always *won.*

She didn't want to *wake* it up.
She didn't want to *rake* it up.

The *rot* was moldy and damp.
The *yacht* was moldy and damp.

Roar loud, he said.
You're loud, he said.

Types of Misarticulation

1. *w/r substitutions.* w/r substitutions represent the most common substitution for consonantal [r]. In some cases, perceived substitutions may not be actual substitutions of [w] for [r]. What is interpreted as a [w] or [w]-like sound may well just be a derhotacized [r] (Shriberg and Kent, 1995).

Phonetic transcription of the error: If it is a sound substitution, [w]. If the quality is somewhere between [w] and [r], then [ɹ], indicating a derhotacized [r], would be a better choice. (See following section on derhotacization of [r].)

2. *j/r substitutions.* With this substitution, a [j]-like sound is produced instead of the consonantal [r].

Phonetic transcription of the error: [j]

3. *l/r substitutions.* This misarticulation is characterized by [l] replacing the consonantal [r], as in [lɛd] for *red.*

Transcription of the error: [l]

4. *Derhotacization of [r] and central vowels with r-coloring.* These distortions/substitutions lack the characteristic r-quality. Clinical impressions range from a "trace of r coloring to almost r" (Shriberg and Kent, 1995, p. 236). According to Shriberg and Kent (1995), derhotacized [r] realizations (transcribed as [ɹ]) represent the most common error of these sounds in school-age children and adults. Derhotacized central vowels also lose their r-quality; [ɝ] is perceived as [ɜ], while [ɚ] sounds like [ə]. The articulatory component necessary to produce the particular [r] resonance is lacking. Fletcher (1992) stated that children often substitute lip rounding for front tongue actions during attempts to produce the rhotics. This results in an [o]- or [ʊ]-like quality.

Therapeutic Suggestions

Phonetic Placement: [r]. Two possibilities offer themselves for phonetic placement therapy with [r]: (1) the apical-alveolar "retroflexed" or (2) the mediodorsal-mediopalatal "bunched" [r] articulation. The retroflexed [r] is often easier to implement because its features can be explained more easily. The choice of retroflexed or bunched [r] will depend on the client and the type of aberrant production presented.

Apico-Prepalatal Retroflexed Articulation. The client is instructed to elevate the front of the tongue so that the tongue tip is pointing behind the alveolar ridge. The tongue tip should come close to the area behind the alveolar ridge but should not touch it. The posterior edges of the tongue are in contact with the upper molars. Selected tongue exercises might be helpful preceding this placement attempt. First, instruct the client to glide the tongue, which is touching the alveolar ridge, forward and backward, "sweeping" the palatal area. Next, instruct the client to execute, with a slightly open mouth posture, the same action but this time *without* touching the palatal area. If, at the same time, the back edges of

the tongue are raised and voicing is added, an r-like quality might be heard when the client moves the tongue slowly backward from the area below the alveolar ridge to the palate.

An additional consideration for the client using w/r substitutions is lip rounding. Although some degree of lip rounding is usually present during retroflexed [r] productions as well, care needs to be taken that this rounding does not trigger [w]. In addition, if the client's productions continue to give a [w] impression, the clinician needs to make sure that the back portion of the tongue is not elevated. Under the condition of a fairly wide open-mouth posture, for example, it will be more difficult for the client to maintain a high-back tongue position.

For j/r substitutions, the elevated tongue tip becomes an important factor. [j] is characterized by a convex shape of the tongue with the midportion of the dorsum coming very close to the midportion of the palate. The retroflexed [r], on the other hand, is marked by a concave shape of the front and mediodorsal portions of the tongue with the tongue tip pointing into the direction of the prepalatal area.

When [l] is substituted for [r], two changes must be achieved for a norm [r]: (1) release the contact between the tongue tip and the alveolar ridge and (2) raise the lateral edges of the tongue so that airflow is directed medially. Tongue exercises noted in the section on the phonetic placement of the apico-prepalatal retroflexed articulation may also prove helpful here.

Mediodorsal-Mediopalatal Bunched Placement. The bunched [r] is produced with the tongue tip down while central portions of the tongue's body are elevated. The characteristic rhotic resonance is created by a voiced medial-sagittal airflow over the relatively broad surface of the tongue. The client should be instructed to lower the tongue tip so that it rests on the top of the lower incisors. The client must also be aware that the lateral edges of the tongue need to touch the upper molars. A practice progression might start with the client articulating [d], noting how the back portions of the tongue touch the molars. Next, the tongue tip should be lowered, leaving the back of the tongue in the same position. Finally, the whole body of the tongue, including the tongue tip, must be moved backward, posteriorly. The necessary change could be aided by gently pushing back the tip of the tongue with a tongue depressor so that the mediodorsal portion of the dorsum becomes more elevated.

To move from [w] to a bunched [r], two steps need to be accomplished: (1) the lips need to be retracted slightly and (2) the elevation of the tongue's dorsum needs to be more anteriorly located. First, have the client try a "small smile" while saying [w]. Next, while prolonging this [w], have the client slowly move the whole body of the tongue forward. Because it is difficult to define production elements of "rhotic resonance," the clinician may need to experiment with varying tongue positions to attain an acceptable [r] quality.

If the client substitutes [j] for [r], organ and place of articulation remain the same; both are considered mediodorsal-mediopalatal consonants. However, the manner of articulation needs to be somewhat modified. When comparing [j] to [r] in this respect, the distance between organ and place of articulation is smaller for [j]. Therefore, for [r], the dorsum of the tongue must be lowered slightly. One could also achieve the larger distance between organ and place of articulation by lowering the jaw during the [j] production. In addition, the medial groove of the tongue is more pronounced for [r]. To achieve this, the client could roll the tongue after having lowered the tongue's dorsum.

If the [r] substitution is [l], the contact between the tip of the tongue and the alveolar ridge must first be released, that is, the tongue tip must be dropped. In addition, the lateral edges of the tongue must be slightly elevated to prevent lateral airflow. Finally, the dorsum of the tongue must be moved back.

Central Vowels with R-Coloring. The central tongue position is the primary articulatory feature of the vowels [ɝ] and [ɚ]. However, their important additional characteristic is r-coloring. This r-coloring is similar to the main feature of consonantal [r]; there are therefore two ways to achieve the r-quality for [ɝ] and [ɚ]: retroflexed or bunched tongue formations. If the vowels are perceived as lacking r-coloring, the individual does not realize either a retroflexed tongue position or an adequate bunching of the central portions of the tongue (Secord, 1981b). If the client is substituting ɜ/ɝ and ə/ɚ, only this r-coloring needs to be added. During the respective vowel productions, the client should either (1) point the tongue tip in the direction of the prepalatal area or (2) push the tongue posteriorly, creating more of a bulge in the tongue's midsection. Instructions at the beginning of the phonetic placement techniques for the retroflexed and bunched [r] sounds may prove helpful.

Sound Modification Methods: [r] and Central Vowels with R-Coloring. Several of the following modification methods utilize sounds that were noted as substitutions for [r]. For example, a client may have a j/r substitution, and [j] is one of the sounds that can be modified to an [r]. Substituting one of these sounds for [r] does not eliminate the possibility of modifying it to a norm [r] articulation. In fact, this may prove to be a relatively effective way to achieve a regular [r].

1. *[d]-[r] Method.* With this sound modification method, the goal is a retroflexed r-sound. The client is instructed to:

a. Produce [d] followed by the central vowel [ʌ]. Normally, the tongue tip drops straight down from the release of the [d] to the vowel.

b. Glide the tongue tip back, pointing into the direction of the prepalatal area. The tongue tip should not touch the palate but rather the movement should follow the release of the [d]; that is, the tongue tip should drop and then move back. The [d] production as a point of departure for [r] also underlines the necessary contact of the posterior edges of the tongue with the molars. This will in turn aid the elevation of the lateral edges of the tongue, which reinforces the [r] resonance.

2. *[l]-[r] Method.* The end product of this sound modification method is again a retroflexed [r]. The steps necessary to modify the articulation from [l] to [r] are outlined in the section on phonetic placement of the retroflexed [r]-sound: l/r substitutions.

3. *[j]-[r] Method.* A higher degree of phonetic similarity exists between [j] and the bunched r-sound than between [j] and the retroflexed production. The steps needed to modify the articulation from [j] to [r] are outlined in the section on phonetic placement of the bunched [r]-sound: j/r substitutions.

4. *[ɝ] or [ɚ]-[r] Method.* Clients who have difficulty with [r] usually show problems with the r-colored central vowels as well. If, however, a clinician decides to work on the consonantal [r] and the client does have acceptable productions of the central vowels with r-coloring, a transfer of this r-coloring would be the method of choice. If the client has [ɝ] and [ɚ] but not [r], a word could be specifically divided to elicit the [r] sound. For example, the client could begin with the

word *purr.* Then, the client tries *purring.* Next, a pause is made in the word: *pu-rring.* Finally, the last syllable is isolated as *ring*: a consonantal [r] is achieved.

CLINICAL APPLICATION

When to Initiate Therapy with R-Problems

A clinical decision must be made if the client has either the r-colored central vowels or the consonantal [r], but not both. Should the clinician initiate "r" therapy? The fact that the r-coloring is somehow present should make this an easy sound to remediate. Or should the clinician wait and watch? The underlying assumption is that if the r-coloring is present in one sound, it will probably generalize to other sounds as well. Do children in fact generalize r-coloring in such a manner? After reviewing the literature of sound generalization research, Elbert and Gierut (1986) established certain "predictions" that can be used by clinicians to reduce the number of sounds to be worked on in therapy. The idea is that if a specific sound is taught, certain features of the newly acquired sound might transfer without therapy to other sounds requiring the same features. One prediction is that if one allophone is acquired, [ɝ] for example, norm production of [r] and [ɚ] will probably be achieved without therapy. In this case, a wait-and-watch decision might be best. However, not every child is able to generalize features from one sound to another. In addition, there may be other factors that will impact our decision making, such as the age of the child, the intelligibility of the child, parental concerns, and peer pressure, to mention just a few. Evaluating the various factors and making clinically valid decisions is an important portion of a speech-language pathologist's clinical skills.

Where to Begin Therapy? Certain clinical decisions will need to be made in respect to therapy. First, should therapy begin with the consonantal [r] or the central vowels with r-coloring? This choice will be based on stimulability probes and the perceptual saliency of the error sound. Perceptual saliency refers to the conspicuousness, the noticeability, of the error sound to listeners. Given a client with a w/r or a j/r substitution and derhotacization of central vowels, the substitutions will probably be more prominent perceptually. Dialect might also play a role in our decision making. If dialect features include derhotacization of central vowels, the consonantal [r] would be our only therapy choice. Second, which type of [r]-production, the bunched or the retroflexed [r], should be the goal of phonetic placement or sound modification techniques? Again, the stimulability of the client will play a role. Placement techniques for both can be implemented and the resulting [r] evaluated. If an acceptable [r] production is achieved in isolation, probes can determine which vowels or words promote the accurate use of the newly acquired sound. The therapeutic goal will be to appraise the client's individual possibilities and determine the most efficient means of changing aberrant productions to acceptable articulations. Every client will present us with a different set of challenges.

Coarticulatory Conditions

The retroflexed [r]-sound offers a challenge when the clinician is trying to determine which vowel sounds might present coarticulatory conditions that assist its production. There are no vowels in General American English with a tongue placement similar to the retroflexed [r]-position. If the retroflexed [r] follows front vowels, especially high-front vowels, at least elevated frontal portions of the tongue are promoted. But combinations with these vowels would necessitate a quick movement from a concave retroflexed [r] to a convex "bunched" tongue shape for the front vowels. On the other hand, the back vowels, with their characteristic posterior elevation of the tongue, are clearly not supportive of any retroflexed articulation. The central vowels without r-coloring, especially if they are pro-

duced with an elevated mandibular position, offer perhaps the best possibility. Next, the front vowels would clearly be better in supporting retroflexed [r] than the back vowels.

Similar coarticulatory conditions would exist for the central vowels and the bunched r-production with its relative centralized elevation of the tongue's dorsum. However, the secondary feature of lip rounding, which often characterizes the bunched [r], is also characteristic of the back vowels. Therefore, if the goal is the bunched [r], the sequence of vowels might be central vowels, back vowels, and finally front vowels.

As noted previously, the articulatory features of [r] may change with the individual and with the context in which the sound occurs. Because of this, clinicians will need to concentrate on the client's possibilities and on the coarticulatory conditions that seem to foster the norm production of these sounds.

Word Examples. Keeping in mind that individual and contextual variations will often dramatically alter the production of [r], the following one-syllable words are given to exemplify one possible vowel sequence that could be used for a child with an [r]-problem. This order is based on the retroflexed [r] as target. The vowel sequence is the one suggested at the beginning of this section. Word examples are given for both the consonantal [r] and central vowels with r-coloring.

Consonantal [r] Words

rub - rough - run - rut - rush - rug - rung
ram - rap - ran - rat - rag - rack - rang
red - wren - rent - wrench - wreck
Ray - rain - rail - raid - race - rake
rim - rib - rip - ridge - rig - Rick - ring
real - read - reach
raw - Ron - rod - rot - rock - wrong
row - robe - rope - roll - road - wrote
room - roof - rude - rule - root

Consonantal [r] Words

Words with the central vowel with r-coloring - [ɝ]	Words with centering diphthongs
her - burr - purr - fur - sir - spur - stir	air - hair - mare - bear - pear*
earn - earth - urge	ear - fear - deer - near - cheer - gear
worm - burn - turn - word - hurt - learn	are - bar - far - jar - car - star
slurp - skirt	oar - more - bore - pour - door
	blur
	lure - tour

MISARTICULATIONS OF [θ] AND [ð]

[θ] and [ð] are among the latest sounds to develop in the speech of children. Often, difficulties in articulating them extend into the beginning school year. Common errors are the substitution of t/θ and d/ð. Other misarticulations include the substitution of the labiodental fricatives [f] and [v] for [θ] and [ð]. Clinicians should also be aware that variations in [θ] and [ð] productions can be a feature of African American Dialect. The realization of these features is conditioned by the position of [θ] and [ð] within the word. These dialectal features are not considered articulation errors.

> See the Dialect Speaker section of Chapter 6 for more information on the influence of word position on [θ] and [ð] variations.

Phonetic Description

[θ] and [ð] can be produced in two ways: as interdental or as addental fricatives. For the interdental realization, the tongue tip is protruded slightly between the front incisors. For the addental articulation, which is phonetically described as apico-dental, the tongue tip approaches the inner surface of the front incisors. The friction that characterizes these sounds as fricatives is created by a restriction of the breath stream between the apex of the tongue and the backside of the upper front teeth. For the interdental productions, this friction occurs between the apex and the cutting edge of the front incisors. For both productions, the tongue remains relatively flat.

Linguistic Function

Frequency of Occurrence. On a frequency of occurrence list for General American English speech sounds, [θ] and [ð] are not neighbors. Whereas [ð] shows up slightly above the middle, occupying a rank order of approximately ten among twenty-four consonants, [θ] is among the last on the list, ranking number twenty-one out of a total of twenty-four (Carterette and Jones, 1974; Mines, Hanson, and Shoup, 1978). Only word-initial [θr] is considered a fairly frequent cluster in General American English (Mader, 1954; Dewey, 1923; French, Carter, and Koenig, 1930).

Phonotactics. Both [θ] and [ð] are found in word-initial and word-final positions. [ð] occurs primarily in word-initial positions, while [θ] occurs approximately half the time in word-initial positions, the other half fairly evenly split between word-medial and word-final positions (Mader, 1954). Table 8.17 lists examples of consonant clusters with [θ] and [ð].

Morphophonemic Function. Word-final clusters that end in [θ] or [ð] can signal (1) plural-

---

*Pronunciation of the words with centering diphthongs may vary from speaker to speaker. Thus, the word *hair* might be pronounced [hɛɝ] or [heɪɝ]. These differences could have an influence on the sequencing of the words.

TABLE 8.17 Consonant Clusters with [θ] and [ð]

WORD-INITIATING		WORD-TERMINATING	
[θr]	thread, three	[tθ]	width, hundredth
		[lθ]	health, wealth
		[nθ]	ninth, month
		[ŋθ]	length, strength
		[ɝθ]	earth, birth
		[ðd]	bathed, breathed
		[ðz]	bathes, breathes

ity, as in mo<u>nths</u> and mou<u>ths</u>; (2) third person singular, as in ba<u>thes</u> and brea<u>thes</u>; and (3) past tense, as in ba<u>thed</u> and brea<u>thed</u>.

Minimal Pairs. Frequent sounds substituted for [θ] and [ð] include [s]-[z], [t]-[d], and [f]-[v]. Table 8.18 lists minimal pairs and sentences with these sounds.

Types of Misarticulation

1. *t/θ and d/ð substitutions.* Examples of these frequent substitutions are [tʌm] for *thumb* and [dɪs] for *this*. This misarticulation involves changes in both place and manner of articulation: The place of articulation is moved posteriorly to the alveolar ridge while the manner of articulation is changed into a stop-plosive.

Phonetic transcription of the error: [t] or [d]

2. *f/θ and v/ð substitutions.* Examples are [fʌm] for *thumb* and [vɪs] for *this*. Although the fricative manner of articulation is similar for [f] and [v] and [θ] and [ð], both organ and place of articulation change. The constriction for the labiodentals [f] and [v] is established between the bottom lip and the upper incisors. The tongue does not play a role in their production. The necessary constriction for [θ] and [ð], though, does involve the tongue; either the tongue tip is protruded slightly be-

tween the teeth for the interdental or the tongue approximates the back of the upper incisors for the apico-dental [θ] and [ð].

Therapeutic Suggestions

Phonetic Placement

Interdental Productions.   [θ] and [ð] are articulated with

1. the tongue tip *slightly* protruded between the upper and lower incisors,
2. the tip of the tongue lightly touching the lower edges of the front teeth,
3. the underside of the tongue resting on the top edges of the lower incisors, and
4. the body of the tongue relatively flat.

The expiratory airflow should be directed over the surface of the tongue between tongue tip and the bottom edge of the front incisors. Specific tongue exercises could be implemented prior to this placement. For example, the client could move the tip of the tongue forward and backward over the bottom edge of the front incisors. Next, with the tip of the tongue placed lightly on the bottom edge of the front incisors, the client lowers the tongue tip minimally during expiration. The goal is to create awareness of the air flow over the surface and tip of the tongue. Because the tip of the tongue is visible during the interdental production, a mirror will provide excellent feedback. Care should be taken that this placement is not established with excessive tongue protrusion. The tongue tip should barely be visible between the teeth.

Apico-Dental Productions.   The tongue tip is placed touching the posterior surface of the front incisors. The body of the tongue should be relatively flat. During expiration, the client

TABLE 8.18 Minimal Pair Words and Sentences Contrasting [θ] and [ð] to [s] and [z]

[θ] VERSUS [s]		[θ] VERSUS [s]		[ð] VERSUS [z]		[ð] VERSUS [z]	
thank	sank	Beth	Bess	then	Zen	clothe	close
thick	sick	faith	face			teethe	tease
thin	sin	path	pass			breathe	breeze
think	sink	mouth	mouse				
thinner	sinner	myth	miss				

[θ] VERSUS [t]		[θ] VERSUS [t]		[ð] VERSUS [d]		[θ] VERSUS [d]	
thank	tank	bath	bat	than	Dan	breathe	breed
thick	tick	Beth	bet	then	den	loathe	load
thin	tin	math	mat	though	dough		
thought	taught	tooth	toot	thine	dine		
		path	pat				

[θ] VERSUS [f]		[ð] VERSUS [v]	
thin	fin	than	van
		that	vat
		thine	vine

The fog was *thickening*.
The fog was *sickening*.

It hurts when children *teethe*.
It hurts when children *tease*.

They walked by the *clothing* store.
They walked by the *closing* store.

She couldn't *breathe* through the testing, so she left.
She couldn't *breeze* through the testing, so she left.

now glides the tongue back slightly until a friction noise is heard. The required posterior movement is minimal. For the client with a t/θ substitution, care must be taken that the posterior movement does not result in the tongue tip coming into contact with the alveolar ridge.

The substitutions t/θ and f/θ can be effectively influenced by employing sound modification methods. Therefore, the descriptions for changing the articulation from [t] and [f]

to an interdental or addental [θ] and [ð] will be found in the following section.

Sound Modification Methods

1. *[t]-[θ] Method.* These two sounds are distinguished by their place and manner of articulation. To move from [t] to [θ], the place of articulation must be moved anteriorly. Also, the manner of articulation changes from a stop to a fricative. The client should be instructed to:

a. *slowly* release [t]. This should result in a frictionlike sound.

b. maintain this frictionlike quality while moving the tongue forward until its tip comes very close to the back of the front incisors. If this constriction is continued, the client should feel the air flowing over the tip of the tongue, forcing its way between the tongue and the back of the upper front teeth.

2. *[f]-[θ] Method.* For this method, organ and place must be modified; the manner of articulation remains the same. The easiest articulation to achieve when modifying [f] to [θ] is the interdental one. Two different ways can be used:

a. During the production of [f], the client pulls the bottom lip away from the upper incisors.

b. The friction sound must continue during the placement of the tongue tip between the upper and lower incisors.

Or during the production of [f], the client is instructed to

a. "split the /f/ in half with his tongue by sticking his tongue between his teeth" (Secord, 1981b, p. 32). Here, the goal is the release of the labiodental placement when the client places the tongue between the incisors.

b. The friction sound must continue during the placement of the tongue.

3. *[s]-[θ] Method.* If the client has an acceptable [s], this seems to be the easiest sound modification method to use because the place of articulation is the only feature distinguishing the two sounds. The goal is an apico-dental [θ]. During the [s] production,

a. glide the tongue forward until the tip almost touches the back of the upper incisors.

b. feel the air flowing between the tongue tip and the back of the teeth.

Coarticulatory Conditions

Due to the high front position of the tongue during [θ] and [ð] realizations, high-front vowels offer perhaps the best coarticulatory conditions following these sounds. The back vowels with the positioning of the tongue toward the back of the mouth would not aid the production. Therefore, a possible vowel sequence is high-front, mid-front, low-front, followed by central vowels, and finally the back vowels moving from low- to mid- to the high-back vowels.

Compared to the voiceless [θ], the voiced [ð] has a much higher frequency of occurrence in General American English. This would suggest that practice with [ð] will be an important aspect of therapy.

Word Examples. The following one-syllable words are ordered from relatively easy to more difficult coarticulatory conditions for a child with [θ] and [ð] problems.

[θ] Words	[ð] Words
theme	thee - these
thin - thick - thing - think	this
	they
theft	them - then - their - there
thank - thanks	
thumb - thud - thug - thump	that - than - that's
	the
third - thirst	though - those
thaw - thought - thawed - thong	

The following section describes phonetic errors that are less frequently encountered. These errors include voicing problems and difficulties with f-sounds, affricates, and consonant clusters.

VOICING PROBLEMS

Voicing problems manifest themselves in the substitution of a voiced for a voiceless cognate, such as [du] for *two,* or a voiceless for a voiced cognate, such as when *ball* is pronounced as [pɑl]. Voicing has phonemic value in General American English. Different word meanings are established by the presence or absence of a voicing component. This can be exemplified by the minimal pairs *face* and *vase* and *tot* and *dot.* Because of its phonemic relevance, a voicing problem should trigger evaluation to determine whether a phonemic disorder exists.

Several authors (i.e., Ingram, 1989b; Grunwell, 1987; Smit and Bernthal, 1983; Smith, 1979) have noted that children still show difficulties with certain aspects of voicing at age 4. The most common pattern is the voiced production of normally voiceless stops, fricatives, and affricates initiating a syllable or word (prevocalic voicing). Thus, *toe* and *soup* may be pronounced as [doᵘ] and [zup]. In addition, voiceless cognates are substituted for their voiced counterparts terminating a word or syllable (postvocalic devoicing), that is, *cub* becomes [kʌp] and *dog* [dɑk]. *Context-sensitive voicing* is a term used to refer to these types of voicing errors (Grunwell, 1987). According to Grunwell (1987), context-sensitive voicing, especially postvocalic devoicing, may continue in some children beyond 3 years of age.

Specific factors that need to be appraised before implementing therapy for difficulties with consonant voicing/devoicing include the frequency of occurrence in the speech of the client and the contexts in which the voicing/devoicing occurs. First, the voicing/devoicing difficulties should occur at a relatively high frequency before therapy is implemented. Second, some specific contextual modifications resulting in devoicing are commonly heard in General American English; these modifications would not be considered

misarticulations. For example, devoicing of final consonants and assimilations of voicelessness are common (Abercrombie, 1967). Devoicing of final consonants can be found most often before a pause. Therefore, devoicing of final consonants could be realized during an articulation test as well as on spontaneous speech samples. Personal clinical experience has shown that final devoicing often occurs on plurals that end in [əz]: *matches* is pronounced as [mætʃəs] and *dishes* as [dɪʃəs]. Assimilations of voicelessness can be either progressive or regressive. During an utterance, these assimilations can often be heard if a voiceless consonant precedes or follows a voiced stop, fricative, or affricate. For example, we pronounce *news* as [nuz]. However, *news* is typically pronounced [nus] in the word *newspaper.* This devoicing of [z] is a regressive assimilation influenced by the following voiceless [p]. While these types of sound change in context are common, they must be evaluated in relationship to their frequency of occurrence for a particular client. If the frequency is so high that intelligibility is somehow affected, even these "normal" modifications may warrant therapy.

Therapeutic Suggestions

Probably all children use some voicing distinctions in their speech. The task is to create an awareness of voicing versus lack of voicing for a particular cognate pair. The following guidelines can be supplemented with auditory discrimination exercises in order to enhance the general awareness of voicing versus devoicing. Minimal pair words that target the particular voicing/devoicing cognate difficulty can also be employed.

This sequencing of auditory discrimination exercises is suggested:

1. General awareness of the presence or absence of voicing could be aided by having

the client listen to two sounds—[s] and [z], for example—and identify which one is voiced. This could be combined with the tactile feedback method, which is explained in the following section.

2. The cognates could be placed in minimally paired words and the client asked to identify voiced versus voiceless sounds at the beginning or end of a word. Word pair discrimination exercises would utilize the particular consonant cognates and the position of these sounds in words that are problematic for the client. If the client has trouble with the devoicing of final stops, word pairs such as *cap* versus *cab* and *lock* versus *log* could be identified.

Tactile Feedback Method. This method develops the client's awareness of the vibratory sensation associated with voicing. This is then contrasted to the lack of vibration present during voiceless sounds. Clients place their fingers on or slightly above the thyroid cartilage during the production of a voiced sound. Attention should be directed to the vibration that is felt. For children, this vibration can be compared to a motor being "on" during voiced versus "off" during unvoiced consonants. This method works fine with fricatives and affricates but is difficult to implement with stop-plosives. The natural tendency to add a vowel after the production of stop sounds can trigger the feeling of vibration on unvoiced stop sounds. Actually, the vibration for the vowel *follows* the stop production, but many children will not be able to discern this. If the clinician decides to implement the tactile feedback method for establishing an awareness of voiced versus voiceless stop-plosives, the child should be instructed to whisper the stop to attain a voiceless realization while saying the voiced cognate with a "big (loud) voice." This should eliminate the voicing influence of the following vowel on the voiceless stop.

Auditory Enhancement Method. This method enhances the humming effect heard during the production of voiced consonants. The client's hands are cupped and placed over the ears. During the production of voiced consonants, the client should hear a humming not present during the production of voiceless consonants. A similar effect can be achieved by plugging each ear with an index finger. Difficulties may arise when using this method to discriminate between voiced and voiceless stops; the instructions noted in the tactile feedback method should be followed here as well.

Whispering Method. If a child produces a voiced consonant and its voiceless cognate is the goal, the clinician can have the child whisper the sound. As with all the previously noted methods, this one is implemented only until the client understands the distinction between voiced and voiceless productions.

Singing Method. This method is implemented for clients who can produce a voiceless consonant but the goal is its voiced cognate. Here, the client "sings" the voiceless consonant. A familiar melody such as "Happy Birthday" is sung with the voiceless consonant combined with the [ʌ] vowel replacing the words: [pʌpʌpʌpʌ pʌpʌ]. If the client actually continues to sing, that is, to produce continuous voicing, the voiceless consonant will become voiced. If this is accomplished, the client is made aware of the voiced production, which can then be isolated from the tune.

Developing Voiced Stop Productions. This technique is actually a sound modification method. The voiced stop-plosives are modified from the nasals, [m], [n], and [ŋ]. Personal clinical experience has shown that this technique is often surprisingly effective if one of the previous methods has failed. During the nasal production, the nostrils are pinched closed. The client releases the air orally. If the voicing of the nasal continues, [b] should result from [m], [d] from [n], and [g] from [ŋ]. The success of this technique depends on the continuation of the voicing component of the nasal sounds.

MISARTICULATIONS OF [f] AND [v]

[f] is one of the earliest fricatives to emerge in the speech of children, and it is usually mastered between 3 and 4 years of age. However, if sound mastery data are examined (see Chapter 5), the voiced [v] is consistently noted as being later in acquisition than its voiceless cognate. When Sander (1972) reinterpreted the Wellman et al. (1931) and Templin (1957) data, he reported that 90 percent of the children had mastered [f] by age 4, compared to only 51 percent for [v]. It was not until age 8 that 90 percent of the children had mastered the voiced [v]. Therefore, approximately four years separate similar levels of competency for [f] versus [v].

What could account for this large difference in the age of acquisition? Although differences exist between the mastery ages of other consonant cognates as well, such large age variations are noted only for [f] and [v]. Perhaps the later acquisition of [v] reflects a much lower frequency of occurrence in General American English when compared to [f]. If it is not a frequent sound, children may simply not be utilizing it, thus, seemingly, extending the mastery age. However, frequency of occurrence data for children (Carterette and Jones, 1974; Mader, 1954) do not support this hypothesis. The frequency of occurrence for [f] and [v] is relatively similar. A second possibility is that it is not the quantity of different words but rather a limited number of highly frequent words with [v] that raise the frequency count. (A similar case can be made for the voiced [ð]. Its relative high frequency of occurrence can be attributed to a small

number of very frequently used words, such as *the*.) Two studies (Denes and Pinson, 1973; Dewey, 1923) may support this hypothesis. These investigators found that *of* [ʌv] was among the ten most frequently used words in General American English. Such words as *have* and *give* would also seem to be fairly common words. The Mader (1954) study also adds some credibility to this hypothesis. If the frequency of occurrence according to the position in the word is examined for first-, second-, and third-grade children, the majority of the [v] sounds occur in word-final positions. These are merely possibilities for explaining the differences between the reported ages of acquisition for [f] and [v]. Whatever the reason, the later age of acquisition for [v] may have clinical implications.

In the previous therapeutic discussions for phonetic errors, it has been assumed that one would proceed clinically from one consonant cognate to the other. Thus, therapy with [s] would closely coincide with [z] work. The acquisition information might cause us to question the validity of this procedure for [f] and [v]. These data suggest that therapy for [f] should be initiated prior to [v]. Depending on the age of the child, it may not be realistic to expect the same level of accuracy for [v]. One of the predictions established by Elbert and Gierut (1986) might be considered here. They stated that if one member of a cognate pair is achieved in therapy, improvement will occur with the other member. Interpreted in light of the acquisition data, therapy would most often begin with [f]. However, we might want to wait and watch to see if [v] would develop on its own. For many children, [v] acquisition appears to take place much later than the mastery of the voiceless [f].

Phonetic Description

[f] and [v] are labio-dental fricatives. A constriction is created by bringing the inner edge

of the lower lip into light contact with the edges of the upper incisors. If this contact is very light, the breath stream can pass between the inner edge of the lower lip and the cutting edge of the upper incisors. Firmer contact between the lower lip and upper teeth might cause the breath stream to flow around the incisors, some of the air being forced out in the region of the canine and premolar teeth. The upper lip remains inactive during [f] and [v] articulation.

Types of Misarticulation

1. *p/f and b/v substitution.* Examples of these substitutions include [pɪŋgɚ] for *finger* or [ʃʌbəl] for *shovel*. Place and manner of articulation have been modified for this substitution. The labio-dental articulation is replaced by a bilabial one while the fricative is changed to a stop-plosive.

   Phonetic transcription of the error: [p] or [b]

2. *Bilabial fricative substitution.* For this substitution, only the place of articulation has been altered from a labio-dental to a bilabial production. The symbols [ɸ] and [β] are used to denote voiceless and voiced bilabial fricatives.

   Phonetic transcription of the error: [ɸ] or [β]

Therapeutic Suggestions

Phonetic Placement. To develop an awareness of the labiodental articulation, the client should "bite down" on the lower lip with the upper teeth. This will probably result in the client touching the outside edges of the lower lip. Because [f] is produced with the inside of the lower lip contacting the the upper incisors, the client should then glide the lower lip along the cutting edges of the upper teeth toward the inside of the lip, letting the lip "pop out" of the bite. When the upper incisors are lightly positioned on the inner edge of the lower lip, the client should blow, allowing air to escape between this narrow slit. If the labio-dental contact is too firm, the jaw can be lowered *slightly.*

If the client realizes a p/f substitution, the presence of airflow should be targeted. Although the airflow for [f] is relatively weak, a light feather or a small piece of tissue placed in front of the mouth should show some movement during the entire [f] production. This could then be contrasted to the lack of movement during the stop phase of the [p] articulation. In isolation, producing [p] causes movement of the feather only at the very end, during the plosive portion of the articulation.

The labio-dental contact is also an important aspect of the phonetic placement for the client who demonstrates a bilabial fricative substitution. Because the substitution and the target sound are both fricatives, if the labio-dental positioning can be established, an acceptable [f] will result. A passive method may assist in this placement. During the bilabial fricative production, the bottom lip is pushed inward with the tip of the index finger. This should position the bottom lip approximately in the right spot for [f]. When a mirror is used, this passive method will allow the client visual feedback regarding the relative positioning of the lower lip and the upper incisors. In addition, auditory feedback is provided when the two different sound qualities are compared.

Sound Modification Methods

[p]-[f] Method. During the stop phase of the [p] production, the bottom lip is pushed inward with the tip of the index finger so that air can escape. The lower lip should be positioned in such a manner that its inner edge approximates the upper incisors. Initially, maintaining the position of the index finger can serve as an aid until the client is aware of the necessary articulatory placement.

Coarticulatory Conditions

Vowels with lip rounding, such as the back vowels (with the exception of [ɑ]), should be avoided when beginning syllable or word practice with a newly acquired [f]. Lip rounding is clearly an unfavorable coarticulatory condition. The central vowels with r-coloring, which are often produced with lip rounding, would not provide a beneficial coarticulatory condition either. When comparing the tongue placement and the relatively closed position of the jaw during normal [f] realizations, the sequence of vowels to be considered might be high-front, mid-front, low-front, followed by the central vowels without r-coloring. The final vowel sequence would start with the low-back vowels followed by the mid-, high-back, and central vowels with r-coloring.

Word Examples. The following one-syllable words are ordered from relatively easy to more difficult coarticulatory conditions for a child with [f] difficulties. One-syllable words beginning with [v] are also included. However, it should be kept in mind that according to the Mader (1954) results, 96 percent of [v] sounds used by school-age children were in the medial and final word positions.

[f] Words	[v] Words
feet - feed - feel - field	
fit - fill - fin - fig - fish - fist	Vic - Vince
fade - fail - face - fake - faint	veil - vein - vase
fed - fell - fence	vet - vest
fat - fan - fast - fact	van - Val - vamp
fun - fudge	
fought - fall - fog - false	vault
phone - phones - fold	vote
foot - full	
food - fool	
fur - fern	Vern - verb

AFFRICATE PROBLEMS

The affricates [tʃ] and [dʒ] develop relatively late in the speech of children. This may be due to the complexity of the production or, possibly, to their low frequency of occurrence in General American English. Several investigations (Carterette and Jones, 1974; Mader, 1954; Shriberg and Kwiatkowski, 1982a) that analyzed the continuous utterances of children and adults consistently rank both [tʃ] and [dʒ] as one of the least frequent consonants. This is further exemplified in Olmsted's (1971) study. In spontaneous speech, only one of the forty-eight children ranging from 36 to 54 months of age attempted [dʒ], and that child produced it in an aberrant manner. Although several of the acquisition studies did not test both [tʃ] and [dʒ], others (Arlt and Goodban, 1976; Prather et al., 1975; Templin, 1957) reported that there is a somewhat later age of acquisition for [dʒ] compared to [tʃ]. Sander's (1972) reinterpretation of the Wellman et al. (1931) and Templin (1957) data demonstrated similar mastery age levels for both the voiceless and voiced affricates. However, a relatively long time span separated the age when the majority of the children (51 percent of the children tested) versus most of the children (90 percent of the children tested) mastered the affricates. At 3;6, 51 percent of the children had mastered both affricates, while it was not until age 7 that 90 percent of the children had reached comparable mastery levels.

Phonetic Description

Although some descriptions of affricates give the reader the idea that they are merely the stops [t] and [d] followed by the fricatives [ʃ] and [ʒ], this is not entirely accurate. Based on palatograms, Kantner and West (1960) reported two factors that differentiate isolated consonant sequences from affricate productions: (1) the initial position of the stop portion and (2) the nature of the movement from the stop to the fricative portion of the affricates. First, the initial stop portion of [ʧ] is articulated closer to the articulatory position for [ʃ]; therefore, it is produced more posteriorly than is normally the case with an isolated [t]. Second, movement from the stop to the fricative portion of the affricate is characterized by the front of the tongue dropping relatively slowly, creating momentarily a constriction that is typical for the [ʃ] sound. This is different from the release of an isolated [t], in which the tongue drops suddenly to a neutral position. The degree of lip rounding during the production of these affricates depends primarily on the speaker and the phonetic context.

As noted, then, an affricate is not merely a stop followed by a fricative production. Its realization varies in characteristic ways from the articulation of an isolated stop followed by a fricative. However, in an attempt to simplify the directions for their use with children, it will often sound as if our goal is merely to fuse the stop with the fricative. In addition, the previously reported differences between affricates versus stop plus fricative productions may prove helpful to clinicians if the resulting sound quality is perceptually still not acceptable.

Types of Misarticulation

1. *t/ʧ and d/ʤ substitution.* These misarticulations are characterized by the substitution of a stop for the affricate production. Examples include [tɝt] for the word *church* or [pədɑməz] for *pajamas*. Because the substituted stop and the stop portion of the affricate are the same, only the slow release of the stop to [ʃ] distinguishes these two speech sounds.

Phonetic transcription of the error: [t] or [d]

2. *ʃ/ʧ and ʒ/ʤ substitution.* A substitution of a fricative for the affricate is exemplified by [wɑʃ] for *watch* and [ʒʌmp] for *jump*. The initial stop portion of the affricate distinguishes this substitution from the affricate production.

Phonetic transcription of the error: [ʃ] or [ʒ]

3. *s/ʧ and z/ʤ substitution.* Examples for this substitution include [pis] for *peach* and [zæm] for *jam*. This realization does not have any initial stop portion, only a fricative element. In addition, the fricative segment is articulated more anteriorly than the normal fricative portion of the affricates.

Phonetic transcription of the error: [s] or [z]

Therapeutic Suggestions

Phonetic Placement. The tongue tip is placed on the posterior edge of the alveolar ridge in a manner similar to [t]. This [t] realization should be released *slowly*. It is important that the client be aware that during the release, the lateral edges of the tongue need to remain in contact with the premolars and molars, similar to a [ʃ] production. In addition, the tongue glides slightly back during the release. The posterior movement of the tongue can be aided by pushing the tongue back with a tongue depressor during the slow release of [t].

One could also begin with [ʃ] to emphasize the tongue placement necessary for the release of the stop portion of the affricate. The client produces [ʃ] and, without moving the body of the tongue, "stops" or "blocks" off the airflow with the tip of the tongue. The resulting stop is then again slowly released.

Sound Modification Methods

[t]-[ʧ] Method. The description for employing this method is similar to the one explained

in the first paragraph of the previous section on phonetic placement. In order to achieve success with this method, it is important that the lateral edges of the tongue remain in contact with the premolars and first molars during the slow release of the [t]. If this is not the case, a [tʰʌ] quality will result rather than [tʃ].

Secord (1981b) suggests telling "the client to practice saying /t/-/ʃ/ slowly at first, then rapidly until they blend and become one sound" (p. 41).

[ʃ]-[tʃ] Method.   The description for utilizing this method is similar to the one explained in the second paragraph of the previous section on phonetic placement.

[s]-[tʃ] Method.   During [s] production, the client should glide the tongue slightly back. When an acceptable [ʃ] quality is achieved, proceed according to the instructions for the [ʃ]-[tʃ] method.

Coarticulatory Conditions

Because of the anterior placement of the tongue for both the stop and the fricative portions of the affricate, the front vowels would seem to offer more coarticulatory support than the back vowels. Consequently, a possible vowel sequence would be high-, mid-, low-front vowels followed by the central vowels and the back vowels. The back vowels, however, offer two advantages: (1) the lip rounding of especially the high-back vowels might provide coarticulatory support for the lip rounding noted in the [tʃ] production, and (2) the back positioning of the tongue for the back vowels might enhance the backward gliding movement of the tongue in its transition from stop-plosive to the fricative portion of the affricate. If this proves to aid the production of [tʃ] in a given case, the vowel sequence might be the high-, mid-, and low-back vowels followed by the central and the front vowels. Clinicians should use probes to

determine which vowel sequence would be more beneficial for their particular client.

Word Examples.   The following one-syllable words are ordered from relatively easy to more difficult coarticulatory conditions for a child with an affricate problem. In this case, affricate-vowel probes demonstrated that the series of back vowels offered better coarticulatory conditions than the front vowels.

[tʃ] Words	*[dʒ] Words*
chew - choose	June - juice
choke - chore - chose	Joe - joke - Joan
chalk - chop - chopped - chops	jaw - jog - jar - job - John - jaws
chirp - churn	jerk - germ
Chuck - chug - chum - chunk	jug - junk - jump - jumped
chat - champ - chance	Jack - jam - jab
check - chair	gem - jet - Jeff
chain - chase	jay - Jane
chick - chin - chill - chips	Jim - Jill
cheek - cheep - cheese - cheat - chief	gee - jeep - Gene - jeans

CONSONANT CLUSTER PROBLEMS

For some children, the acquisition of consonant clusters may extend into the beginning school years. Weiss et al. (1987) reported that it was not until children were 7 years of age that all consonant clusters were realized in a regular manner. Children also seem to go through certain stages in acquiring consonant clusters (see Chapter 5). Consonant cluster reduction and substitution are two processes that describe these stages. One of the earliest stages in a child's attempt to produce consonant clusters is consonant cluster reduction. This is exemplifed by the production of [dʌm] for *drum*. Typically, though not always, the marked member of the cluster is the one that is deleted (Ingram, 1989b). According to Greenlee (1974), the next phase in acquiring clusters is consonant cluster substitution, which is demonstrated when [dwʌm] is realized for *drum*. The last phase is the norm articulation of the consonant cluster.

At the word level, most consonants of General American English can be phonotactically members of a consonant cluster. Consonant clusters at the end of a word are often used to signal certain linguistic functions such as plurality (exemplified by the word *dogs*), third person singular tense (as in *kicks*), past tense (as in *kicked*), and possessives (as in *Jack's*). At the spontaneous speech level, any consonant cluster may occur. Therefore, the treatment of consonant clusters will often be one stage of a therapy program. In addition, children may be referred for therapy who can produce the individual sounds of a cluster but have difficulty with clusters containing those sounds. Depending on the number and type of consonant clusters affected, this may reduce the intelligibility of the child's speech considerably. The following guidelines are given to aid in the treatment of consonant clusters.

Therapeutic Suggestions

In General American English, consonant clusters consist of either two or three consonants in word-initial position and from two to four consonants in word-final position. Consonant clusters with only two consonants are typically easier to produce than those with three or four consonants. In addition, before therapy with consonant clusters begins, all members of the consonant cluster should be sounds that the child can produce accurately. For example, if a clinician is working on [k] clusters but the child cannot produce [r], then [kr] clusters should be avoided.

Production of Word-Initial Clusters

Epenthesis. During the acquisition of clusters, children often insert a schwa between the two consonants. This is a process referred

to as epenthesis. The same process can also be used to aid a client's production of a cluster. If the cluster is [sk], as in the word *skate,* the client starts with [sə -keɪt]. At first, the word should be slowly pronounced so that the schwa is somewhat prolonged. After a period of practice, the client attempts to shorten the schwa vowel gradually. This can often be achieved by increasing the tempo of the entire word. The end result should be a smooth transition from the first to the second consonant.

Pausing. For this method, a pause is inserted between the first and second member of the consonant cluster. Using the previous example, [sk] becomes [s] (pause) [keɪt]. After a period of practice, the client again shortens the pause between the two consonants. Personal clinical experience has shown that visual feedback in the form of a drawn line or gestures can often aid children in shortening this pause. For example, a long line is drawn which can be successively shortened, or the clinician can start with hands outspread moving them closer and closer together to indicate a shorter pause. Due to the natural pause that occurs between two syllables, this method is especially effective for consonant clusters that occur across syllable boundaries, such as [ns] in *answer* or *pencil.*

Production of Word-Final Clusters

Prolonging the First Sound. This method is best suited for clusters whose first element can be easily prolonged, such as the fricatives, affricates, nasals, or liquids. The first sound is prolonged for about two seconds and is then followed by the second element of the cluster, as in the word *nest,* "sssssssssss-t" for [st]. With repeated practice, the prolongation of the first sound is then successively shortened.

Pausing. This technique presents itself as a possibility if the first element of the consonant cluster is a stop-plosive. The instructions are similar to those described under initial consonant clusters.

Production of Word-Medial Clusters. Many word-medial clusters, especially two-consonant clusters, occur across syllable boundaries, as in *base-ball* or *an-swer*. Other clusters are to be found initiating a syllable, as in *ze-bra* or *A-pril*. Although common pronunciations do not syllabify these clusters between the two elements, for therapeutic purposes they could be artificially divided into *zeb-ra* or *Ap-ril*. The previously mentioned pausing method could be easily implemented by inserting a pause between the two syllables. This pause could first be lengthened and then shortened as the client gains stability of production.

Coarticulatory Conditions

Three variables should be considered when working on consonant clusters: (1) the length of the cluster, (2) the position of the cluster in the word, and (3) the coarticulation between the specific elements of the cluster.

The *length of the cluster* refers to how many individual consonants form the cluster. Typically, the fewer the consonants, the easier the cluster will be for the client. Therefore, consonant clusters with two elements should be attempted prior to three-element clusters.

The *position of the cluster* in the word refers to whether the cluster initiates the word, terminates it, or occurs somewhere in the middle. While most clinicians will probably begin with clusters initiating the word, medial clusters offer some positive features. The "natural" pause between two syllables can be used to separate the cluster into two discrete elements: For example, the [ns] cluster in *pencil* is divided into *pen-cil*. Again, this pause is at first prolonged and later shortened. Such a procedure gives the client, within a relatively natural word situation, time to produce the

transition between the elements of the cluster. Inserting a pause can also be used for clusters that typically are not syllabified between the two elements of the cluster. If the consonant cluster [st] is selected, practice could include *Eas-ter, toas-ter,* and *roos-ter,* for example. If the client can produce the cluster without a pause between the syllables, it can then be transferred to the word-initiating position. The client would be instructed to whisper the first part of the word, saying the last *ster* portion in a louder voice. This does necessitate that the syllable boundary is now changed from between the cluster, s-t, to initiating the cluster, st-. However, if the client can make this transition, the consonant cluster stands now at the beginning of a word, *stir*. A similar technique can be used to gain word-final consonant clusters. In this case, the last *er* portion of the word is whispered, which results in *East, toast,* and *roost* productions.

A disadvantage to using the clusters medially is that the client has to deal with a two-syllable rather than a one-syllable word. If more difficulty is noted when the client has to articulate a two-syllable word, this technique loses its appeal. Both word-initiating and -terminating consonant clusters should then be practiced in one-syllable word contexts, for [st] in words such as *star* and *stone* or *nest* and *lost,* for example. Here, word-initiating clusters would probably be easier than word-terminating clusters. As with all stages of therapy, the clinician needs to establish which sequence offers more favorable effects for each individual client.

The third factor that needs to be considered is the coarticulation between the elements of the cluster. Given a specific target sound within the cluster, certain sound combinations will be easier to produce than others. For example, if the target sound is [s], consider the consonant cluster [sk], as in *skate,* versus [sp], as in *spot*. For [sk], the tongue must move quickly from a front approximation of the articulators to a stop closure involving the back of the tongue. With [sp], on the other hand, the [p] element can be articulated with very little or no tongue movement from the [s] position. When the coarticulation features are considered, [sp] appears easier to articulate than [sk].

Certain consonant clusters might also need to be carefully evaluated based on the original misarticulation. For the child who originally demonstrated a lateral [s], clusters with [l], a lateral sound, might trigger the old misarticulation, for example. Or, for the child who originally had a [t] for [k] substitution, the word-final cluster [kt], as in *kicked* or *locked,* might prove troublesome.

In addition, specific techniques used to elicit the norm production may be reinforced by the selection of specific consonant clusters. If the [t]-[s] method was used to establish [s], the cluster [ts] used at the beginning of therapy might reinforce the [s] production. Similarly, a clinician who has established an acceptable [r] realization by means of the [d]-[r] method might use the consonant cluster [dr] to aid in stabilizing [r] during the initial stages of therapy.

The preceding guidelines have been provided to guide, not dictate, clinical decision making. The choice of the cluster and the sequencing of clusters within the therapy program will depend on the needs and the articulatory possibilities of the individual client. However, one of the tasks of a clinician is to understand and consider the factors that could have a positive or negative influence on the production of a specific target sound. This understanding will increase the efficacy of therapy.

SUMMARY

This chapter dealt with the phonetic (traditional or motor) approach to the treatment of articulation disorders, which is based on placement of the articulators in such a manner as to achieve an acceptable articulation of the sound in question. First, a sequence for therapy was outlined, beginning at the sound level and systematically moving to more complex articulatory conditions. Dismissal criteria were also suggested in the first portion of this chapter.

Misarticulations of several consonants were discussed in detail in the second portion of this chapter. The consonants chosen represented the most frequently misarticulated speech sounds: misarticulations of [s] and [z], [ʃ] and [ʒ], [k] and [g], [l], [r], the central vowels with r-coloring, and [θ] and [ð]. Other sound problems included voiced and voiceless substitutions, misarticulations of [f] and [v], the affricates [tʃ] and [dʒ], and consonant clusters. When applicable, phonetic placement as well as sound modification techniques were described. In addition, effects of coarticulation were treated for each of the noted problems.

Any successful application of this approach to articulation therapy presupposes a firm knowledge base concerning not only the phonetic characteristics of the sound's norm realization but also the misarticulated sound. An attempt has been made to provide both within this chapter.

CHAPTER 9

TREATMENT OF PHONEMIC ERRORS

CHAPTER OUTLINE

- Treatment Principles
- Minimal Pair Contrast Therapy
- Cycles Training
- Metaphon Therapy
- Phonemic Disorders with Concurrent Language Problems: Therapeutic Suggestions

- The Child with an Emerging Phonological System: Therapeutic Suggestions
- Treatment of Multiple Vowel Errors
- Summary

This chapter focuses on phonologically based approaches to treatment. Fey (1992) lists three basic principles underlying most of these approaches:

1. *Groups of sounds* with similar patterns of errors are targeted. In direct contrast to treating individual sounds in a sequential order, patterns of errors are noted and selected targets are chosen for therapy.

2. *Phonological contrasts* that were previously neutralized are established. Many of the phonologically based treatment methods use minimal pairs to contrast phonemic oppositions. If these distinctions can be made, one assumes that the child will generalize this knowledge to other phonemic contrasts.

3. A *naturalistic communicative context* is emphasized. Work on individual sounds or nonsense syllables is, strictly speaking, not a part of phonologically based therapy techniques.

This chapter describes several of these treatment approaches. Although each uses a somewhat different analysis system to describe the patterns of errors, most of them employ minimal pairs in their remediation program. These *minimal pair contrast therapies* have been grouped together; their differences, however, will be discussed. Other treatment techniques, such as *cycles training* and *metaphon therapy*, which incorporate different concepts into their methodology, will also be addressed. The last portion of this chapter contains some guidelines for combining phonologically based approaches with other treatment necessities. This includes their integration with language therapy, exemplified by the child with co-occurring phonemic and language disorders and the child with an emerging phonological system. Finally, phonologically based approaches will be discussed in relationship to *vowel therapy* in children with multiple vowel errors.

As discussed earlier, the production of speech sounds, the speech form, and the contrastive use of phonemes within the phonological system, speech function, are closely related. In addition, the phonological system interacts with other language areas. Although phonologically based approaches emphasize the function of phonemes, both the production of speech sounds and the relationship of phonology to other language areas should not be overlooked. This chapter attempts to integrate some of these factors with a discussion of intervention techniques for phonemic disorders.

TREATMENT PRINCIPLES

Several principles underly the treatment of phonemic errors in phonologically based approaches. First, the phoneme as a basic unit differentiating between word meanings is at the core of these therapies. Consequently, intervention begins at the word level. This differs considerably from the traditional or motor approach, which typically begins with the production of the respective sound(s) in isolation. In addition, word materials used to treat phonemic errors are structured in a very specific manner. Phonemes are usually arranged contrastively between words, resulting in "minimal pairs"—two distinct words that differ by only one phoneme value.

Second, treatment focuses on the phonological system of the child. An analysis of the child's phonology as an integrated system results in knowledge of (1) the inventory and distribution of speech sounds, (2) the syllable shapes and phonemic contrasts utilized, and (3) the error patterns displayed. All of these factors become important when the child's phonological system, not the individual speech sound, is at the center of the remediation process.

Third, groups of sounds or sound classes, rather than just individual speech sounds, are targeted. Children with phonemic disorders often have difficulties with several phonemes. Their aberrant realizations may extend to whole classes of sounds, such as fricatives, for example. This makes it impossible for the child to establish phonemic contrasts; neutraliza-

tion of phonemic oppositions therefore occurs. Phoneme-based remediation focuses on more than one sound or, perhaps, on an entire class of sounds at the same time. Several sounds may be targeted simultaneously, as in the cycles training approach (Hodson and Paden, 1991), or two sounds may be used to demonstrate phonemic oppositions, as in minimal contrast therapy (Blache, 1982; Blache, Parsons, and Humphreys, 1981; Cooper, 1985; Ferrier and Davis, 1973; Fokes, 1982; Lowe, Mount-Weitz, and Schmidt, 1992; Weiner, 1981; Weiner and Ostrowski, 1979). With phonologically based therapies, it is assumed that generalization will occur to other sounds or sound classes.

There are important differences between the traditional-motor approach (which is often used to treat phonetic errors) and phonologically based remediation methods (which target phonemic errors). Traditional-motor approaches represent therapy for *speech form,* the production of speech sounds. In contrast, phonologically based remediation methods target *phonemic function,* the contrastive use of phonemes to establish meaning differences. However, in the actual therapy situation, it is often impossible to separate these two different approaches to therapy entirely. Form and function constitute an interactive unity that might impact our treatment of children with phonemic difficulties.

MINIMAL PAIR CONTRAST THERAPY

Minimal pair contrast therapy refers to the therapeutic use of pairs of words that differ by one phoneme only. These minimal pairs are used to establish contrasts not present in the child's phonological system. For example, an analysis reveals that a child does not differentiate between stops and fricatives, that is, all fricatives are produced as homorganic stops (e.g., [s] → [t], [f] → [p]). One type of minimal pair therapy might use [f], representing the fricatives, and [p], exemplifying stops, in word pairs such as *fin* and *pin,* to establish this opposition. The underlying principle is that by establishing the contrast between [f] and [p], generalization will occur to other stops and fricatives.

Distinctive Feature Therapy

What Is Distinctive Feature Therapy? Distinctive feature therapy is based on the concept of distinctive features as bundles of phonetic components that establish and distinguish between phonemes. Many different distinctive feature therapies have been described (e.g., Blache, 1982, 1989; Costello, 1975; McReynolds and Bennett, 1972; McReynolds and Engmann, 1975; Singh, 1976; Weiner and Bankson, 1978), and it should be noted that distinctive feature therapy does not need to employ minimal pairs. Often, this type of therapy follows a sequence similar to the phonetic

> The foundations of distinctive feature theory are discussed in Chapter 4. Analysis procedures using distinctive features are contained in Chapter 7.

or traditional motor approach. For example, some of the earlier distinctive feature approaches (McReynolds and Bennett, 1972) used nonsense syllables that contrasted two distinctive features. Weiner and Bankson (1978) developed a program that attempted actually to teach a feature, in this case, [+ frication]. Distinctive feature therapy has been included in this section as it can be effectively combined with minimal pairs (see Blache, 1982, 1989; Blache, Parsons, and Humphreys, 1981). In this case, distinctive feature therapy uses minimal word pairs that exemplify the binary (+ and –) function of a certain distinctive feature.

When to Use Distinctive Feature Therapy. Deciding which specific therapy approach to choose amounts to a series of selection procedures. First, there should always be a specific

reason why one approach is chosen over another. For example, why use the distinctive feature approach? Therapy selection should not be based on what is currently in vogue; rather, it should be the best possible means of helping the individual client. The selection should also consider the efficacy of the intervention procedure chosen.

Are there certain clients who would benefit more from distinctive feature therapy than others? Distinctive feature analysis is based on the features of phonemes and their subsequent realization. Therefore, substitutions of one phoneme for another can be effectively established and the contrasting distinctive features recognized. However, the analysis procedure does not provide a means of examining sound distortions or omissions. Consequently, for clients who demonstrate a relatively large number of sound distortions or omissions, distinctive feature therapy would probably not be the intervention method of choice. Distinctive feature therapy would certainly be more suitable for a client who primarily substitutes one sound for another, that is, for the client who does not use phonemes contrastively.

The efficacy of an intervention procedure is indicated by research that has examined its effects. Several investigators (Costello, 1975; McReynolds and Bennett, 1972; Weiner and Bankson, 1978) report that when distinctive feature therapy was implemented, children generalized from the features of the sounds they were being taught to other sounds. However, the degree of occurring generalization was found to be variable. In addition, the number of subjects was very limited (a total of five subjects). For these subjects, though, it appears that distinctive feature therapy proved to be effective.

How to Select Target Sounds for Distinctive Feature Therapy. If distinctive feature therapy is the method of choice, additional decisions need to be made. One important decision for

See the section on Distinctive Feature Analysis in Chapter 7. Figure 7.12 and Table 7.3 provide example summaries of distinctive feature analysis.

any therapy planning involves the target selection. Which distinctive features should be chosen for beginning therapy? Based on a distinctive feature analysis used to analyze a client's patterns of errors, the following information is available:

- all target phonemes and substitutions
- the distinctive features representing the target phonemes
- the distinctive features representing the substitutions
- a summary of feature changes and the number of affected phonemes

Target selection is based on (1) the identification of those features that neutralize phonemic contrasts and on (2) the relative frequency with which these features occur. Concerning the identification of features that neutralize phonemic contrasts: Assume that the target phoneme is /s/ (+ strident, + continuant) and the substitution is /t/ (– strident, – continuant); stridency and continuancy are therefore features affecting /s/ in its contrastive function. Concerning the relative frequency of occurrence of these features: If these two features, strident and continuant, are also neutralizing contrasts of several other phonemes—such as /f/, /v/, /z/, and /ʃ/—this high degree of occurrence would impact the selection of the target.

After having established which distinctive features are neutralizing phonemic contrasts and which are occurring to a relatively high degree, a further decision must be made. The analysis will often reveal that several distinctive features are affecting phonemic contrasts. How does one select which feature to work on, or should therapy begin with many different features? Distinctive feature protocols (Blache, 1989; McReynolds and Engmann, 1975;

Weiner and Bankson, 1978) suggest that training should initially be restricted to one distinctive feature. If several distinctive features demonstrate a relatively high frequency of occurrence, the distinctive feature that affects a whole class of sounds, such as all fricatives, or a group of sounds, such as all voiced stops, should be selected. Distinctive feature therapy is based on the assumption that the establishment of one contrast will generalize to other sounds. By selecting a distinctive feature common to a larger number of sounds, the therapeutic impact will be larger.

After having selected a specific distinctive feature, a sound pair contrasting this binary feature must be found. When looking for such a pair, the clinician should keep several principles in mind:

1. One sound must contain the feature chosen and the other must lack this feature.
2. Typically, one sound chosen is not within the child's inventory while the other sound is.
3. The two sounds selected must exemplify a phonemic contrast not realized by the child. For example, if the child has a t/k substitution, the phonemic contrast between /t/ and /k/ is not present. These two phoneme contrasts might then be selected.
4. Priority should be given to sound pairs that represent a change in the *least* number of features. Therefore, a sound pair that is distinguished by only one or two feature differences has priority over sound pairs with more feature differences. For example, /l/ and /w/ differ by eight distinctive features; /s/ and /t/ differ by two features. For this purpose, /s/ and /t/ would be a better choice.
5. Consideration must be given to the age of the child and the developmental level of the child's phonemic system. Earlier developing sounds should have priority over later developing sounds (Blache, 1989).

Examination of the development of children's phonological systems shows that individual variation is the rule rather than the exception. Table 9.1 provides developmental guidelines to aid in the selection process. The reader is also referred to Chapter 5 and Bauman-Waengler (1994b).

CLINICAL APPLICATION

Target Selection Using Distinctive Features

A child who is 4;3 has no fricatives in his phonemic inventory; his stops include [p], [b], [t], and [d]. The continuant feature has been chosen as a therapy goal.

Distinctive Feature Chosen = [Continuant]		
(+) and (–) features	Phonemes	Target Possibilities in Child's Inventory (Early Sounds)
[+ continuant]	[h], liquids, glides, fricatives	[h], [l], [w], [f]
[– continuant]	nasals, stops, affricates	[p], [b], [t], [d] [m], [n]

Number of features distinguishing:

[h] and [p] = 5	[h] and [b] = 6	[h] and [t] = 6	[h] and [d] = 7
[h] and [m] = 6	[h] and [n] = 7		
[l] and [p] = 6	[l] and [b] = 5	[l] and [t] = 5	[l] and [d] = 4
[l] and [m] = 5	[l] and [n] = 4		
[w] and [p] = 8	[w] and [b] = 7	[w] and [t] = 9	[w] and [d] = 8
[w] and [m] = 7	[w] and [n] = 8		
[f] and [p] = 2	[f] and [b] = 3	[f] and [t] = 3	[f] and [d] = 4
[f] and [m] = 5	[f] and [n] = 6		

Best choice for target: [f] and [p]

TABLE 9.1 Early to Late Sounds: Approximate Development

EARLY SOUNDS

Nasals	Typically, [m] and [n] develop before [ŋ].
Stops and [h]	[p], [b], [t], and [d] are early stops; [k] and [g] later ones. The appearance of [k] and [g] may extend into the development of early fricatives. [h] appears around the time of early stop development.
Glides	[w] is usually earlier than [j].
Liquids	[l] develops earlier than [r]. For some children, [r] may be among the later developing sounds.
Fricatives	[f] is an early fricative, often appearing much earlier than [v].

LATER SOUNDS

Fricatives	The sibilants [s], [z], [ʃ], are late, while [ʒ], [θ], and [ð] often belong to the latest developing sounds.
Affricates	Typically [tʃ] and [dʒ] develop after, or approximately at the same time, the fricatives [ʃ] and [ʒ] appear.

Source: Summarized from Bauman-Waengler (1994).

How Is Distinctive Feature Therapy Used? After two target sounds have been chosen, word pairs that contain these target sounds need to be found. Typically, target sounds are placed in the word-initial position. The word selection is based on common usage, that is, whether the word is fairly common and might be used by the child. For the nonreading child, the word should be clearly portrayed in a picture. (Real words might in effect be nonsense syllables if the child does not understand them. Care should be exercised when selecting words and pictures.) Based on the previous clinical application, *fin-pin, fig-pig,* and *fill-pill* would be possible examples. After minimal pairs are chosen, the following steps are suggested (Blache, 1989):

Step 1: Discussion of Words. The therapist must be certain that the concepts portrayed are known to the child. To confirm this, the child can be asked to point to the picture named and questions can be asked about it. For example, if the chosen word pair was *fig-pig,* the clinician could ask, "Which one is a fruit?" or "Which one is an animal?"

Step 2: Discrimination Testing and Training. In this phase, the client's discrimination between the two sounds is tested. The therapist repeats the two words in random order while the child is instructed to point to the respective picture. If the response is correct seven consecutive times, the therapist can be reasonably certain that the client is differentiating between the two sounds.

It is advised that if the criterion level of seven correct discriminations in a row cannot be reached, poor auditory discrimination or memory skills may be the cause. These skills will then need to be addressed before continuing with the program.

Step 3: Production Training. This phase is directed toward the elicitation of the minimal-pair words. The child is instructed to be the teacher, saying the words while the therapist points to the correct picture. In the selection of the target sound for the minimal pairs, the child can produce one of the sounds chosen while the other is not in the child's inventory. If the target sound is stimulable, the child will probably be able to contrast the minimal pair. If the target sound is not stimulable, which is typically the case, the child will say one word of the pair incorrectly. For example, in the previous example, [f] and [p] were selected. The child could produce [p] but not [f]. If the child says [pɪn] for *pin* and [pɪn] for *fin,* the therapist will point to *pin* both times, that is, will point to a word not intended by the child. Blache (1989) states, "The therapist then uses traditional cues to elicit the distinctive feature property" (p. 368). If the child cannot articulate the sound correctly, a traditional or motor approach could be implemented to achieve the sound at the *word level.* The word level is emphasized as the minimal unit of distinctive feature therapy. Immediate reinforcement should follow the correct sound production.

Step 4: Carryover Training. Once the target word can be accurately articulated, the following sequence is suggested:

MODEL	EXAMPLE
"a" + word	a pig, a fig
"the" + word	the pig, the fig
"Touch the" + word	Touch the pig, Touch the fig
"Point to the" + word	Point to the pig, Point to the fig
longer expressions + word	That is a big pig, That is a big fig

A home program is also implemented to practice the target words. Parents serve as motivators and monitors. In these cases, though, not correction but rather praise for the child's acceptable productions is emphasized.

These steps follow a fairly traditional approach to therapy. The unique aspect of distinctive feature therapy lies in the selection of the target sounds. A distinctive feature is selected and sounds are chosen that represent + and – parameters of that distinctive feature. Although the distinctive feature therapy outlined here is phonologically based, traditional-motor techniques are also employed if the sound was not stimulable.

CLINICAL APPLICATION

Distinctive Features with H. H.

The distinctive feature analysis for H. H. (see Chapter 7, Figure 7.13 and Table 7.4) indicated that anterior, high, continuant and strident features are very frequent. Each of the four features affects six phonemes. The continuant, anterior, and high features also distinguish earlier developing sounds such as [f] and [k]. If continuant is chosen, the following targets are possible:

[ð] and [d]: one feature difference

[f] and [b]: three feature differences

[s] and [t]: two feature differences

[z] and [t]: three feature differences

Although [ð] and [d] demonstrate the fewest feature differences, [ð] is a late developing sound. That is also the case with the pairs [s] and [t] and [z] and [d]. The pair [f] and [b] might be a better choice, especially because H. H. can produce an acceptable [f] in certain contexts (*telephone* on the articulation test).

If anterior or high are chosen, the following are possible targets:

[ʃ] and [s]: two feature differences

[k] and [t]: four feature differences

[d] and [g]: four feature differences

Although [ʃ] and [s] have the lowest number of distinguishing features, [k] and [t] are earlier developing sounds. Stimulability of the sounds would play a role in the final decision.

Minimal Opposition Contrast Therapy

What Is Minimal Opposition Contrast Therapy?
Minimal opposition contrast is another method in which minimal pairs are employed

as the beginning unit of therapy. However, the selection of the sounds for the minimal pairs is based on a different principle from that utilized for distinctive feature therapy. Two sounds with as many articulatory similarities as possible are selected. Articulatory similarities are typically measured according to the phonetic production features of place, manner, and voicing. In minimal opposition contrast therapy, the sounds chosen differ in only one or two production features.

Although minimal opposition contrast is considered a phonologically based approach, the parameters for establishing these contrasts are phonetic in nature: Differences between phonetic production features are employed to determine the minimal contrast. Both speech "form," exemplified by the phonetic production features, and "function," the utilization of phonemic contrasts, are united for this therapy approach.

When to Use Minimal Opposition Contrast Therapy.
Which clients seem to be good candidates for this remediation plan? The minimal opposition contrast procedure targets the substitution of one phoneme for another. Sound distortions and omissions cannot be adequately addressed using phonemic contrasts. Therefore, clients who display a large number of sound distortions and omissions would probably not benefit from this therapy.

In contrast, those who primarily display phonemic substitutions are the best choices for minimal opposition contrasts. In addition, Lowe (1994) states that "The minimal opposition procedure is most appropriate for clients who are stimulable for the target sound" (p. 190). Hodson (1992) supports this view and adds that it appears inappropriate to set up a potentially frustrating situation by requiring differential productions of word pairs until the child can spontaneously and effortlessly say the target sounds within the pairs.

Before considering the minimal opposition contrast approach, clinicians will want to know if any data document its successful therapeutic use. Saben and Ingham (1991) found that therapy based on minimal opposition contrasts alone produced little progress in two clients. However, these subjects improved when a traditional motor approach was implemented together with the minimal opposition contrasts. So, then, does minimal opposition contrast seem a viable therapy method? There is as yet not much information available to answer this question. Based on very limited data, one would have to conclude that this procedure might work better if combined with a traditional motor approach.

How to Select Target Sounds for Minimal Opposition Contrast Therapy.

When establishing the target sounds for minimal pairs, the following principles should be kept in mind (Lowe, 1994):

1. Phonemic substitutions form the basis for target selection. The norm production and the substitution(s) should first be analyzed.

2. The place, manner, and voicing features for both the target sound and the substitution should be considered and the differences

> Place-voice-manner analysis for the various consonants can be found in Chapter 7.

counted. For example, if the child demonstrates an f/v and a d/v substitution, the number of differences between the two substitutions should be listed. The production features that primarily distinguish [f] from [v] are voicing; those that differentiate between [d] and [v] are manner and place.

3. The sound substitutions chosen should reflect the least number of differences in production features. Therefore, [f] and [v] would be selected because they demonstrate only one production feature difference; [d] versus [v] differs in two production features.

4. The age of the child and the developmental level of the child's phonemic system should be evaluated. Earlier sounds have priority. For example, when place, manner, and voicing characteristics are analyzed, both t/s and p/b substitutions represent differences of one production feature. However, [b] is earlier than [s]. Therefore, the [p]-[b] contrast is probably the better choice.

5. Sound substitutions that affect the child's intelligibility most should have priority over those with little negative effect on intelligibility. This choice is primarily related to the frequency of occurrence of the two sounds. Therefore, if two sound substitutions demonstrate an equal number of differences in production features, priority should be given to the sound that impacts the intelligibility of the child the most.

6. Stimulable sounds have priority over those that are not stimulable.

This procedure can be exemplified in the following manner. A 5;6-year-old child demonstrates the following substitutions: w/r, θ/s, ð/z, d/ʤ, t/ʧ, and w/ʃ. The production differences are as follows:

Substitution	*Main Production Differences*		
w/r	w = labial	glide	voiced
	r = palatal	liquid	voiced
θ/s	θ = dental	fricative	voiceless
	s = alveolar	fricative	voiceless
ð/z	ð = dental	fricative	voiced
	z = alveolar	fricative	voiced
d/ʤ	d = alveolar	stop	voiced
	ʤ = postalveolar	affricate	voiced
t/ʧ	t = alveolar	stop	voiceless
	ʧ = postalveolar	affricate	voiceless
w/ʃ	w = labial	glide	voiced
	ʃ = postalveolar	fricative	voiceless

Based on the number of production differences, two possibilities exist for target sounds: θ-s or ð-z. Both sound pairs are acquired at about the same time. Given that both sounds are stimulable, the best selection of target sounds would probably be [θ] and [s], because [s] has a higher frequency of occurrence and will, therefore, have more of an impact on the child's intelligibility.

How Is Minimal Opposition Contrast Therapy Used? The two target sounds selected are placed in minimal pair words with the chosen sounds at the beginning: *think-sink, thing-sing,* or *sick-thick,* for example. However, there are often few words that are appropriate for children. Therefore, it has been suggested that if meaningful minimal pairs cannot be found for contrastive phonemes, near-minimal pairs should be used (Elbert and Gierut, 1986). **Near-minimal pairs** are pairs of words that differ by more than one phoneme, and the vowel preceding or following the target sound remains constant in both words. For example, *sir-third* or *thorn-sore* would be considered near-minimal pairs.

Many of the treatment protocols of minimal opposition contrast therapy include discrimination, imitation, and spontaneous production of the word pairs using methods similar to those found in distinctive feature therapy. The following treatment suggestions are summarized from Lowe (1994).

Therapy is structured so that the child is placed in a situation in which the production of the sound substitution results in a communication breakdown. This breakdown focuses attention on the contrastive function of the phoneme in question. The child will probably attempt to repair the communicative situation by producing the intended target sound in an appropriate manner.

After having identified the substitution and minimal pairs appropriate to the age and interests of the child, the following procedure is implemented:

1. Familiarize the client with the minimal pair words by showing pictures of each word, describing the attributes of each concept, or actually providing concrete objects as examples.

2. Show several exemplars of each word. The client must pick up the picture named by the clinician. In the [θ-s] example with the minimal pair *thing-sing,* the clinician could show different types of "things" versus various people singing.

3. Reverse roles: The client must name one of the words and the clinician picks up the appropriate picture.

4. Substituted sounds result in the clinician picking up the picture actually named, not the one the child intended. A communicative breakdown has occurred due to inaccurate realization of the target sound.

5. Opportunity is given for the child to make some form of repair (attempts somehow to produce the sound in a different manner). The clinician rewards the attempt by picking up the intended picture.

CLINICAL APPLICATION

Selecting a Target for Minimal Opposition Contrast Therapy

The following substitutions are noted in the speech of the child H. H.

SUBSTITUTION	MAIN PRODUCTION DIFFERENCES
[ʧ] → [t]	place, manner
[ʤ] → [d]	place, manner
[k] → [t]	place
[g] → [d]	place
[f] → [b]	manner, voicing
[θ] → [b]	place, manner, voicing
[ð] → [d]	place, manner
[ʃ] → [d]	place, manner, voicing
[ʃ] → [s]	place
[s] → [t]	manner
[z] → [t]	manner, voicing

[r] → [w]   place, manner
[l] → [w]   place, manner

Four substitutions are candidates for this approach: [k-t], [g-d], [ʃ-s], and [s-t]. Stimulability of the sounds would need to be ascertained before target sounds could be selected. If all are stimulable, [k] and [t] would be a good choice because they are early developing sounds.

Maximal Oppositions Approach

What Is the Maximal Oppositions Approach? This treatment method is similar to distinctive feature and minimal opposition contrasts in that minimal word pairs are used as the beginning unit of training. However, in direct contrast to minimal opposition contrasts, in which target sounds that are productionally similar are selected, the maximal oppositions approach chooses sounds that are productionally very different. Differences in production were originally defined (Elbert and Gierut, 1986; Gierut, 1989) according to the number of variations in place, manner, or voicing between the two sounds. If possible, sounds were then selected that demonstrated differences in all three production features.

In the meantime, the conceptual framework for this therapy has changed somewhat. Currently, the term *maximal oppositions* refers to differences in distinctive features. These differences vary along two dimensions: (1) the number of unique features that differentiate between the two phonemes and (2) the nature of the features, that is, if differences are major or nonmajor class features. The Chomsky-Halle (1968) system, which defines major class features as consonantal, sonorant, and vocalic, is used.

The concept of maximal oppositions training was first introduced by Elbert and Gierut (1989) in response to their continuum of productive phonological knowledge (see Chapter 7). A series of investigations (Dinnsen and Elbert, 1984; Elbert, Dinnsen, and Powell, 1984; Gierut, 1985) examined the relationship between "most" and "least" phonological knowledge and the amount of generalization that occurred within the phonological system of children. In one of these studies, findings indicated that children treated in the order of least to most phonological knowledge showed generalization across the overall sound system (Gierut, 1985). In other words, if treatment focused first on sounds that the child could not produce (consistent "error" productions) and only later targeted sounds that appeared in some contexts (inconsistent "error" productions), the most generalization occurred. On the other hand, if the order of treatment proceeded from most to least phonological knowledge, generalization was very limited. These findings led to the development of the maximal oppositions approach.

When to Use the Maximal Oppositions Approach. Which clients benefit most from maximal oppositions training? By examining the children in the series of investigations conducted to demonstrate this method, (Gierut, 1990, 1992), most subjects had at least six sounds that were excluded from their phonetic and phonemic inventories. This suggests that clients who would benefit the most from this intervention strategy would be those with moderate to severe phonological disorders.

The maximal oppositions technique has been described in several research investigations in which its efficacy has been tested on several children. Gierut (1989) reported that after three different word pairs contrasting maximal oppositions had been presented, the child learned sixteen word-initial consonants and restructured his phonological system. Other studies (Gierut, 1990, 1991, 1992; Gierut and Neumann, 1992) supported these findings. When minimal versus maximal oppositions approaches were therapeutically contrasted, more generalization occurred using maximal contrasts (Gierut, 1990). Other studies challenged one of the basic principles of minimal pair therapy, the selection of sounds based on the concept of "substitution" and "error" sounds (Gierut, 1991, 1992; Gierut and Neumann, 1992). If both sounds used to establish word pairs were *not* in the child's inventory, this proved to be as effective, or at times even more effective, than teaching one sound versus its substitution. In the last of the series of investigations, word pairs comparing two previously unknown phonemes that differed by maximal and major class features were found to be the preferred way to change the phonological system of the child (Gierut, 1992). Research findings seem to support the efficacy of maximal oppositions therapy.

How to Select Target Sounds for the Maximal Oppositions Approach.   Between the earlier and the later versions of maximal oppositions therapy, the procedure for target selection changed (Elbert and Gierut, 1986; Gierut, 1989, 1992). Only the later selection procedures will be outlined here.

Two sounds not in the child's inventory (i.e., two unknown sounds) are selected. In addition, these two sounds should be maximally different according to their distinctive features. Two parameters are used to determine the maximum distinctive feature differences: (1) the number of unique distinctive features that differentiate the two sounds (more distinctive feature differences = maximum feature distinction) and (2) the nature of the feature, that is, whether it is a major or nonmajor feature class (major class features = maximum feature distinction). Major class features are:

[+ vocalic]	differentiates vowels and liquids *from* stops, fricatives, affricates, and nasals
[+ consonantal]	differentiates stops, fricatives, affricates, nasals, and liquids *from* vowels, glides, and [h]
[+ sonorant]	differentiates nasals, liquids, glides, and [h] *from* stops, fricatives, and affricates

The following example (Subject 11 from Gierut, 1992) is given to illustrate the selection process used in maximum feature distinctions.

Inventory	Sounds Not in Inventory	Major Class Difference
m, n, ŋ, w, j, h, p, b, t, d,	r, l k, g	yes, between r, l versus k, g
f, v, ʧ, ʤ	s, z, ʃ, ʒ, θ, ð	yes, between r, l versus s, z, ʃ, ʒ, θ, ð

Major class differences are evidenced between /r/ and /l/ and several other phonemes. Because both /r/ and /l/ are [+ voice], the voiceless consonants [– voice] would demonstrate more distinctive feature differences. When feature differences are counted between the noted voiceless consonants and /r/ and /l/, the following number of distinctive feature differences emerges:

[r] and [k] = 5	[l] and [k] = 7
[r] and [s] = 3	[l] and [s] = 3
[r] and [ʃ] = 3	[l] and [ʃ] = 5
[r] and [θ] = 2	[l] and [θ] = 2

Note: The categories sonorant, consonantal, and vocalic are not counted again when figuring the number of distinctive features.

Therefore, considering both major class distinctions and the differences in distinctive features, the target phonemes would be /l/ and /k/. These phonemes would then be utilized to form minimal pairs such as *lane-cane, leg-keg,* and *lamp-camp.*

How Is the Maximal Oppositions Contrast Approach Used? The perception of, or discrimination between, the phonological contrast is not directly trained; rather, treatment includes two phases, *imitation* and *spontaneous production,* for each sound pair. However, it should be noted in this context that this treatment protocol originated from a research project comparing different word pairs and their impact on changes within the phonological system of children. For clinical purposes, practitioners may want to implement additional activities to serve the needs of individual clients.

Imitation Phase. Minimal pair picture cards are presented and the client asked to repeat the clinician's model of the pictures. Several different activities can be used to maintain interest, such as matching or sorting pictures during imitative production, moving a car around one space on a track each time the word is imitated, playing various card games with the pictures, and so on. This phase of treatment continues until 75 percent imitative accuracy over two to maximally seven consecutive sessions is achieved.

Spontaneous Phase. Word pairs are now produced by the client without the clinician's model. Again, various activities can be found to keep the child's interest. This phase continues until 90 percent accurate production without a model over three to maximally twelve consecutive sessions is achieved.

Phonological Process Therapy

What Is Phonological Process Therapy? Phonological processes are currently the most widely used systems to assess error patterns in

---

CLINICAL APPLICATION

Selecting Target Sounds with the Maximal Oppositions Approach

The following results are provided for H. H.

INVENTORY	SOUNDS NOT IN INVENTORY	MAJOR CLASS DIFFERENCE
m, n, ŋ		
w, j, h	r, l	
p, b, t, d	k, g	yes, between r, l versus k, g
f, v, s*	ʧ, ʤ, z, ʃ, θ, ð	yes, between r, l versus z, ʃ, ʒ, ʧ, ʤ, θ, ð

Major class differences are evidenced between /r/ and /l/ and several other phonemes. Because both /r/ and /l/ are [+ voice], the voiceless consonants [– voice] would render more distinctive feature differences. When feature differences are counted between the noted voiceless consonants and /r/ and /l/, the highest number of feature differences exists between /l/–/k/ and /l/–/ʧ/ (seven different features). Therefore, previously noted word pairs for /l/ and /k/ or word pairs such as *lane* versus *chain* and *Lynn* versus *chin* could be used in this maximal oppositions approach.

*[f] and [v] were each produced correctly one time during the articulation test; [s] was used as a substitution for [ʃ].

---

the speech of children (Howell and Dean, 1991, 1994). As an assessment tool, its practical application is often traced back to David Ingram's (1976, 1989b) *Phonological Disability in Children.* Since that time, several assessment protocols and tests founded on the concept of phonological processes have been developed (e.g., Bankson and Bernthal, 1990; Dean, Howell, Hill, and Waters, 1990; Grunwell, 1985a; Hodson, 1986; Ingram, 1981; Khan and Lewis, 1986; Lowe, 1996; Shriberg and Kwiatkowski, 1980; Weiner, 1979). Although some therapy methods, such as cycles training or metaphon therapy, utilize phonological process *assessment* to determine training goals, a phonological process *therapy* as such does not exist. Typically, a phonological process is selected and minimal pair contrasts are then employed. If the child can produce the minimal pair distinctions, the phonological process has been suppressed.

In order to bridge the gap between the assessment of phonological errors (see Chapter 7) and their treatment, the following section will describe how minimal contrasts can be established when specific phonological processes have been selected as intervention targets.

When to Use Phonological Process Therapy. Which clients would benefit the most from specific phonological process therapies using minimal contrasts? For the young client whose phonological system is characterized primarily by the persistence of only a limited number of phonological processes, the phonological process therapy approach is probably a viable option. However, for the child who is unintelligible or who demonstrates a wide variety of phonological processes, other approaches that will be discussed in the following sections (cycles training, maximal oppositions, metaphon therapy) may offer better possibilities.

As mentioned earlier, phonological processes are frequently used to assess patterns of phonemic errors. However, would minimal

contrast therapy targeting specific phonological processes also influence their reduction? Weiner (1981) tested this hypothesis with two children using minimal contrasts therapy in game activities. Accurate production was required or a breakdown in communication would occur. For example, in attempting to reduce the frequency of occurrence of final consonant deletion, *bow* and *boat* were contrasted. The child had to gather a certain number of pictures of *boat* from the clinician. If the child said *bow* although *boat* was intended, the clinician would pick up the picture of *bow*. A communicative breakdown had ensued. With this intervention method, a reduction of specific phonological processes was achieved, which generalized to nontrained words as well. Based on the results of this one study, phonological process therapy seems to enhance suppression of phonological processes. However, far more research is needed, especially in light of the newer developments maximal feature distinctions seem to offer.

How to Select Target Sounds with Phonological Process Therapy. Which phonological processes should be chosen for therapy, and how does this choice impact target selection? Phonological processes should be chosen based on

- their relative frequency of occurrence,
- the effect this process has on the client's intelligibility, and
- the age and phonological development of the child.

Good candidates for process selection are those that occur most often in the speech of the child because they will probably affect intelligibility to a higher degree. However, certain phonological processes will have more of an impact on intelligibility than others. For example, the process final consonant deletion affects many different sounds, whereas velar fronting is typically limited to a t/k sub-

---

It is fairly easy to construct minimal pairs with the substitution processes. For example, when treating velar fronting, minimal pairs contrasting /t/ and /k/ could be used. However, syllable structure processes are a bit more difficult. Final consonant deletion could be treated by contrasting words that contain a final consonant versus those that do not, for example, *bow* versus *boat*. Minimal pairs could also be constructed for consonant cluster reduction—*street* versus *treat*—and for unstressed syllable deletion—*before* versus *four*. On the other hand, reduplication does not seem to lend itself very effectively to the use of minimal pairs.

stitution. Therefore, if a decision must be made between final consonant deletion or velar fronting, final consonant deletion would probably be the process to work on first. Finally, the age of the child must be considered. There are phonological processes that are normally suppressed at an early age, such as reduplication, and others that continue to operate until the end of the preschool years, such as stopping of /θ/ and /ð/. Therefore, earlier processes are typically targeted before later processes.

> For a list of the most common processes and the approximate age of suppression, see Chapter 5.

An example: A 4;6-year-old child demonstrates a high frequency of occurrence of final consonant deletion, consonant cluster reduction, gliding (/r/ → /w/), and stopping of /θ/ and /ð/. Based on his age and the impact on intelligibility, final consonant deletion would be a good choice for beginning therapy. The others are "late" processes that would probably not affect the intelligibility of a 4-year-old.

After an appropriate phonological process is selected, word pairs must be found for the beginning phase of minimal contrast training. The child's phonetic inventory and the stimulability of specific sounds will often guide the selection. Table 9.2 offers examples for a number of phonological processes.

How Are Minimal Pairs Used with Phonological Processes?

There are many ways these minimal pairs can be used in a therapy situation. Several of them have been discussed in the sections on distinctive feature therapy and minimal and maximal oppositions training. These activities can be as varied as the clinician's imagination but should always incorporate the client's interest and level of ability. Also, communicative function should stand in the foreground of any activity.

CLINICAL APPLICATION

Selection of a Phonological Process

Consonant cluster reduction, final consonant deletion, and stopping are the most prevalent processes in H. H.'s speech. Consonant cluster reduction is a relatively late process and would, therefore, not be a good candidate for therapy selection. Final consonant deletion would probably impact the intelligibility of H. H's speech the most. Minimal pairs should be found that would contrast a word with a final consonant using a sound that H. H. can realize versus no final consonant. For example, [b] and [t] can be articulated in an acceptable manner but are deleted in word-final position. Selected minimal pairs would be exemplified by *meat* versus *me, boat* versus *bow,* or *tube* versus *two.*

CYCLES TRAINING

What Is Cycles Training? This approach was developed by Hodson and Paden (1983, 1991). It is referred to as cycles training because the phonological patterns that are to be remediated are trained successively during specific time periods known as cycles. For example, certain patterns are trained for a given period of time in Cycle 1, others in Cycle 2.

This approach is unique for several reasons. First, there is no predetermined level of mastery for phonemes or phoneme patterns within each cycle. Therefore, clients do not have to reach 75 percent or 90 percent accuracy of any phoneme or pattern realization to move to the next cycle. The targeted patterns within the cycle are used to stimulate *emergence* of a specific sound or pattern, not *mastery* of it. The underlying premise for this procedure is based on the known observation that phonological acquisition is gradual. The cycles approach is an attempt to approximate closely the way phonological development normally occurs, as a gradual process. Second, several sounds are targeted within

TABLE 9.2 Examples for Constructing Minimal Pairs Using Phonological Processes

SUBSTITUTION PROCESSES

Underlying Principle:	Construct word pairs with the target sound and the substitution. If the target sound is not stimulable, a traditional approach may be necessary to achieve correct production of the sound within a specific word context.
Velar Fronting:	t/k and d/g substitutions: word pairs need to be found contrasting /t/ and /k/ and /d/ and /g/. Examples: *tea* versus *key, tape* versus *cape. Dumb* versus *gum, dull* versus *gull.*
Palatal Fronting:	s/ʃ substitution: word pairs need to be found contrasting /s/ and /ʃ/. Examples: *sip* versus *ship, sell* versus *shell.*
Stopping of /s/ and /z/	t/s and d/z substitutions: word pairs need to be found contrasting /t/ and /s/ and /d/ and /z/. Examples: *toe* versus *sew, tee* versus *sea.* *D* versus *Z, do* versus *zoo.*
Gliding /r/ → /w/	w/r substitution: word pairs need to be found contrasting /w/ and /r/. Examples: *wed* versus *red, weed* versus *read.*

UNUSUAL PROCESSES

Stops Replacing Glides /j/ → /d/	d/j substitution: word pairs need to be found contrasting /d/ and /j/. Examples: *yacht* versus *dot, yarn* versus *darn.*
Denasalization of /n/ → /d/	d/n substitution: word pairs need to be found contrasting /n/ and /d/. Examples: *knot* versus *dot, near* versus *deer.*

PROCESSES AFFECTING GROUPS OR CLASSES OF PHONEMES

Underlying Principle:	Select contrast pairs containing sounds that the child can produce or are stimulable.
Final Consonant Deletion	Start with word pairs with and without final consonants, such as *bow* versus *boat.* If generalization does not occur, present word pairs contrasting another final consonant against no final consonant. Example: Child can produce [m, n, t, d, l, f, v, p, b] but not in word-final position. First, present contrasts such as *toe* versus *toad, low* versus *load.*
Consonant Cluster Reduction	Use singletons within the child's inventory to structure reduced consonant clusters contrasted to standard consonant clusters. Example: Cluster reductions are noted on several consonant blends. Child can produce [b], [p], [k], and [l] but says [kaᵘn] for *clown,* [peɪ] for *play,* [bu] for *blue.* Begin with [pl] and contrast word pairs such as *plan* versus *pan, peas* versus *please.*
Stopping of Fricatives	Select a stimulable fricative, which is then contrasted with the homorganic stop. Example: Child is stimulable for [f] but uses p/f substitution in most contexts. Use word pairs such as *fig* versus *pig, fin* versus *pin.*

UNUSUAL PROCESSES

Initial Consonant Deletion	Start with word pairs contrasting one initial consonant versus no initial consonant. If generalization does not occur, present word pairs with another initial consonant.

UNUSUAL PROCESSES Continued

	Example: Child can produce [p, b, t, d, h, w, m, n] but inconsistently deletes these sounds at the beginning of a word. Use word pairs such as *beet* versus *eat*, *bee* versus *E*.
Sound Preference Substitutions	Select a stimulable sound and use it in a contrasting word pair with the sound preference. Child produces [s], [z], [ʃ], [tʃ], and [dʒ] as [t]. The child is stimulable for [ʃ]. Contrast word pairs such as *two* versus *shoe*, *top* versus *shop*.

---

one cycle. While some of the patterns from Cycle 1 might be "recycled" in the next phase, new sound patterns are also introduced. Third, this approach targets very specific clients: It is explicitly designed for highly unintelligible children. The goal of cycles training is to increase intelligibility within a relatively short period of time. A by-product is the acquisition of certain sounds and patterns.

When to Use Cycles Training

Which clients benefit most from cycles training? This therapy targets a specific group of clients: highly unintelligible children. "This approach was *not* designed for children with mild speech disorders" (Hodson, 1989, p. 331). Although *highly unintelligible* is not explicitly defined, these children seem to be in the profound to severe range on the Assessment of Phonological Processes—Revised (Hodson, 1986). Utterances of the children in the profound category were characterized by extensive omissions, some phoneme substitutions, and a very restricted repertoire of consonants. Utterances of the children in the severe category had fewer omissions, but more substitutions and consonant classes were still limited (Hodson and Paden, 1991).

Is cycles training a viable therapy? According to the authors, it was developed, tested, and refined at experimental clinics in which this approach was utilized with over 200 clients (Hodson and Paden, 1991). Hodson (1992) further states that "Most clients have been dismissed from our clinic as essentially intelligible in less than 1 year" (p. 252). This would seem to indicate that the cycles approach is an effective treatment method. However, enough research has not yet been conducted to confirm these statements. Bankson and Bernthal (1998c) summarize by saying, "While the authors have a wealth of clinical experience to support this approach to intervention, published data, particularly of a comparative nature, are lacking" (p. 346). Research is needed to verify the efficacy of this treatment approach.

How to Select Target Sounds with Cycles Training. The following are guidelines for potential target patterns or phonemes for Cycle 1 training: primary potential target patterns/phonemes.

1. *Early Developing Phonological Patterns.* These patterns are typically present in very young normally developing children. Highly unintelligible children should be assessed to determine their individual

abilities in the following categories. Deficiencies in the following categories would be potential targets for Cycle 1 training.

- *Syllableness.* Two- and three-syllable equal stress word combinations such as *cowboy* or *cowboy hat.* This category is evaluated according to whether the vowel nuclei exist, not in respect to the accurate production of all sounds.
- *Word-initial singleton consonants.* Includes CV structures with the following phonemes: /m, n, p, b, t, d, w/.
- *Word-final singleton consonants.* Includes VC structures with the following phonemes: /p, t, and/or k, m, n/.
- *Other word structures.* Both CVC and VCV words are found in the child's speech.

2. *Posterior/ Anterior Contrasts*
The child's speech is examined to see if either alveolar or velar sounds are absent.

3. */s/ Clusters*
The child's speech is examined to see if /s/ clusters are produced. Based on clinical experience, the authors have found that word-final /s/ clusters are the most facilitating for these children. Singleton /s/ is not targeted until a later cycle.

4. *Liquids*
The child's speech is examined to see if /l/ and /r/ are produced. If absent, these phonemes should be stimulated during each cycle.

5. *Nasals*

6. *Velars* (if stimulable)

7. *Glides*

If the child does not have one or more of these patterns or phonemes, any of the aforementioned categories would be acceptable targets for Cycle 1. Target selection of specific

phonemes also depends on the client's stimulability. The clinician should select the client's most stimulable sounds or patterns so that the child can experience immediate success. Unacceptable targets include /ŋ/, /θ/, /ð/, the syllabic /l/, and weak syllable deletion.

An example: A child demonstrates a high frequency of occurrence of the following processes: final consonant deletion, consonant cluster reduction, velar fronting, gliding (w/l and w/r substitutions), and stridency deletion. Going down the list of potential primary targets noted above, the following emerge:

1. word-final singleton consonants
2. CVC structures
3. s-clusters
4. liquids
5. velars

Patterns eliminated: Word-final singleton consonants were not considered a Cycle 1 target because the child did produce [p], [t], [m], and [n] in the word-final position.

The child was not stimulable for stridents.

Patterns targeted: 1. CVC structures to stimulate the understanding of final consonants

2. liquids

3. velars

Because the child was not stimulable for stridents, /s/ clusters, which would normally be a primary target, were delayed until a later cycle.

How Is Cycles Training Used? *Establishing a cycle.* Each phoneme within a pattern should be targeted for *sixty minutes per cycle.* If therapy is thirty minutes per session, two times a week, then the first phoneme would be targeted for one week of therapy. After completion of the first phoneme, a second one is initiated for the next sixty minutes. All remaining phonemes are presented consecutively for sixty minutes each. If the goal is a specific phonological pattern rather than an individual phoneme, at least two exemplars of the pattern should be presented in two consecutive sixty-minute time intervals before moving on to the next phoneme or pattern. For example, if the pattern targeted is CVC structures, then two different CVC word types should be utilized, CVCs with final voiced stops versus final nasals. Only one phonological pattern or phoneme should be targeted during any *one* session. In Cycle 1, all the patterns determined from the assessment are presented consecutively. Typically, this cycle contains between three and six different patterns or phonemes.

Preparing word cards for therapy. Words are used as the minimal unit of production practice, and word cards that picture each of the chosen concepts are developed. Chosen words should be monosyllabic and incorporate facilitative phonetic environments. For example, words containing sounds that are produced at the same place of articulation as the substitute sound should be avoided. Thus, *cat, can, kite,* and *goat* should not be used if the child has a t/k substitution (Hodson, 1989). Object and action words are preferred. Obviously, the words should also be appropriate for the vocabulary level of the child.

Structuring the remediation session. The following format is given for each therapy session:

1. *Review.* The child reviews the preceding session's word cards.
2. *Auditory bombardment.* Amplified auditory stimulation is provided for one to two minutes while the clinician reads approx-

imately twelve words that contain the target pattern for this session.

3. *Target word cards.* The client draws, colors, or pastes pictures of three to five target words on large index cards. During this phase, the child repeats the words modelled by the clinician.

4. *Production practice through experiential play.* During experiential play (e.g., fishing, bowling), clinician and child take turns naming the pictures. The clinician provides models and/or tactile cues (such as touching the upper lip of the child to indicate an alveolar sound or the throat to indicate a velar production) so that the child achieves 100 percent success on the target patterns. (This is why it is essential that target words are carefully selected). Opportunities are also given to engage in conversation to determine if the pattern is beginning to emerge spontaneously.

5. *Stimulability probes.* The child's stimulability is assessed for potential targets of the next session. For example, if /s/ clusters are prospects for the next session, the child is asked to model several words that contain different /s/ clusters. The most stimulable /s/ cluster is then targeted for the next session.

6. *Auditory bombardment.* Step 2 is repeated.

7. *Home program.* The parent or school aide participates in a two minutes per day home program that consists of reading the week's listening list (Step 2) and the child naming picture cards of the production practice words.

METAPHON THERAPY

What Is Metaphon Therapy?

Metaphon therapy orginated in the 1980s as a result of dissatisfaction with minimal pair management strategies for phonologically disordered children. In the experience of its developers, Janet Howell and Elizabeth Dean, the use of minimal pair contrasts was often not causing the necessary changes in the child's phonological system. This led to questioning the metaphonological skills of these children. In other words, what do children with phonological disorders know about sounds? The concept of metaphon therapy was born.

Similar to cycles training, metaphon therapy has evolved out of clinical experience and incorporates different approaches that are merged into two therapy phases. However, the framework established to guide therapy is obviously different from that proposed by cycles training. Metaphon therapy is based on metalinguistic awareness. **Metalinguistic awareness** is the ability to think about and reflect on the nature of language and how it functions (Pratt and Grieve, 1983). Specifically, metaphon therapy is structured to develop children's metaphonological skills. Metaphonology is defined as the ability to pay attention to, and reflect upon, the phonological structure of language (Howell and Dean, 1991, 1994).

The nature of metaphonological and general metalinguistic ability is neither clear-cut nor universally agreed upon. Metaphon therapy is based on the assumption that metalinguistic and specifically metaphonological awareness develops alongside language; as children's language systems grow, so do their metalinguistic skills. Although highly dependent on the experimental task that must be fulfilled, some evidence of metalinguistic knowledge has been found in 2- and 3-year-old children (Chaney, 1992; Gleitman, Gleitman, and Shipley, 1972). Metaphonological awareness seems to be present during the preschool years (e.g., Leopold, 1948; Pease, 1986; Reid, Grieve, Dean, Donaldson, and Howell, 1993; Sinclair, Jarvella, and Levelt, 1980).

However, is there evidence that supports the notion that children with phonological disorders have problems with metaphonological skills? Using different metaphonological tasks, several investigations have demonstrated that children with phonological disorders do generally not perform as well as normally developing children of a similar age (e.g., Bird and Bishop, 1992; Howell, 1989; Kamhi, Friemoth-Lee, and Nelson, 1985; Magnusson, 1983, 1991; Magnusson and Naucler, 1987; Stackhouse, 1985; Stackhouse and Snowling, 1983).

Metaphon therapy also assumes that phonologically disordered children fail to realize the communicative significance of the phonological rule system. Their difficulties do not pertain to producing speech sounds in a normal manner but to their failure to acquire the rules of the phonological system. Howell and Dean (1991, 1994) postulate that the best way to help these children change their rule systems is to provide them with information that will encourage them to make their own changes and thus impact their speech output. The following are seen as prerequisites for this to occur:

1. The child must have knowledge that change is required.
2. The child must have knowledge that change can be made.
3. The child must have information that can be used to assist change.

The phases of metaphon therapy are constructed in an attempt to provide this knowledge.

When to Use Metaphon Therapy. Which clients can benefit the most from metaphon therapy? Howell and Dean (1991, 1994) target preschool children because it is at this age that metaphonological knowledge is developing. The existing case studies have several features in common: Most of the children presented had very restricted phonetic inventories; all the children had unusual or idiosyncratic processes, such as initial consonant deletion; and all the children had a wide variety of phonological processes operating in their speech. Based on these results, one could conclude that metaphon therapy would be a good match for children who have moderate to severe phonological disorders and who have at least two or three processes that predominate their speech patterns.

Does metaphon therapy work? Both the first and second editions of Howell and Dean's book (1991, 1994) provide the results of an efficacy study that evaluated several aspects of metaphon therapy. Originally, thirteen children participated in the study; according to the second edition, the number of subjects now totals fifty. Preliminary results indicate that metaphon therapy does indeed work. First, the results indicate a reduction in the use of specific phonological processes pre- and posttreatment. Second, changes in the phonological system were accelerated beyond the expected level according to chronological development. Because the children in this study were not divided into treatment versus no-treatment groups, two different measures of language were used to verify whether treatment, not development, was actually responsible for the changes. Pre- and posttreatment scores for phonological processes were compared to those obtained from a second nontreated language area, which was measured by the British Picture Vocabulary Scale (Dunn, Dunn, Whetton, and Pintilie, 1982). While significant differences could be verified between pre- and posttreatment phonological process scores, the scores from the British Picture Vocabulary Scale remained the same, verifying that treatment, not development, had caused the noted changes. Third, while some subjects demonstrated a reduction in the targeted phonological processes, for others the

change was more generalized, causing a reduction in processes that were unrelated to those specifically targeted in treatment. Based on these results, metaphon therapy appears to be a viable therapeutic option, but more controlled studies are needed.

How to Select Target Sounds for Metaphon Therapy. Dean and Howell (1991, 1994) use the *Metaphon Resource Pack* (Dean, Howell, Hill, and Waters, 1990) as the basis for their assessment procedure. Seventy words (forty-four monosyllabic and twenty-six multisyllabic) are elicited; thirteen different phonological processes are identified. A frequency of occurrence of each process can be calculated. However, this quantitative measure is based on *selected* target words and is not indicative of the overall frequency of occurrence within the sample. Process Specific Probe material is provided for each of the thirteen processes to further evaluate the extent to which the process is operating in the child's speech. The child's phonetic inventory is another important aspect of the selection process.

Howell and Dean provide the following general considerations that influence the choice among the processes to be treated:

1. Processes selected for treatment should not be those that are seen in normally developing children of the same age.
2. Variable use of a simplifying process, which may be evidence of spontaneous change in the child's phonological system, should be given priority in the selection process.
3. The effect the operation of the phonological process has on the intelligibility of the child is important. Processes that cause more disruption, such as stopping of fricatives or atypical processes, should be given priority.
4. The sounds available to the child, both spontaneously and on an imitative basis,

play a role in the selection process; sounds that are not in the inventory but can be imitated are usually given priority.

An example: A child, age 4;4, demonstrates the following processes with an occurrence of over 50 percent:

Velar fronting	Word-initial and -final positions
Stopping of fricatives	All positions
Stopping of affricates	All positions
Initial consonant deletion	Limited to fricatives
Initial consonant cluster reduction/deletion	All contexts
Phonetic inventory:	[m, n, ŋ]
	[p, b, t, d, k, g]
	[w, j]
	[l]

Based on the child's age, velar fronting, stopping of fricatives, and initial fricative deletion were all potential target processes. Consonant cluster reduction could be seen as a consequence of the child's lack of fricatives and of the limited phonetic inventory. Velar fronting was chosen as the first target because the child did show evidence of suppression of this process in some contexts. Initial fricative deletion was selected as the second target on the grounds that the introduction of fricatives might generalize, eliminating the stopping of fricatives as well.

How Is Metaphon Therapy Used? There are two therapy phases. Phase 1 is designed to develop the awareness of the properties of sounds. This is done in a motivating setting where success is facilitated. Phase 1 is the most important phase because it forms the basis for the application to more realistic communicative settings emphasized in Phase 2.

Phase 1 Therapy: Developing Phonological Awareness. The primary aim of Phase 1 is to capture the child's interest in sounds and the en-

tire sound system. Although this is a natural activity of normally developing preschoolers, Howell and Dean (1991, 1994) believe that such awareness has not been possible for the phonologically disordered child. Child and clinician explore the properties of sounds together, how sounds differ from each other (i.e., place, manner, and voicing distinctions), and the importance of realizing these distinctions.

Phase 1 therapy is divided into four levels: concept level, sound level, phoneme level, and word level. Although the emphasis is somewhat different depending on whether the target selection is a substitution or a syllable structure process, each client moves through each of the levels with each process. Throughout Phase 1, the child remains a listener only.

Therapy for Substitution Processes

Concept Level. During the discussion and exploration of sounds with the child, it is essential that there is a shared understanding of the vocabulary and concepts utilized. At the concept level, child and clinician play games that involve this vocabulary when talking about different classes of sounds. At this level, individual speech sounds are not contrasted; rather, some of their characteristics—such as long versus short, front versus back, and noisy versus whisper—are considered. The child plays games such as matching long and short socks, ribbons, or strings; putting bricks at the front or back of the house; and growling noisily and in a whisper to identify the respective characteristics as a preparation for later place, manner, and voicing comparisons of actual speech sounds. One-hundred percent success should be achieved at this level. Therapy at this level may be brief, depending on the child's success.

Sound Level. In this phase, the previous achievements are transferred to the description of sounds in general. Games might involve musical instruments, noise-making rattles, shakers, and vocalizations made by the therapist and child, such as lions "roaring," people "singing," and cars "racing." The aim is to show that all sounds can be classified according to the dimensions specified in the concept level, that is, long–short, front–back, and noisy–whisper.

Phoneme Level. After having achieved success at the first two levels, the client is now ready to move on to activities involving speech sounds. The child and clinician take turns producing a range of sounds that vary along the three dimensions previously indicated. Individual sounds are not yet the focus; rather, all sounds from one class are contrasted with sounds from another (e.g., different stops are contrasted with various fricatives). The respective speech sounds may be produced spontaneously or in response to a visual referent (a card with a mnemonic of the property in question). See Figure 9.1 for an example of Mr. Noisy and Mr. Whisper. At this level, speech sound activities can also be paired with those introduced at the concept level—for example, first the matching of long and short strings and then the identification of long and short sounds.

Word Level. After the phoneme level, minimal pairs of words containing the targeted contrast are introduced. The client is asked to make a judgment about whether the sound is, for example, long or short, front or back, or noisy or whispered. Although the client is only a listener at this level, some discussion about the sound properties are included. For example, a noisy (voiced) sound is identified and then knowledge of other "noisy" sounds is questioned. Later, other minimal pair words may be introduced. In addition, visual referents used in previous levels may be placed

Mr. Noisy

Mr. Whisper

FIGURE 9.1 Examples of Mr. Noisy and Mr. Whisper

Source: Reproduced with permission from *Treating Phonological Disorders in Children: Metaphon-Theory to Practice* (p. 12), by Janet Howell and Elizabeth Dean, 1994, London: Whurr Publishers.

on the back of the card to provide additional feedback about the target item.

Therapy for Syllable Structure Processes

Concept Level. For syllable structure processes, such as initial or final consonant deletion, other concepts will be introduced, such as "beginning" and "end," for instance. These could be exemplified by the engine at the beginning of the train and the caboose at the end, or the nose of the alligator at the beginning and the tail at the end. If cluster simplification is the target, suitable contrasts could consist of the concepts of one horse in front of the wagon, two engines pulling the train, or three dogs pulling the sled.

Syllable Level/Word Level. At this stage, syllables representing the targeted contrast are utilized. For initial consonant deletion, for example, V and CV structures with nonsense syllables could be introduced with the analogy of a train with no engine versus one with an engine. Because it will not always be appropriate and motivating to stay with nonsense syllables, some words might be selected as well.

Phase 2 Therapy: Developing Phonological and Communicative Awareness. Phase 2 of therapy has three aims:

1. to transfer the metaphonological knowledge gained during Phase 1 to real communicative situations
2. to build up the client's communicative awareness to the point of recognizing when speech output and the intended meaning are at variance with one another
3. to develop phonological awareness to the degree that output repair can result so that the intended meaning can be conveyed

The link between Phases 1 and 2 is established by incorporating Phase 1 activities into Phase 2. Phonological awareness needs to be well developed before Phase 2 will be successful. Both Phase 1 and Phase 2 activities are essential for the core activity.

Core Activity. The core activity is structured so that clinician and client are taking turns in producing minimal pair words. Howell and Dean (1994) establish word cards as "secret messages"; however, different activities could be invented that are specifically developed for the individual client's interests. If the child says the word pictured on the card accurately, positive feedback is given and expanded into a relevant discussion. For example: "Right, that was a noisy sound. I bet you know lots of other noisy sounds." If, however, the child produces one of the minimal pair words incorrectly, intending the other word, the clinician picks the word that was said, not the intended one. This may stimulate the child to produce a spontaneous repair. The clinician never comments directly on the child's inappropriate production of a particular word but draws the child's attention to the salient features of the contrast: "That was a noisy sound. Should it have been a whisper sound?" Phase 1 activities can be used prior to or after the core activity.

There are no instructions regarding the child who repeatedly does not produce the sound or sound pattern in question correctly. One assumes that one goes back to Phase 1 activities. Therefore, for children who are not stimulable for a particular sound and remain unstimulable throughout Phase 1, Phase 2 could prove to be frustrating. In a later portion of the text, Howell and Dean suggest, based on the child's increased metalinguistic awareness, a discussion of the reasons for the loss of contrast. "Referring to sounds in a way which allows children to discuss them allows specific exploration of the reasons why a child has failed to convey meaning" (Howell and Dean, 1994, p. 110).

The last phase moves the minimal word pairs into sentences such as "Put the picture of the pea/key in the box," and "Draw a picture of the pea/key on the board." Situations that facilitate communication and promote repairing communicative breakdowns are important variables. It is also stressed that a supportive environment is an essential ingredient of this therapy.

PHONEMIC DISORDERS WITH CONCURRENT LANGUAGE PROBLEMS: THERAPEUTIC SUGGESTIONS

Phonological disorders often co-occur with language disorders. Tyler and Watterson (1991) estimated a co-occurrence rate in preschoolers of between 60 to 80 percent. Based on data from 178 children with developmental phonological disorders, Shriberg and Kwiatkowski (1994) found that between 50 percent and 70 percent of these children had co-occurring expressive language problems while 10 percent to 40 percent evidenced a delay in language comprehension as well. Other studies (Bishop and Edmundson, 1987; Shriberg, 1991; Shriberg, Kwiatkowski, Best, Hengst, and Terselic-Weber, 1986) support these statistics. Thus, most of the children seen clinically for a phonological disorder will also demonstrate other language problems.

The relationship between phonology and other areas of language is a complex one. A synergistic model of language (Schwartz, Leonard, Folger, and Wilcox, 1980; Shriner, Holloway, and Daniloff, 1969) proposes an intricate web of interdependencies between various aspects of language. This view has been tested by several investigations that examined specific remediation interactions between phonology and syntax in children with phonological disorders (Fey et al., 1994; Hoffman, Norris, and Monjure, 1990; Matheny and Panagos, 1978; Panagos, Quine, and Klich, 1979; Paul and Shriberg, 1982; Tyler and Watterson, 1991).

One hypothesis tested was whether treatment of one area, either phonology or syntax, would impact the other. Matheny and Panagos (1978) found a positive interaction between phonology and syntax; that is, instruction in either phonology or syntax resulted in gains in the other area also. With a slightly different conceptual basis, Hoffman, Norris, and Monjure (1990) examined the impact of a whole language approach versus phonological instruction alone on the language abilities of two children. Language abilities were measured by a comprehensive language test, an articulation test, an index of phonological processes, and a narrative task. Both children's overall language skills increased. As might be expected, the child with a whole language approach showed greater improvement in expressive language skills (as measured by the narrative task) while the child with phonological instruction demonstrated more improvement in phonological skills (as measured by the articulation and phonological processes tests). These results seem to indicate that phonological intervention does impact other language areas and that language-based treatment might also have a positive influence on the child's phonological system.

However, other investigations have not supported these results (Fey et al., 1994; Tyler and Watterson, 1991). Based on their findings, Tyler and Watterson (1991) suggested that children with more severe deficits may not evidence generalization from one language area to another, whereas children with mild to moderate difficulties may benefit from therapy with either a phonological or a language-based approach. Fey and colleagues (1994), in a carefully controlled investigation with twenty-six children ages 44 to 70 months, examined the impact of two different types of language instruction on the phonological abilities of their subjects. Although the grammar of these children was affected by the training, there was no direct effect on the children's phonological skills. One of the conclusions of Fey and colleagues (1994) is that

> the strategy of trying to improve intelligibility by focusing intervention on grammar (or even broader discourse patterns) is not defensible at this time…. For most children who have impairments in both speech and language, we believe that some clinical attention must be focused directly on both areas. (p. 605)

Although more research is needed on the interaction of phonology with other language areas, it is currently safe to say that (1) most children with phonological disorders will also demonstrate language difficulties and (2) intervention will need to target both phonology and additionally deficient language areas. To achieve this, a specified amount of time could be allotted to each deficient area: phonology, morphosyntax, semantics, or pragmatics. It would, of course, be more time-efficient if some language therapy goals could be unified. In the following section, some suggestions will be offered on how specific phonological remediation goals could be combined with noted morphosyntactic and semantic problems. Although divisions into morphosyntax and semantics, for example, are made to aid organization, it should always be kept in mind that a complex interaction exists between all language components. The next section addresses only some of the more common difficulties observed in children with language impairments.

Connecting Phonology to Morphosyntax

Morphological skills in children with specific language impairment (SLI) have been examined in many studies. However, in order not to confound the results, children with phonological disorders have purposely been excluded. In this context, it should be noted that children with phonological disorders may represent only a subset of children with specific language impairment. Nevertheless, the findings can probably be generalized to include children with phonological disorders, especially in light of the additional production difficulties with specific morphemes these children display.

Various morphological problems in children with SLI have often been observed (e.g., Bishop, 1994; Eyer and Leonard, 1994; Johnston and Schery, 1976; Khan and James, 1983; Leonard, 1994; Leonard, McGregor, and Allen, 1992; Oetting and Horohov, 1997; Oetting and Rice, 1993; Paul and Shriberg, 1982; Rice and Oetting, 1993; Rice, Wexler, and Cleave, 1995). Based on findings of several of these investigations, Leonard, McGregor, and Allen (1992) summarized the grammatical morphemes that were used less frequently by SLI children. These results are listed in Table 9.3.

If this list of grammatical morphemes is examined according to their production difficulties, it becomes clear that phonologically disordered children might have problems actually producing some of them. Plurality, past tense -ed, possessive, and third person singular, for example, very often result in word-final consonant clusters. If the child deletes final consonants or reduces consonant clusters, the grammatical function of these morphemes will be lost. Even for the child displaying pri-

TABLE 9.3 Problematic Morphemes for Children with Specific Language Impairment

GRAMMATICAL MORPHEME	EXAMPLES
Present progressive -*ing**	swimming, eating
Plural -*s*	coats, shoes
Preposition *on*	on the table, on top
Possessive *'s*	Daddy's, dog's
Regular past tense -*ed*	walked, stopped
Irregular past tense	caught, drank
Regular third person -*s*	he hits, she throws
Articles *a* and *the*	a sweater, the man
Copula	He is tall, She's happy
Auxiliary *be*	They are singing, She's talking

Source: Adapted from Leonard, McGregor, and Allen, 1992.

*This grammatical morpheme is least likely to reveal a difference between children with and without language disorders, although in some studies, children with language impairments also evidenced difficulty.

marily substitution processes, these morphemes may not be realized accurately. In order to preserve morphemic contrasts, attention must be given to final consonants and consonant clusters when working with the child with a phonological disorder.

Remediation Suggestions

1. If a therapy goal is final consonant deletion, words that incorporate specific grammatical morphemes in contrasting word pairs could be targeted. The use of such pairs will depend on the sounds in the client's inventory and the targeted sound(s), but, whenever possible, aspects of morphology could be included, especially grammatical morphemes. The following are given as examples:

Grammatical morpheme	Examples
Plurality	toe-toes, key-keys, shoe-shoes
Possessive	Joe-Joe's, Ray- Ray's, ma-ma's
Regular past tense	row-rowed, lay-laid, show-showed
3rd person singular	I go-he goes, I do-he does

2. If a therapy goal pertains to consonant cluster reduction or deletion, contrastive word pairs like these incorporate grammatical morphemes:

Grammatical morpheme	Examples
Plurality	boat-boats, cup-cups, wheel-wheels
Possessive	cat-cat's, Dad-Dad's, dog-dog's
Regular past tense	walk-walked, kiss-kissed
3rd person singular	I walk-he walks, I drink-he drinks
Irregular past tense	drink-drank, hold-held

3. In sentences that are more conversationally based, minimal pair words could be used systematically to represent other grammatical morphemes:

Grammatical morpheme	Examples
Copula	She is sad versus She is mad He is tall versus He is small
Auxiliary	He is shopping versus He is hopping She is kissing versus She is hissing
Preposition *on*	on the toe versus on the go on his hat versus on his bat

4. In sentences that are more conversation-ally based, subject and object pronouns could be systematically used:

	Examples
Subject pronouns	She is here versus He is here
	She opened the door versus Lee opened the door
	She has the tea versus She has the key
	He helped the man versus We helped the man
Object pronouns	Give it to Jim versus Give it to him
	The tea belongs to her versus The key belongs to her

5. Length and complexity of the utterance also needs to be considered because syntactical complexity has an effect on productional accuracy (Panagos, Quine, and Klich, 1979; Schmauch, Panagos, and Klich, 1978). The more complex the syntax, the more likely a child will demonstrate a breakdown in articulatory accuracy. Although one therapeutic goal may be to increase the length and complexity of a child's utterances, this should always be evaluated in respect to the interaction between production accuracy and syntactic complexity.

Connecting Phonology to Semantics

The majority of research on the semantic limitations in children with language impairments has focused on their use of nouns (Leonard, 1988; Rice, 1991). Such studies have found that language-impaired children are slow in using their first words, and subsequent vocabulary development occurs at a slower rate than in normally developing children. More recent literature has also examined the use of verbs in language-impaired children (Conti-Ramsden and Jones, 1997; Fletcher and Peters, 1984; King and Fletcher, 1993; Paul, 1993; Rice, 1994; Rice and Bode, 1993; Rice, Wexler, and Cleave, 1995; Watkins, Rice, and Moltz, 1993). These studies suggest that verbs and verb-related grammatical properties may be a particular problem for children with language impairments.

Remediation Suggestions

1. Although minimal pair words typically incorporate nouns ("things" are easier to picture), various verbs could also be targeted. These could be selected in accordance with the child's targeted sound or process. Some examples:

Velar fronting   t/k substitution
take-rake, tan-can, taught-caught

Stopping of fricatives   t/s
tea-see, toe-sew, tip-sip

Final consonant deletion
shoe-shoot, ray-rake, say-sail, go-goat

Initial consonant deletion
eat-beat, add-sad, add-mad

2. When targeted sounds emerge in the child's speech, expand vocabulary with new words containing the target. Research on the acquisition of newly acquired words in normally developing children (Leonard, Schwartz, Morris, and Chapman, 1981; Schwartz and Leonard, 1982) indicates that children appear to learn more easily and quickly new words that begin with consonants they have used previously in other words. Therefore, if a targeted sound is emerging in the child's speech, the clinician could try to utilize new practice words that also expand the vocabulary of the child.

THE CHILD WITH AN EMERGING PHONOLOGICAL SYSTEM: THERAPEUTIC SUGGESTIONS

As previously noted, the term *emerging phonological system* refers to a time period when sounds are beginning to be used to form conventional words, in other words, to the emergence of expressive language. By age 2, normally developing toddlers begin to combine single words into two-word utterances. However, this communicative development seems to lag behind in some 2-year-olds. Children whose comprehension abilities are considered normal but who fail to achieve a fifty-word vocabulary and two-word combinations by age 2 are referred to as "late talkers," toddlers with "slow expressive language development or delay" (Paul and Jennings, 1992; Reed, 1994; Rescorla and Schwartz, 1990), or as children with "specific expressive language impairment" (Paul, 1989; Rescorla and Ratner, 1996). It has been estimated that approximately 10 percent to 15 percent of the total 2-year-old population meet these criteria (Rescorla, 1989). While half of them seem to outgrow this delay, the other half will continue to demonstrate language problems at age 3 and beyond (Paul, 1991; Paul, Looney, and Dahm, 1991; Rescorla and Schwartz, 1990).

When children with slow expressive language development are compared to norm children of similar ages, their vocalizations occur less often (Paul and Jennings, 1992; Rescorla and Ratner, 1996). In addition, the phonetic profiles of these children show a reduced repertoire of consonants and syllable shapes (Paul and Jennings, 1992). Inventory constraints are especially notable in word-final positions (Rescorla and Ratner, 1996).

To evaluate the child's emerging phonological system, an independent analysis was suggested in Chapter 6. Such an analysis does examine the child's productions of individual words, but the utterances are not compared to the adult model. At this point in the child's development, it is far more important to note the child's actual usage of specific sounds within words. To this end, two types of data need to be collected: (1) the inventory of speech sounds and (2) the syllable shapes used.

General remediation strategies for children with slow emerging language development include developing expressive language skills, specifically expanding the number of vocabulary items, the consonant inventory, the syllable shapes, and finally the use of two-word utterances (Paul, 1995). At this stage of the child's development, therapy must represent a unified package. Therapy to promote phonological skills needs to be combined with increasing the child's lexicon. The use of specific syllable shapes will also be a consideration when selecting which words to target. Remediation for the child with an emerging language system must account for the interdependencies that exist between all language areas.

The following suggestions provide some points to consider when choosing the first words for children with small expressive vocabularies. The consonant inventory and the syllable shapes the child uses will be especially important variables in this selection process.

Combining Phonology with Semantics: Developing a Lexicon

1. First, the child's consonant inventory needs to be considered. Early vocabularies are influenced by the phonological composition of the word. Words that are easier for children to produce are more likely to be included in their early vocabularies (Leonard, Schwartz, Folger, Newhoff, and Wilcox, 1979; Stoel-Gammon and Cooper, 1984). In addition, children appear to learn more easily and quickly new words that begin with consonants they have used previously in other words

(Leonard, Schwartz, Morris, and Chapman, 1981; Schwartz and Leonard, 1982). Therefore, new words that contain sounds already in the child's inventory should be targeted.

An example:

The child's inventory contains the following sounds:

[m, n]
[p, b, t, d]
[h, j]

Depending on the child's present lexicon, the following might be good word choices:

me, no-no
puppy, baby, bye-bye, teddy, toe
happy, yes

2. The child's present use of syllable shapes needs to be considered. Early syllable shapes include V, CV, CVCV, and CVC. The therapist selects words with syllable shapes the child already uses, possibly including other early syllable shapes. In doing so, it should be kept in mind that the therapy goal is to *expand* the child's use of syllable shapes; therefore, early syllable shapes not in the child's repertoire should also be stimulated.

An example:

If the child primarily realizes V, CV, and CVCV syllable shapes:

mama might be easier than *mom*
papa might be easier than *dad*
puppy or *doggie* might be easier than *dog*
kittie might be easier than *cat*
baby might be easier than *doll*

3. When expanding the child's consonant inventory, the normal developmental sequence should be the guiding principle. Children with slow emerging language seem to acquire consonants in the same order as normally developing children, only at a slower rate (Paul and Jennings, 1992). Therefore, early sounds that are not yet in the child's inventory should be targeted. For the child with only a few expressive words, Paul (1995) suggests introducing the sound by first using a babbling game activity rather than by putting it directly into words. The clinician begins by imitating the child's vocalizations. Once a reciprocal babbling exchange is established, the clinician introduces the new consonant into the babbling activity. Paul (1995) emphasizes that the goal of this activity is not to get the child to produce that particular sound but to increase the consonant inventory. Therefore, any new consonant, even if it is not the one modelled by the clinician, should be rewarded.

4. New words should be similar to those used first by normally developing children. These include, for example, names of important people in the child's environment, names for objects the child directly acts upon, labels for objects that move and change, actions, games, and routines in which the child is an active participant (Owens, 1992; Pan and Gleason, 1997). Table 9.4 provides some examples of children's earliest words.

5. After having evaluated the child's inventory and use of syllable structures, words from a wide variety of grammatical classes should be selected. Although nouns dominate young children's early speech, children's vocabularies include words from a variety of grammatical classes from the beginning (Bloom, 1973; Nelson, 1973; Pan and Gleason, 1997). Therefore, not just nouns should be targeted but also words that can be used to talk about the *relations* between objects. These relational words express more communicative functions and can be readily combined with other words into two-word utterances (Lahey, 1988; Lahey and Bloom, 1977). Table 9.5 lists some of the words Lahey and Bloom (1977) and Lahey (1988) proposed for a first lexicon. These one- or two-syllable words include both nouns and relational words and represent early syllable shapes.

TABLE 9.4 Children's Earliest Words: Examples from the Vocabularies of Children Younger than 20 Months

Sound effects
  baa baa, meow, moo, ouch, uh-oh, woof, yum-yum
Food and drink
  apple, banana, cookie, cheese, cracker, juice, milk, water
Animals
  bear, bird, bunny, cat, cow, dog, duck, fish, kitty, horse, pig, piggy
Body parts and clothing
  diaper, ear, eye, foot, hair, hand, hat, mouth, nose, shoe, toe, tooth
House and outdoors
  blanket, chair, cup, door, flower, keys, outside, spoon, tree, tv
People
  baby, daddy, gramma, grampa, mommy, [child's own name]
Toys and vehicles
  ball, balloon, bike, boat, book, bubbles, plane, toy, truck
Actions
  down, eat, go, sit, up
Games and routines
  bath, bye, hi, night-night, no, peekaboo, please, shhh, thank you, yes
Adjectives and descriptives
  allgone, cold, dirty, hot

Source: From "Semantic Development: Learning the Meaning of Words," by B. Pan and J. Berko Gleason, in *The Development of Language* (4th ed.) (p. 132), edited by J. Berko Gleason, 1997, Boston: Allyn & Bacon. Copyright © 1997 by Allyn & Bacon. Reprinted by permission.

At this stage in the child's development, articulation patterns will very often not mirror adult pronunciation. However, the therapy focus for these children is on expanding the use of consonants, syllable shapes, and words, not on norm production. Therefore, any word approximations produced by the child should be rewarded, not corrected. For example, if the word is *down* and the child says [daᵁ] or [taᵁ], this word approximation

should be rewarded. Even if the child produces the final [n] in another word, that does not mean the child can produce [n] under different coarticulatory conditions in a new word. The goal during this phase of therapy is to stimulate word production, not articulatory "correctness."

TREATMENT OF MULTIPLE VOWEL ERRORS

There is an abundance of information available about children's difficulties with consonant articulation and their remediation. In contrast, vowel problems have not received the same degree of attention. This has been generally justified by the fact that vowels are mastered at an early age in the child's development. Therefore, children with phonological disorders will probably show few vowel errors. However, this assumption stands in contrast to the documented vowel errors that have been noted in many case studies and in the literature (e.g., Beebe, 1957; Clark and Goldstein, 1996; Haas, 1963; Hargrove, 1982; Ingram, 1981; Khan, 1988; Leonard and Leonard, 1985; Pollock and Keiser, 1990; Pollock and Swanson, 1986; Renfrew, 1966; Reynolds, 1987, 1990; Stoel-Gammon and Herrington, 1990).

Although vowels are normally among the earliest sounds acquired, it appears that some phonologically disordered children demonstrate difficulties with regular vowel realizations. Using the Pollock and Keiser (1990) data as an estimate for the frequency of occurrence, one of their fifteen phonologically disordered children had distinct difficulties with vowel productions. This child's speech showed that approximately half of the vowels were in error. Vowel difficulties may well belong to the clinical profile of some children with phonological disorders.

When several studies containing vowel data from children with phonological disorders are reviewed, two patterns seem to emerge (Stoel-Gammon and Herrington,

TABLE 9.5 Words for a First Lexicon

CONTENT CATEGORY	RELATIONAL WORDS		SUBSTANTIVE WORDS
	Relational words that are not object specific	Relational words that are more specific to objects but still relate to many objects	
Rejection	no		
Nonexistence or disappearance	no, all gone, away		
Cessation of action	stop, no		
Prohibition of action	no		
Recurrence of objects and actions on objects	more, again, another		
Noting the existence of or identifying objects	this, there, that		
Actions on objects		give, do, make, get, throw, eat, wash, kiss	
Actions involved in locating objects or self		put, up, down, sit, fall, go	
Attributes or descriptions of objects		big, hot, dirty, heavy	
Persons associated with objects (as in possession)			person names

Source: From "Planning a First Lexicon: Which Words to Teach First," by M. Lahey and L. Bloom, 1977, *Journal of Speech and Hearing Disorders, 42,* p. 350. Copyright © 1977 by the American Speech-Language-Hearing Association. Reprinted by permission.

1990). First, there are children with extremely limited vowel inventories. These children's vowel productions seem to resemble those of the babbling period with lax, nonhigh vowels predominating (Khan, 1988; Leonard and Leonard, 1985; Pollock and Swanson, 1986). A second group demonstrates relatively large vowel inventories but a high incidence of vowel errors, that is, a large number of vowel substitutions (Hargrove, 1982; Ingram, 1981; Stoel-Gammon and Herrington, 1990). The sequence of vowel acquisition in this group of children appeared to be similar to the one for younger normally developing children. In both groups of children with vowel problems, the vowels represented by the corners of the vowel quadrilateral were mastered earlier.

There is very little information available on deviant vowel systems. Although several authors state that some children with phonological disorders do have deviant vowel systems (e.g., Grunwell, 1987; Hodson and Paden, 1991; Lowe, 1994; Renfrew, 1966), neither assessment nor remediation procedures are described in these texts. However, more recently, Pollock (1991) described an assessment procedure for identifying vowel errors. In addition, Leonard and Leonard (1985) and Khan (1988) documented the gains that could be made when therapy focused on expanding the vowel inventory of children. Klein (1995) appears to be one of the first to describe therapy for vowel problems in some detail. If a child's vowel inventory is severely restricted or if the child's speech contains a high proportion of vowel substitutions, remediation focusing on vowel distinctions should be implemented.

How disordered should a vowel system be to warrant therapy? Three types of diagnostic information for vowel analysis are suggested: (1) the vowel inventory, (2) the accuracy of production, and (3) error patterns. Examination of the vowel inventory will determine whether the child has a limited or near normal inventory. Data on the accuracy of vowel production will be important when assessing children with a fairly complete vowel inventory but a high proportion of vowel substitutions. The third piece of diagnostic information, error patterns, will be especially valuable when planning therapy. Figure 9.2 is a matrix that can be used to record the vowel inventory of the child. The use of this matrix is similar to the consonant matrix presented in Chapter 7. Accurate and irregular vowel realizations can be recorded directly on the matrix. This will provide the inventory and the number of occurrences of accurate productions. Error patterns can also be identified by comparing the substitutions to the norm productions.

The Child with a Very Limited Vowel Inventory: Therapeutic Suggestions

According to the rather limited data available, it appears that the vowel system of these children is characterized by only two or three vowels. These vowels are lax and nonhigh vowels such as [ɑ], [ɛ], [æ], or [ʌ]. Such lax, nonhigh vowels are typical for the babbling period. If it can be assumed that the vowel development in these children parallels that of normally developing children, vowel acquisition data should provide some remediation guidelines. Stoel-Gammon and Herrington (1990) group vowel acquisition into three categories, which were determined after reviewing several studies in respect to the accuracy and the general order of acquisition of vowels

Vowel Matrix

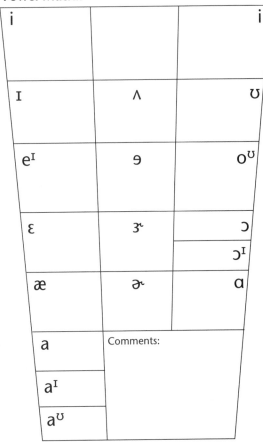

FIGURE 9.2 Vowel Matrix

in children (Hare, 1983; Irwin and Wong, 1983; Paschall, 1983; Wellman, Case, Mengert, and Bradbury, 1931):

Group 1
Vowels that are mastered relatively early   i, ɑ, u, o, ʌ

Group 2
Vowels acquired somewhere between early and late (some investigations reported early acquisition, others later)   æ, ʊ, ɔ, ə

Group 3
Vowels that are mastered relatively late   e, ɛ, ɪ, ɚ, ɝ

Using One Known and One Unknown Vowel in Minimal Pairs.

1. *First, the child's vowel inventory needs to be compared to those vowels that are mastered relatively early.* A vowel from Group 1 that is productionally very different from one of the child's vowels is selected. For example, if the child has [ɑ], a lax, low-back vowel, the tense high-front vowel [i] would be a good candidate.

2. *Next, the two vowels should be contrasted in minimal pairs.* Whenever possible, consonants from the child's inventory should be used.

Examples

Not in Inventory	In Inventory
me	ma
beet	bought
team	Tom
hee	haw

3. Other early vowels in minimal contrasts with the original vowel are introduced. Using the example with [ɑ], another productionally distinct vowel would be [u].

Examples

Not in Inventory	In Inventory
moo	me, ma
boo	bee
moon	mean
new	knee

Using Two Unknown Vowels in Minimal Pairs

1. This variation of maximal oppositions uses two unknown vowels in minimal pairs. Two vowels that are not in the child's inventory should be chosen, if possible, from Group 1. The vowels should again be as productionally different as possible (a distinctive feature analysis could be used to determine the maximal feature distinctions). If the child's inventory includes [ɑ] and [ʌ], [i] and [o] might be selected. These sounds are placed in minimal pairs.

Examples

bean-bone
peek-poke
knee-no
eat-oat

2. *Two different unknown vowels are then targeted.* The selection process should consider the general order of vowel acquisition.

The Child with a High Proportion of Vowel Substitutions: Therapeutic Suggestions

Children with a high proportion of vowel substitutions usually show a relatively intact vowel inventory. An error pattern analysis can be helpful in selecting the target vowels. Although identification of vowel processes will provide the clinician with an overall pattern of errors (e.g., the child primarily "lowers" or "fronts" vowels), it is not especially helpful in selecting vowels to target for therapy. Therefore, in the following therapy suggestions, a substitution analysis is utilized as a means of determining the vowels to be targeted for remediation.

This analysis procedure contrasts the target vowel to the substituted vowel. A list of all vowel substitutions together with their relative percentage of occurrence is generated. One possible target could be inconsistent vowel substitutions. For example, the following substitutions are noted:

ɛ/æ, frequency of occurrence = 30 percent,

ɪ/æ, frequency of occurrence = 35 percent, and

correct production of [æ], frequency of occurrence = 35 percent.

In this case, the [æ] would be selected as one vowel because of the demonstrated inconsistent substitutions. One of the substitutions for [æ] would be selected as the second vowel. In addition, the substitution chosen should be as productionally different as possible from the target. These two vowels would then be utilized as the vowel nuclei of minimally paired words. Using these criteria, [æ] and [ɪ] would be a good choice. These two vowels are then placed in minimal word pairs.

Examples

mat-mitt
bag-big
pan-pin
ham-him

A second possibility is to target a vowel that is used as a substitution for several different vowels. The following exemplifies this scenario:

Target Vowel	Substitution
i	ɪ
eᴵ	ɑ
ɛ	ɑ
æ	ɑ
ʊ	u

In this case, [ɑ] is used as a substitution for [eᴵ], [ɛ], and [æ]. Therefore, [ɑ] would be contrasted with either [eᴵ], [ɛ], or [æ]. Clear production differences should be given priority when selecting the targeted vowel. Contrasting [ɑ], a lax, low-back vowel to [eᴵ], a diphthong with a mid-high tense onglide, would provide such distinct differences. These two vowels would then be placed in minimal pairs.

Examples

tall-tail
cop-cape
top-tape

Therapy proceeds from vowels with dissimilar to more similar production features. In this example, [ɑ] and [ɛ] would be the next vowels targeted as the nuclei for minimal pairs.

SUMMARY

In this chapter, several different intervention approaches for the treatment of children with phonemic disorders have been described. Some of these remediation programs use minimal pair contrasts as the beginning unit of remediation, for example, distinctive feature therapy, minimal opposition contrasts, maximum oppositions, and therapy designed to reduce the use of phonological processes. Other remediation techniques are unique, such as cycles training and metaphon therapy. These two therapy protocols, which have been developed and refined through actual clinical experience, forge together a combination of methods that can be effectively utilized to treat phonological disorders in children.

Discussion of the treatment approaches has been designed to answer specific questions. First: When should this therapy be chosen? Which clients could best be treated with this approach? Guidelines that broadly separate clients who might be better versus poorer candidates for each particular approach were given. Documented research on therapeutic efficacy of each model has also been provided. Second, selection of beginning targets and clinical applications have been supplied to exemplify the transition from assessment to intervention. Third, intervention methods have been outlined in some detail to indicate the utilization of each approach in a therapy setting.

The last portion of this chapter explored and suggested some special applications of phonological therapy. Phonological remediation principles with children displaying concurrent language difficulties and those with emerging phonological systems exemplified the merging of phonological intervention strategies with other language areas such as morphology and semantics. Finally, treatment principles for children with disordered vowel systems were presented to demonstrate how minimal pair contrasts can be structured within a remediation program.

Throughout this chapter, assessment results and their connection to therapy goals have been emphasized. Whenever possible, a direct link has been made between the assessment results outlined in Chapter 7 and the therapy procedures in this chapter. Several clinical applications have been provided to demonstrate the assessment-treatment connection, which is essential for professional speech-language services.

CHAPTER 10

ARTICULATORY/PHONOLOGICAL DISORDERS IN SELECTED POPULATIONS

CHAPTER OUTLINE

- Developmental Apraxia of Speech: A Disorder of Speech Motor Control
- Motor Speech Disorders: Cerebral Palsy
- Clefting: Cleft Palate and Cleft Lip
- Mental Disability

- Hearing Impairment
- Motor Speech Disorders: Acquired Apraxia of Speech
- Motor Speech Disorders: The Dysarthrias
- Summary

This chapter provides an overview of articulatory and phonological characteristics of selected populations. They represent a number of different disorders with specific speech problems as one of the hallmarks of their symptom complexes. Many comprehensive books have been written on each of these disorders. Therefore, the following synopsis represents only selected aspects of the main characteristics and the diagnostic-treatment principles for each of the disorders relating to articulatory and/or phonological impairment. Each individual discussion is organized into four sections: (1) definition and general features, (2) articulatory/phonological characteristics, (3) clinical diagnostics, and (4) therapeutic implications.

DEVELOPMENTAL APRAXIA OF SPEECH: A DISORDER OF SPEECH MOTOR CONTROL

Definition and General Features

The term *developmental articulatory dyspraxia* was first used by Morley, Court, and Miller

(1954) to describe a small group of children with articulation disorders that differed from other children with known speech sound realization difficulties. These children have subsequently been labelled as having *developmental apraxia of speech* (Rosenbek and Wertz, 1972), *congenital articulatory apraxia* (Eisenson, 1972), and *developmental verbal apraxia* (Edwards, 1973), to mention a few. Currently, either the term **developmental apraxia of speech (DAS)** or **developmental verbal dyspraxia (DVD)** is used to refer to children who evidence a lack of motor control of the oral mechanism for speech production which is not attributable to other problems of muscular control (Hall, Jordan, and Robin, 1993). Difficulty in sequencing speech sounds is central to the disorder. **Sequencing errors** are defined as disruptions in the production of the correct ordering of speech sounds or syllables (Hall et al., 1993).

An exact delineation of symptoms of this disorder as well as the DAS concept itself are highly controversial. Early reports delineating the symptoms (Rosenbek and Wertz, 1972; Yoss and Darley, 1974a) were authored by individuals who had worked with acquired apraxia of speech in adults. They pointed out similarities and differences between the specific articulatory problems noted in adults with acquired apraxia of speech and children with so-called developmental apraxia of speech. The most important similarity between these two groups of clients pertains to the lack of sequential volitional control of the oral mechanism (Hall et al., 1993). However, the major difference is that a neurological basis for comparable speech symptoms could never be verified in children with developmental apraxia of speech (Aram, 1984; Ferry, Hall, and Hicks, 1975; Rosenbek and Wertz, 1972). Some authors (e.g., Aram, 1984; Hall et al., 1993) even argue against the assumption that an underlying neurological impairment is indeed the cause of developmental apraxia of speech.

Many have disputed the concept of, and supporting evidence for, developmental apraxia of speech. For example, after a complete review of the literature, Guyette and Diedrich (1981) state that "The diagnosis 'developmental apraxia of speech' is neither appropriate nor useful" (p. 44). Love (1992), on the other hand, believes that "despite the serious questions raised about etiology, pathology, and validity of the reported signs and symptoms of the DVD syndrome, it remains an appropriate and useful diagnostic category of childhood motor speech disability" (p. 95). Shriberg, Aram, and Kwiatkowski (1997a) state,

> For clinical needs, DAS appears to provide a tentative explanatory label for children who have severe, irregular, and persistent speech disorders, in contrast to the mild-to-severe, regular, and typically self-limiting error patterns of the common form of developmental phonological disorders.... (p. 274)

This statement furnishes a good point of departure for further discussion. It exemplifies the tentative nature of the label while also suggesting the clinical necessity of differentiating the speech characteristics of DAS children from those evidenced by children with developmental phonological disorders. If one accepts the label DAS, both groups of children do have certain characteristics in common: The onset is early in the developmental period and the course is long-term, often extending into adulthood (Shriberg et al., 1997a). Its estimated prevalence of occurrence is approximately 1 to 2 children per 1,000 (Shriberg et al., 1997a).

Articulatory/Phonological Characteristics

Several studies have reported speech characteristics of children with suspected DAS. However, some of these reports refer to case studies describing only one or two children. Other investigations cannot be compared because uniform criteria were not used when selecting the subjects. Therefore, when interpreting the data, it should be remembered that methodological differences exist between the studies. With this in mind, the following speech characteristics are offered for children with DAS (Hall et al., 1993):

1. *More errors made in the sound classes involving more complex oral gestures.*

Thus, consonant clusters, fricatives, and affricates evidence a larger percentage of difficulty (Crary, 1984; Rosenbek and Wertz, 1972).

These same sound classes are also troublesome for children with developmental phonological disorders, although Jackson and Hall (1987) suggest that the DAS children may be acquiring these sounds at a much slower rate, only at older ages, and possibly only after intensive remediation procedures.

2. *Unusual errors not typically found in children with speech sound disorders.*

These errors include sound additions, prolongations of vowels and consonants, repetitions of sounds and syllables (Rosenbek and

Wertz, 1972; Yoss and Darley, 1974a), and unusual substitutions, such as glottal plosives and bilabial fricatives (Aram and Glasson, 1979).

3. *A large percentage of omission errors.*

Several investigators have found that sound and syllable omissions are the most frequent type of errors noted in DAS children (LaVoi, 1986; Rosenbek and Wertz, 1972). However, Yoss and Darley (1974a) related the percentage of omissions to the complexity of the speech tasks. Polysyllabic words demonstrated more syllable omissions, while spontaneous speech included sound omissions. Other reports indicate that the high degree of omissions may be age-related, with younger children evidencing more and older children fewer omission errors (Aram and Glasson, 1979; Jackson and Hall, 1987).

4. *Difficulty producing and maintaining appropriate voicing.*

DAS children may voice unvoiced sounds and devoice voiced sounds (Aram and Glasson, 1979; Morley, 1959; Yoss and Darley, 1974a). These errors have also been verified by acoustic analyses (Robin, Hall, and Jordan, 1987).

5. *Vowel and diphthong errors.*

Several studies have identified vowel and diphthong errors in DAS children (e.g., Davis, Marquardt, and Sussman, 1985; Rosenbek and Wertz, 1972). Pollock and Hall (1991) specifically describe the vowel errors of five school-age children with DAS. All of these children had difficulty with tense-lax vowel contrasts, while four of the five evidenced diphthong reduction.

6. *Difficulty sequencing speech sounds and syllables.*

According to Hall et al. 1993, sequencing problems are central to this disorder. Difficulty with sequencing seems to increase as the complexity and/or length of the utterance increases (e.g., Ferry, Hall, and Hicks, 1975; Hardcastle, Morgan-Barry, and Clark, 1987). In addition, sound transpositions within a word,

or metatheses, have been frequently cited in descriptions of DAS (Aram and Nation, 1982; Rosenbek and Wertz, 1972). It is not clear whether the frequency of metathetic errors is in fact higher for this population than for children with developmental phonological disorders (LaVoi, 1986; Parsons, 1984).

7. *Difficulties with nasality and nasal emission.*

Conflicting reports exist as to whether problems with nasality and nasal emission constitute an error pattern noted in children suspected of DAS. Based on extensive clinical experience, Hall et al. (1993) summarize by saying, "We find that, at some point, most children exhibiting DAS have problems with hypernasality, hyponasality, or nasal emissions. Sometimes this is quite subtle, in most instances, it is variable and inconsistent in occurrence" (p. 35).

8. *Groping behavior and silent posturing.*

Groping behavior is an ongoing series of movements of the articulators in an attempt to find the desired articulatory position. **Silent posturing** refers to the positioning of the articulators for a specific articulation without sound production. Both groping behaviors and silent posturing have been noted in the speech of DAS children (e.g., Hall, 1989; Murdoch, Porter, Younger, and Ozanne, 1984). Hall et al. (1993) state that silent posturing may be seen primarily in younger children while groping behavior is found later, in older children with DAS.

9. *Prosodic impairment*

General and more specific difficulties with prosody have often been reported in the speech of DAS children (e.g., Hall, 1989; Morley, 1972; Robin, Hall, Jordan, and Gordan, 1991). In a recent series of studies by Shriberg, Aram, and Kwiatkowski (1997a, 1997b, 1997c), inappropriate stress was found to be the only linguistic domain which differentiated DAS children from those with delayed speech development.

Although all of these error patterns have been reported in the speech of children with DAS, not all of them occur in all DAS children. Inconsistency and variability of errors is probably the most frequent pattern characterizing this disorder. DAS children are often highly unintelligible. Another common feature is the lack of progress these children make in spite of a considerable amount of therapy over a longer period of time.

Clinical Implications: Diagnostics

Generally, a broad cluster of symptoms is assumed to represent DAS, including speech, nonspeech, and language deficits. But the all-important qualification is that "Not *all* symptoms must be present; no *one* characteristic or symptom *must* be present; and the typically reported symptoms are not *exclusive* to developmental apraxia of speech. Compounding the problem is the observation that children change over time" (Jaffe, 1984, p. 170). Assessment, therefore, must be organized in a way that allows us to look at a wide range of symptoms.

> Studies seem to indicate that two groups of DAS children, which present similiar symptoms but different prognoses, exist (Fawcus, 1971; Milloy, 1985; Morley, 1972; Morley and Fox 1969). One group consists of children with moderate or severe articulation disorders that do not resolve over time. The second group of children show comparable symptoms but develop mature articulatory skills by approximately age 10 (Milloy, 1985). Milloy (1985) used the term *immature articulatory praxis* (IAP) to describe the second condition, hypothesizing that this condition was a maturational disorder that resolves as the children grow older. IAP was found in many children with moderate learning disabilities and a correlation existed between the degree of immaturity these children presented and the severity of their language deficit.

The following assessment procedures are recommended for the child who is suspected of demonstrating DAS:

- hearing screening
- language testing
- thorough speech-motor assessment, including diadochokinetic rates
- articulation test
- language sample
- additional tests to examine the sequencing of sounds and syllables as well as their consistency

Hearing screening is a portion of every assessment; however, it should be evident that the child with suspected DAS does not have a hearing loss as the basis for the noted articulatory problems. Language testing is also an important dimension of the assessment process. Although some research studies have used the absence of receptive language problems as one of the criteria for inclusion in the group of children with suspected DAS, others report both expressive and receptive language difficulties co-occuring with DAS (e.g., Hall, Hardy, and LaVelle, 1990; Hall, Robin, and Jordan, 1986; Lohr, 1978). Formal and informal assessment of language should always be used to gain a more complete understanding of the language proficiency of these children.

A speech-motor assessment needs to include sequential volitional movements of the oral muscles for both speech and nonspeech tasks. Oral diadochokinetic rates in nonspeech and speech activities should be evaluated as well (Haynes, 1985; Love, 1992; Love and Fitzgerald, 1984). Such information helps to document the structural and neuromuscular adequacy of the oral peripheral mechanism. Its functional adequacy for nonspeech and speech tasks should be described and compared.

An articulation test and language sample can be used to appraise several speech parameters: types of errors, any unusual errors, voicing problems with consonants, vowel and diphthong errors, difficulties with nasality and nasal emission, and prosodic problems. Differences between productions of one-word responses and those requiring increased articulatory length or complexity need to be ascertained. Groping behavior and/or silent posturing are additional areas that require close observation.

There are tests and protocols specifically designed to assess DAS children. Examples include the Screening Test for Developmental Apraxia of Speech (Blakely, 1980), The Apraxia Profile (Hickman, 1997), the Milloy Assessment of Praxis (MAP) (Milloy, 1985), and Tests for Apraxia of Speech and Oral Apraxia-Children's Battery (Blakely, 1977). The Screening Test for DAS examines expressive language, vowels and diphthongs, oral-motor movement, verbal sequencing, articulation, motorically complex words, transpositions, and prosody. However, critical reviews of the test (Guyette and Diedrich, 1981; Jaffe, 1984; Thompson, 1988) have demonstrated serious flaws in terms of design, standardization, scoring guidelines, and standards of test construction.

Clinical Implications: Therapeutics

An established set of therapeutic approaches for the treatment of DAS does not exist. This is not surprising when one considers the limited understanding of the cause, nature, and differential diagnostic markers for DAS. Even after a careful diagnostic evaluation of the appraisal data, only *suspected* DAS can normally be assumed. Based on the assumption of suspected DAS, many different remediation approaches have been suggested. The following is a synopsis of the treatment suggested by Hall et al. (1993). It is based on the analysis of outcome measures from many different remediation programs as well as their clinical experience.

1. *Intensive services are needed.*

Children with suspected DAS require an extraordinarily high amount of intensive therapy carried out on an individual basis. The child, the child's caregivers, and the clinician must be dedicated to this concept. Hall et al. (1993) recommend a summer program in which the children are in residence for six weeks, receiving four hours of therapy per day, five days a week.

2. *Remediation should progress systematically through hierarchies of task difficulty.*

Where to begin with remediation and how to progress will depend on the assessment data from each individual child. Hall et al. (1993) evaluate the child's strengths and progress in very small, carefully manipulated steps. They analyze what the child can do successfully and proceed from there. Therefore, the consonant inventory, distribution as well as syllable shapes will be important information when evaluating where to begin with therapy. Speech sounds that can be successfully articulated are combined into syllable structures already present in the child's speech. These are then gradually expanded to include a few monosyllabic words of high utility and, possibly, carrier phrases.

3. *Remediation stresses sequences of movements.*

Careful incremental increases in sequencing movements and the "memory" for such movements are important. Articulation "memory" should be based on internalized tactile-kinesthetic-proprioceptive information relating sounds that are heard to specific motor patterns. Chappell (1973) suggests increasing the demand for memory retention by interrupting the child between requests for response sequences.

4. *Many repetitions of speech movements are required in drill-oriented sessions.*

Hall et al. (1993) use three to ten repetitions of each stimulus. Stimuli range from

CV utterances to multisyllabic words. Each set of repetitions is interrupted by the client returning to a neutral or resting position to reduce perseverative behavior.

5. *The clinician must determine the need for auditory discrimination tasks.*

Not all children need enhancement of auditory discrimination skills. The clinician should determine if, based on assessment data, the individual client needs work in this area.

6. *Remediation should emphasize self-monitoring.*

Self-monitoring should be emphasized as early as possible within the remediation program (Yoss and Darley, 1974b). Some suggest that tactile and kinesthetic self-monitoring be trained (Weiss, Gordon, and Lillywhite, 1987).

7. *Input from multiple modalities is needed.*

Multisensory input appears helpful to many children with suspected DAS. Various types of cuing have been introduced and can be utilized to meet the specific needs of these children. All of the cueing techniques represent visual and/or tactile cues used to help the child articulate certain sounds or sound sequences (see the following Clinical Application for sources).

8. *Remediation should include manipulation of prosodic features as an integral part of the total remedial program.*

Whenever possible, rhythm, intonation, stress, and rate manipulation should be integrated into the therapy program from the beginning. The areas that specifically need to be targeted should be revealed by the diagnostic data. However, there are some children who do not seem capable of manipulating articulatory and prosodic features simultaneously. If this occurs, an articulatory goal is established first and prosody added later to articulation tasks that are relatively easy for the client.

9. *If necessary, the clinician should teach compensatory strategies.*

Compensatory strategies include slowing the overall rate of speech, increasing the use of pauses between words and syllables, vowel prolongation, and the intrusion of a schwa vowel between consonants in a cluster. Hall et al. (1993) state that compensatory strategies may be a necessary portion of therapeutic measures but should be generally seen as only a stage of remediation to facilitate a child's progress. When the compensatory strategies are no longer necessary, productions without them should become the goal.

10. *The clinician must provide successful experiences.*

Treatment should begin at a level at which children can succeed. Therefore, it is important that the clinician understand the child's baseline level of articulatory functioning and the strengths that this individual demonstrates. Children with suspected DAS, especially, need success with speech goals to keep them motivated throughout the typically long and slow remediation process.

CLINICAL APPLICATION

Additional Therapeutic Techniques—Developmental Apraxia of Speech

The following additional therapy techniques have been used with children exhibiting Developmental Apraxia of Speech.

Technique	Sources
Melodic intonation therapy	Albert, Sparks, and Helm (1973); Doszak, McNeil, and Jancosek (1981); Helfrich-Miller (1984); Krauss and Galloway (1982); Sparks, Helm, and Albert (1974).

Technique	Sources
Cueing techniques	
Touch-cue method	Bashir, Grahamjones, and Bostwick (1984).
Signed target phoneme	Shelton and Graves (1985).
Adapted cuing techniques	Klick (1985).
Cued speech	Cornett (1972).
Jordan's gestures	Jordan (1988, 1991).
Multiple phonemic approach	Bradley (1989); Davis, Marquardt, and Sussman (1985); Marquardt and Sussman (1991); McCabe and Bradley (1975).
Sign/total communication	Air, Wood, and Neils (1989); Culp (1989); Ferry, Hall, and Hicks (1975); Harlan (1984); Jaffe (1984).

MOTOR SPEECH DISORDERS: CEREBRAL PALSY

Definition and General Features

Cerebral palsy (CP) is a nonprogressive disorder of motor control caused by damage to the developing brain during pre-, peri-, or early postnatal periods (Dillow, Dzienkowski, Smith, and Yucha, 1996; Hardy, 1994; Love, 1992). The condition results in a wide variety of motor disabilities, dysarthria among them. Given that there are about 400,000 children living with cerebral palsy, this disorder constitutes the most common developmental motor impairment (Best, Bigge, and Sirvis, 1994; Kudrjavcev, Schoenberg, Kurland, and Groover, 1983; Love, 1992), occurring about 3 times in every 1,000 births (Bigge, 1991). The lack of volitional speech motor control is among its central clinical features. However, cerebral palsy's symptom complex, characterized by a host of neurological malfunctions, is far more than disordered articulation. Rather, in addition to general movement and coordination problems, primarily caused by spastic conditions of muscles and increased tendon reflexes, "these dysfunctions include disturbances in cognition, perception, sensation, language, hearing, emotional behavior, feeding, and seizure control" (Love, 1992, pp. 49–50).

The treatment of cerebral palsy requires a team approach to the problem, which is typically a cooperative effort of a physician specializing in these disorders, a physical and occupational therapist, a psychologist, a social worker, and a speech-language pathologist. Clinical management by the speech-language pathologist requires special considerations which differ considerably from those employed in the treatment of other children with articulatory/phonological disorders. Clinical management can only be effective if the complexity of the disabling condition is understood. This includes, among other important factors, being able to evaluate the intricate interrelationships between respiration, phonation, resonance, and articulation in normal individuals versus individuals with cerebral palsy.

Articulatory/Phonological Characteristics

Speech-related dysfunctions in cerebral palsy include respiratory, phonatory, articulatory, prosodic abnormalities and velopharyngeal inadequacies (Dillow et al., 1996; Hardy, 1994; Love, 1992). Cerebral palsy encompasses many different types and degrees of speech-related problems. To facilitate an understanding of the various articulatory/phonatory characteristics, a distinction is usually made between three types of involvement commonly found in cerebral palsied individuals:

1. spasticity
2. dyskinesia
3. ataxia

Among cerebral palsied clients, spastic involvement is the most frequently found. Four major types of spastic involvement are recognized: spastic hemiplegia, spastic paraplegia, spastic diplegia, and spastic quadriplegia. With *spastic hemiplegia,* the arm and leg on one side of the body show signs of spastic paresis. *Spastic paraplegia,* which is relatively uncommon, is characterized by involvement of the legs only. In *spastic diplegia,* all four limbs are affected but the lower limbs show more involvement than the upper limbs. All four limbs are about equally involved in *spastic quadriplegia.* Spastic diplegics and quadriplegics are more likely to have speech disorders than are hemiplegics or paraplegics. Respiratory, phonatory, resonatory, and articulatory symptoms include:

Respiratory difficulties:

reduced vital capacity resulting in inadequate breath support for phonatory and articulatory purposes.

Laryngeal dysfunction:

responsible for harsh voices and, when coupled with respiratory aberrations, result in short phrasing and prosodic disturbances.

Velopharyngeal inadequacies:

with the consequence of hypernasality.

Articulatory deficiencies:

affecting especially the production of fricatives and affricates as well as translating into

an overall laborious, slow rate of speech. Muscle weakness, articulatory instability, and inaccuracy in finding target articulation points are also noted (Love, 1992).

Dyskinesias in cerebral palsy are best exemplified by athetoid conditions marked by unilateral or bilateral disturbances of posture, tonus, and motion. They have been reported to be far less frequent than spastic involvement within the cerebral palsied population (Erenberg, 1984; Love, 1992), but their effects on speech performance are often even more severe. More often than not, the degree of limb dysfunction mirrors the impairments of the speech mechanism. Many athetoid clients show dysfunction of every physiological component contributing to speech:

Respiratory difficulties:

breathing might be rapid and irregular (Davis, 1987), showing a lack of thoracic respiratory movement or even "reverse breathing," in which the sternum is flattened instead of lifted during inspiration.

Laryngeal dysfunction:

general hypertonicity, which can immobilize the phonatory process altogether, can be more pronounced than in spastic involvement. If any voice results, it is commonly marked by an especially strained quality, hard glottal onset, and reduced intensity and prosody realizations.

Velopharyngeal inadequacies:

slow velar activity often results in hypernasal effects.

Articulatory deficiencies:

abnormally large jaw movements during articulation; tongue movements are restricted and for articulatory purposes highly dependent on jaw activity (Kent and Netsell, 1978). This results in distortions of consonant as well as vowel productions (positioning of the mandible during speech can somehow establish necessary differences in tongue height, but not in anterior-posterior tongue movements for the production of front versus back vowels).

Ataxia is infrequent among cerebral palsied clients (Hardy, 1983; Pharoah, Cooke, Rosenbloom, and Cooke, 1987). This is probably why "systematic studies of the speech of ataxic dysarthric children have not been reported" (Love, 1992, p. 66). The main symptom of ataxic involvement is incoordination of essentially hypotonic muscle action. Based on clinical observation, it appears that the speech characteristics of ataxic cerebral palsied individuals are very similar to those of adults with ataxic dysarthria (Love, 1992). The following characteristics are noted in children and adults with ataxia:

Respiratory difficulties:

shallow inspiration and lack of expiratory control.

Laryngeal dysfunction:

harsh voice productions, reduced range of prosodic feature realization.

Velopharyngeal inadequacies:

hypernasality is not typical.

Articulatory deficiencies:

imprecise consonants and vowel distortions, inconsistent sound substitutions and omissions, and a general dysrhythmia (Darley, Aronson, and Brown, 1975; Ingram, 1966; Ingram and Barn, 1961).

Table 10.1 summarizes the three different types of cerebral palsy.

Several studies have verified that children with cerebral palsy demonstrate speech errors of temporal and motor control (Crary and Comeau, 1981; Farmer and Lencione, 1977;

McMahon, Hodson, and Allen, 1983). Based on this evidence, Milloy and Morgan-Barry (1990) describe the following phonological processes which relate to these difficulties:

Phonological Processes
Related to temporal coordination:

voicing difficulties, including devoicing of initial consonants or voicing of unvoiced sounds, variable realizations of voiced-voiceless cognates, prevocalic voicing, consonant cluster reductions, final consonant deletions, stopping of fricatives or frication of stops, weak syllable deletions.

Related to motor control, errors of phonetic placement:

fronting, backing, stopping, gliding, lateral realization of apical and coronal fricatives, vowelization of [l] and [r], nasalization.

Clinical Implications: Diagnostics

The primary communicative impairment of children with cerebral palsy is clearly motor speech in nature. But these children present a variety of clinical pictures which has to do with both the type and the severity of involvement. On the other hand, all cerebral palsies share some common factors that directly relate to basic functions subserving speech, namely problems with respiration, phonation, resonation, and articulation. It is important to assess kind and degree of interference each of these systems may have on speech.

Problems with *respiration* may lead to:

difficulties initiating vocalization, difficulties sustaining vocalization, variations in loudness which may affect word and sentence stress, inability to sustain vocalization for multisyllabic words or longer sentences, loss of expiratory support at end of utterance.

TABLE 10.1   Summary of Types of Cerebral Palsy

TYPE OF C P (WITH SUB-TYPES)	SITE OF TRAUMA	MUSCULAR INVOLVEMENT	SPEECH DISORDER
1. Spasticity a. hemiplegia	Pyramidal tract monolateral lesion of fibres	Hypertonicity of upper and lower limbs on one side	Speech usually auditorily acceptable although there may be developmental delay
b. paraplegia	Uncertain, probably bilateral lesion	Hypertonicity of lower limbs; may extend to torso musculature	Possible problems of respiration and breath control for speech
c. diplegia	Uncertain, probably bilateral lesion	All four limbs involved, lower limbs more severely affected; may extend to torso and neck muscles	Variable, depending on extent of neuromotor disability; may show dysprosody with problems of articulation
d. quadriplegia	Bilateral lesion within pyramidal tract	Equal degree of spasticity in all four limbs	Articulatory problems and dysphonia in varying degrees of severity
2. Dyskinesia (athetosis)	Basal ganglia	Impairment of voluntary movements due to either extreme muscle tone or extreme flaccidity Involuntary continuous muscle movement occurs	Speech defects, very variable in severity, generally slow, with poor articulation, and problems of phonation, stress and rhythm
3. Ataxia	Cerebellum	Incoordination of movement with inability to maintain posture and balance	Speech mainly defective; articulation problems and dysrhythmia evident

Source: From "Developmental Neurological Disorders," by N. Milloy and R. Morgan-Barry, in *Developmental Speech Disorders* (p. 112), edited by P. Grunwell, 1990, Edinburgh: Churchill Livingstone. Reprinted by permission of the publisher Churchill Livingstone.

Problems with *phonation* may result in:

interruptions in phonation, breathy voice, harsh voice, pitch and intensity variations, problems in coordinating voicing and articulation.

Problems with *resonation* may result in:

various degrees of hypernasality, variations in nasality within an utterance, lack of intelligibility due to nasality problems.

Problems with *articulation* may result in:

difficulties in achieving speech sound productions, sound distortions, disorganized phonological systems, possibly leading to

problems with language and learning to read.

When assessing the child with cerebral palsy, it is essential to remember that the smooth integration of all systems subserving speech is a real problem for these children. Therefore, the assessment and treatment of cerebral palsied children must account for far more than just speech sound production difficulties.

The high diversity of possible involvements requires an encompassing evaluation. In addition to respiratory, phonatory, resonatory, and articulatory limitations and possibilities, data from the following areas should be supplemented:

- cognitive skills
- sensory and perceptual abilities beginning with an audiological evaluation
- client's emotional behavior
- feeding/eating characteristics
- language competence

Often, the speech-language pathologist will become part of an early intervention team for infants who have been identified with cerebral palsy. As a member of this team, the speech-language pathologist will be asked to assess prespeech skills as prerequisites for the development of articulation skills. These prerequisites include:

1. Head control with stability of the neck and shoulder girdle. Such stability provides later control and mobility of oral structures.
2. A coordinated pattern of respiration and phonation.
3. A variety of feeding experiences to enhance normal feeding patterns.
4. Babbling practice (Air et al., 1989).

As one example, the *Pre-Speech Assessment Scale* (Morris, 1975) is a tool that can assist the speech-language pathologist in appraising pre-

speech behavior. This scale examines postural tone and movement, response to sensory stimuli, feeding, biting, chewing, sucking, swallowing, respiration, phonation, and sound play.

Clinical Implications: Therapeutics

As always, the selection of appropriate therapeutic measures to influence the communicative abilities of cerebral palsied clients, especially to guide and improve development in young cerebral palsied children, is a direct outgrowth of the specific diagnostic results. Established methods for the treatment of various "types" of cerebral palsy amount only to guidelines for elementary orientation.

There are, nevertheless, general principles that apply to all remediation efforts with young cerebral palsied clients. First, some prespeech prerequisites must be met, the aforementioned head control and the coordination of respiratory patterns with voice production, for example. The necessity of coordination between breathing and phonation for future articulation work is self-evident, but a certain degree of posture control is equally indispensable. Another, although controversial (Jaffe, 1984), prerequisite pertains to the inhibition of certain chewing and swallowing behaviors, specifically the chewing reflex, which might interfere with oral-motor activities for articulatory tasks. Neurodevelopmental therapy—for example, the so-called Bobath approach to the treatment of infants with cerebral palsy—favors heavily the early reduction of abnormal oral reflexes within a prespeech program (Bobath, 1967; Bobath and Bobath, 1972).

The next therapeutic phase within the general principles for remediation efforts with young cerebral palsied children pertains to communication and speech-language stimulation. In infants, it might start with

---

Capute (1974) reports that about 50 to 60 percent of the cerebral palsied population show some degree of mental retardation, with the rest of these individuals demonstrating intelligence within normal limits. Impaired language development, learning difficulties, and academic problems often occur in children with cerebral palsy (Haynes and Pindzola, 1998). In addition, an audiological evaluation is a necessity for cerebral palsied children. Athetotics in particular have higher auditory detection thresholds, poorer speech reception thresholds, and poorer speech discrimination than normal children (DiCarlo and Amster, 1974).

Box 10.1_____

Selected References for the Assessment and Treatment of Prespeech Behaviors and the Assessment of Feeding

ASSESSING AND TREATING PRESPEECH BEHAVIORS

Harding, C. G. (1983). Setting the stage for language acquisition: Communication development in the first year. In R. M. Golinkoff (Ed.), *Transition from prelinguistic to linguistic communication.* Hillsdale, NJ: Lawrence Erlbaum Associates.

Morris, S. (1987). Therapy for the child with cerebral palsy: Interacting frameworks. *Seminars in Speech and Language, 8,* 71–86.

Proctor, A. (1989). Stages of normal noncry vocal development in infancy: A protocol for assessment. *Topics in Language Disorders, 10(1),* 26–42.

Proctor, A., & Murnyack, T. (1995). Assessing communication, cognition, and vocalization in the prelinguistic period. *Infants and Young Children, 7(4),* 39–54.

Rosetti, L. (1994). *Communication intervention: Birth to three.* San Diego: Singular Publishing Group.

ASSESSING AND THERAPY FOR FEEDING

Alexander, R. (1987). Oral-motor treatment for infants and young children. *Seminars in Speech and Language, 8,* 87–100.

Alexander, R. (1987). Prespeech and feeding development. In E. McDonald (Ed.), *Treating cerebral palsy.* Austin, TX: PRO-ED.

Hall, S., Circello, N., Reed, P., & Hylton, J. (1987). *Considerations for feeding children who have a neuromuscular disorder.* Portland, OR: CARC Publications.

Jaffe, M. (1989). Feeding at-risk infants and toddlers. *Topics in Language Disorders, 10,* 13–25.

McGowan, J., & Kerwin, M. (1993). Oral motor and feeding problems. In K. Bleile (Ed.), *The care of children with long-term tracheostomies* (pp. 157–195). San Diego: Singular Publishing Group.

vocal play and babbling practice. Box 10.1 offers references that provide more detail in the areas of assessment and treatment of pre-

speech behaviors, speech-language stimulation, and feeding.

For the older child with cerebral palsy, a basic consideration is the facilitation of desired movements while inhibiting the abnormal reflex patterns. Before a speech-language clinician can address the coordination of respiration, phonation, resonation, and articulation, the child must be able to maintain some reflex-inhibiting postures which the physical therapist will recommend. Because this is usually one of the primary goals of the early intervention team, the child should already have developed some skills in this area. If the child can inhibit abnormal reflexes and realize certain movements required for speech, articulation training can be initiated.

Traditionally, therapy began with establishing temporal coordination and motor control of the speech musculature. Goals were to increase the speed, range, and accuracy of movement of the tongue, lips, and jaw (Westlake and Rutherford, 1961). These goals were then integrated with the maintenance of body and head tonus as well as with respiration, phonation, and resonation (Barlow and Farley, 1989). Oral exercises usually preceded phonetic placement. Selection of the target sound was guided by stimulability, consistency, and visibility and whether the sound was an early or late developing sound. Therefore, stimulable, visible sounds that were produced in some contexts accurately and were early to be acquired were normally given priority (Love, 1992).

However, there were those who felt that groups of sounds rather than a single sound should be treated (Hardy, 1983). Based on guidelines drawn up by Hardy (1983) and Crary (1993), the following procedures are offered:

1. *Consonants that are realized correctly in prevocalic positions but are misarticulated in postvo-*

calic positions should be treated first. Generally, postvocalic errors will be more easily remedied if the child can produce the sound in a prevocalic position.

2. *Distortions should be treated before substitutions,* especially those distortions that fall short of the target because of motor involvement. Prognosis should be better if the child can almost produce the sound, although distorted, rather than deletes or uses a substitute for the sound.

3. *Training articulatory omissions and substitutions that fall short of the target because of motor involvement should be delayed.* Compensatory articulatory efforts for sounds that are difficult to produce should be trained instead. The child will usually have already developed some type of compensatory sound realization. The duty of the clinician is to refine this production as much as possible.

4. *A multiple auditory-visual stimulation approach* is preferred over auditory stimulation alone.

5. *Voice–voiceless distinctions should be trained by slowing the speech process* and then concentrating on the production of the voicelessness of the sound. This is important because cerebral palsied children have a tendency to substitute voiced for voiceless consonants.

6. *It is important to remember that some cerebral palsied children cannot achieve "normal" articulation.* In these cases, *reasonable compensations* are the goal; they can be very efficient for communicative purposes.

Occasionally, the physical handicap is so severe that effective verbal communication cannot be achieved at all. If that is the case, *augmentative communication,* that is, the use of any means (gestural, boards with words or pictures, electronic devices) to promote meaningful communicative exchange, must be implemented (Beukelman, Yorkston, and Dowden, 1985).

CLINICAL APPLICATION

Communication Augmentation

Communication augmentation refers to any approach designed to support, enhance, or augment the communication of individuals who cannot use speech in all situations (Beukelman, Yorkson, and Dowden, 1985). Augmentative approaches have as a goal the expansion of the symbolic communication capabilities of nonspeaking individuals. Common types of augmentation include manual communication, communication boards, and electronic or computer-based aids. For individuals with motor involvement, such as cerebral palsied children, the augmentation system must be chosen with special care. The American Speech-Language-Hearing Association Ad Hoc Committee on Communication Processes and Non-Speaking Persons (1980) identifies three components for the assessment of augmentative communication:

1. The appropriateness of augmentative communication must be appraised. Not all nonspeaking individuals can benefit from such a system (Bryen, Goldman, and Quinlisk-Gill, 1988; Owens and House, 1984). For the child with cerebral palsy, for example, cognitive and speech motor abilities will need to be weighed in relationship to augmentative means.
2. The appropriateness of the augmentative communication mode must be appraised. A decision must be made as to which type or types of augmentative system is appropriate for the individual. Of particular importance are the motoric abilities of the client (Shane and Wilbur, 1980; Silverman, 1980). Restricted motor skills often limit the types of system that can be utilized. This will be a major consideration when evaluating augmentative communication for the child with cerebral palsy.
3. The appropriate symbol system or systems must be found. Cognitive ability, visual acuity, and the receptiveness of the environment all need to be thoroughly assessed within this category (Chapman and Miller, 1980).

Although augmentative communication may prove to be the only possibility for some children with cerebral palsy, the selection and implementation of such a system for children with severe motoric limitations remain a challenge.

CLEFTING: CLEFT PALATE AND CLEFT LIP

Definition and General Features

Occurring in 1 of about 700 births (Brogan and Woodings, 1976), palatal and (upper) lip clefts are among the most frequent congenital anomalies (American Cleft Palate-Craniofacial Association and Cleft Palate Foundation, 1997). **Clefting** refers to a division of a continuous structure by a cleavage, a split prominently caused by a failure of the palate to fuse during fetal development (Shprintzen, 1995). Examples of clefting are cleft palate and cleft lip. Both the hard and soft palates and the lips form normally uninterrupted structures within their anatomical boundaries. If clefting occurs, a gap severs their unity, dividing the roof of the mouth (which also constitutes the floor of the nasal cavity) and/or the upper lip sagittally into separated left and right portions.

Palatal clefts have several etiologies that cause a failure of the regular median fusion of the embryo's oral-facial structures between the eighth and twelfth weeks of gestation. In addition, there is also the possibility of a rupture of already fused oral-facial elements (Kitamura, 1991). Contrary to common understanding, no single cause for clefting exists; "clefting is…a clinical outcome of many possible diseases" (Shprintzen, 1995, p. 5).

Although there are many classification systems, the recommendations by Harkins et al. (1960, 1962) from the American Cleft Palate Association (now the American Cleft Palate–Craniofacial Association) have been most frequently adopted (Bzoch, 1997).

1. Clefts of prepalate
   - Cleft lip: unilateral, bilateral, median, prolabium (central segment of upper lip), congenital scar
   - Cleft of alveolar process: unilateral, bilateral, median, submucous
   - Cleft of prepalate: any combination of foregoing types, prepalate protrusion, prepalate rotation, prepalate arrest (median cleft)

2. Clefts of the palate
   - Clefts of soft palate: extent, palatal shortness, submucous
   - Clefts of hard palate: extent, vomer attachment, submucous

3. Clefts of prepalate and palate

4. Facial clefts other than prepalate and palate

Unilaterality or bilaterality of hard palate clefts refers to their presence on one or both sides of the hard palate, median clefts to their presence at the midline. These clefts are along a line where the lower edge of the nasal septum attaches to the palate. *Submucous clefts*, on the other hand, are characterized by an intact mucous membrane covering a cleft. This cleft may be separated muscular portions of the soft palate and/or a cleavage of the posterior bony portions of the hard palate. A V-shaped indentation in this area might be felt with the finger. Another sign of the probable existence of a submucous cleft is a divided uvula, a *bifid uvula*. Quite in contrast to unilateral and bilateral clefts, submucous clefts seldom cause feeding problems or abnormal speech.

Articulatory/Phonological Characteristics

Children with cleft palate may exhibit developmental and/or compensatory articulatory and phonological disorders (Bzoch, 1997; Lynch, 1986). Developmental speech-language delays are similar to those found in children without clefts, but they occur more frequently in children with cleft palates (Schonweiler, Schonweiler, Schmelzeisen, and Ptok, 1995; Trost-Cardamone, 1990a). Therefore, children with developmental delays are characterized by articulatory and phonological skills that resemble those of younger normally developing children. Developmental delays cannot always be said to be completely independent from the underlying condition. Consonant cluster reductions, for example, a frequent occurrence in children with speech-language delays, can often be traced to placement or omission errors that are disorder-specific in children with palatal clefts.

Compensatory errors pertain to specific errors of organ/place of articulation that may occur in patients who have inadequate closure of the velopharyngeal valve or a cleft or fistula in the hard palate (Witzel, 1995). They have also been described as "compensatory adjustments" (Morley, 1970). These sound substitutions or distortions are produced more posterior and inferior in the vocal tract by posterior positioning of the tongue, associated true and false vocal fold adduction, or abnormal positioning of the arytenoid cartilage and epiglottis. Due to difficulties with velopharyngeal closure, these errors are thought to be a compensatory attempt to modify the airstream below the velopharyngeal valve. But compensatory errors are not always a direct result of velopharyngeal incompetence. Velopharyngeal incompetence may actually result from compensatory articulation due to limited movements of the velopharyngeal valve during productions of specific sounds. Table 10.2 lists the types of compensatory articulation error (Trost, 1981; Witzel, 1995).

Although specific sound production difficulties have often been noted in the speech of cleft palate children, they may not be entirely phonetic in nature. Children with cleft palate may also evidence difficulties with the organization of phonemes within their language system, that is, they may demonstrate phonological disorders (Broen and Moller, 1993; Chapman, 1993; Chapman and Hardin, 1992;

Estrem and Broen, 1989). Early delays in phonological development were exemplified by a high frequency of deletion of final consonants, syllable reduction, and backing. However, at the age of 4 to 5 years, these problems were less apparent.

Clinical Implications: Diagnostics

Obviously, the initial diagnosis of clefting in a newborn—its nature, site, and extent—is a medical task. So is the beginning of its management, typically involving at least a pediatrician, an orthodontist, and an otolaryngologist. But clefts are a matter of long-term care requiring a team of specialists for successful assessment and management. Speech-language pathologists are important members of this team. Their primary job is to assess the child's communicative status and development. This is a challenging task. Not only are all clefts different (including their various effects on verbal communication) but also the personalities of the children and their caregivers are very different in their ability to cope with the situation and its clinical consequences. However, the biggest diagnostic challenge might be the developmental aspects of the disorder, that is, the changing nature of the appraised findings. Today's status will differ from tomorrow's because of natural growth factors, the necessary corrective measures of medical intervention, and compensatory prospects. Diagnostics involving children with clefts is a truly ongoing process.

The areas of diagnostic concern again underline the necessity of a team approach to the clinical management of cleft palate children. For example, they are all prone to intermittent middle-ear infections and their concomitant conductive hearing loss. This means that an otolaryngologist and an audiologist need to be involved to closely monitor the condition and hearing ability of all children with palatal clefts. The findings are

TABLE 10.2 Compensatory Articulation Errors

COMPENSATORY ARTICULATION	PRODUCTION CHARACTERISTICS	SUBSTITUTION FOR:
Glottal stop	Adduction of true vocal folds; greater air pressure may even result in false vocal fold adduction.	Stop-plosives
Laryngeal stop	Abnormal positioning of epiglottis. Epiglottis comes in contact with pharynx.	Stop-plosives, consonants
Laryngeal fricative	Abnormal positioning of epiglottis. Epiglottis approaches pharynx.	Fricatives
Laryngeal affricate	Epiglottis briefly contacts pharynx, then constricts the airstream.	Affricates
Pharyngeal stop	Dorsum of tongue moves posteriorly, contacting the pharynx, causing a buildup and release of air.	Stop-plosives
Pharyngeal fricative	Dorsum of tongue moves posteriorly toward the pharynx; constricts airstream, causing frication.	Fricatives
Pharyngeal affricate	Dorsum of tongue briefly contacts pharynx; then constricts the airstream.	Affricates
Posterior nasal fricative	Posterior dorsum of tongue and soft palate are positioned to generate friction at VP valve; always accompanied by nasal air emission.	Fricatives
Posterior nasal affricate	Posterior dorsum of tongue and soft palate are positioned to create both stopping and friction; always accompanied by nasal air emission.	Affricates
Middorsum palatal stop	Middorsum of tongue contacts the hard palate at approximate place for [j].	[t], [d], [k], and [g]
Middorsum palatal fricative	Middorsum of tongue approaches the hard palate to create friction.	Fricatives
Middorsum palatal affricate	Middorsum of tongue contacts the hard palate followed by frication.	Affricates

important for the speech-language clinician because "evidence indicates that children with recurrent middle ear problems are slower to acquire speech production skills" (Broen and Moller, 1993, p. 230).

The central diagnostic issue pertains to the velopharyngeal port incompetency (VPI)—to its phonatory, resonatory, and articulatory effects. VPI applies to both structural abnormalities and neuromuscular inadequacies. Whereas structural abnormalities will largely be corrected by surgical and/or prosthetic measures, some functional deficits in respect to speech often remain, resulting in hyperna-

sal resonance, nasal air emission, sound distortions, and sound substitutions. The latter two are characterized by these children's tendency to *articulatory backing,* a compensatory measure of cleft palate children to produce speech sounds more posteriorly in the oral cavity than is normally the case (Trost, 1981). Velopharyngeal incompetency impairs the intraoral pressure buildup necessary for the norm production of many speech sounds— primarily stops, sibilants, fricatives, and affricates, the so-called pressure consonants. Nasals and semivowels such as [w] and [j] remain relatively intact.

CLINICAL APPLICATION

Clinical Test Battery for Children with Cleft Palates

Bzoch (1997) recommends the following clinical test battery:

Language Testing:

Audiometric Evaluation

Nasal emission test	A simple airflow paddle held under the nose (Bzoch, 1979), a small mirrored surface, or a headset listening device is sufficient to enhance the auditory and visual perceptions of nasal airflow. Ten two-syllable words, each containing two [p] or [b] sounds, are used in this test.
Hypernasality test	This measure uses ten one-syllable words beginning with [b] and ending with [t]. The subject repeats each word twice. On the second repetition, the examiner pinches the nares closed. A perceptual judgment of hypernasality is indicated if words shift in quality between the first and second repetition.
Hyponasality test	This measure uses ten one-syllable words beginning with [m] and end with [t]. The subject repeats each word twice; on the second repetition, the examiner pinches the nares closed. On this test, there *should be a shift in quality* between the first and second repetition.
Phonation test	[i], [ɑ], and [u] are prolonged for ten seconds. The examiner notes any aspirate or hoarse phonation. Also, if the client cannot sustain phonation for ten seconds, this would indicate a habituated breathy voice. This can be confirmed by the conversational speech sample.
Articulation test	Special tests examining typical errors noted in the speech of children with cleft palate are available. These include, for example, the *Iowa Pressure Test* (Morris, Spriestersbach, and Darley, 1961) and *Bzoch Error Pattern Diagnostic Articulation Test* (described in Bzoch, 1979).
Screening nasometer test	This test is used for children from 2 to 6 years of age. Procedures can be found in many sources. A few examples include Dalston (1997); Dalston, Warren, and Dalston (1991); Fletcher (1970); and Kay Elemetrics Corporation (1988).

One of the most striking features characterizing the speech of children with cleft palates with velopharyngeal incompetence is the substitution of glottal stops for stop-plosives, a maladaptive compensatory articulatory behavior triggered by the impossibility of accumulating the intraoral pressure required for the regular production of these pressure consonants. During this substitution, the standard positioning of the articulators is sometimes retained. For example, for [p], the lips are closed and suddenly opened simultaneously with the release of the glottal stop. This often results in an impression of a slightly distorted yet acceptable [p] production. In addition to the articulatory consequences of VPI, dental anomalies and problems with occlusion of the mandibular and maxillary arches often contribute to the aberrant articulation of children with cleft palate.

"The primary clinical task for the speech-language pathologist is to assess the child's phonological status and then infer the effects of structural deviations on the phonological behavior observed" (Trost-Cardamone and Bernthal, 1993, p. 317). Such a task will differ considerably from child to child, mostly according to age and linguistic/cognitive levels of the individual client, but it always involves:

1. speech sampling and analysis, including sound inventory and phonological pattern development
2. stimulability probes
3. intelligibility judgments
4. oral-facial examination

Each of these assessment areas has been discussed previously in some detail (see Chapters 6 and 7). Procedures do not differ significantly with the cleft palate child.

One important aspect of the diagnosis with these children is to find, and distinguish between, error patterns that are developmental in nature and those that, as a result of the cleft, have a structural or physiological basis. Some patterns are sometimes seen in children with cleft palate but are not typical for children with structurally and functionally intact oral and pharyngeal mechanisms. The following list is provided by Trost-Cardamone and Bernthal (1993):

1. *Consonant distortions associated with nasal emissions.*
   There are three error patterns associated with nasal emission. It is important to distinguish between them because different interventions may be in order for each.
   - *Nasal emission due to a persistence of velopharyngeal inadequacy.* This is characterized by nasal emission distortion during production of all pressure consonants and pervasive hypernasality accompanying production of vowels and the vocalic consonants [l], [r], [j], and [w].

- *Nasal emission due to oronasal fistulae.* An oronasal fistula is an opening between the oral and nasal cavity. Although some can be easily eliminated surgically, others are too large for successful closure. There is a relationship between the location of the fistula and the consonants affected. Posteriorly located fistulae (near the juncture between the hard and soft palate) affect primarily [k] and [g] with little influence on anteriorly produced consonants. When the fistula is anteriorly located, [t], [d], [s], [z], [p], and [b] are likely to be distorted.
- *Nasal emission that is speech sound specific.* This may occur in the absence of clefting or velopharyngeal impairment. It does not affect a class of sounds and is rarely associated with hypernasality. Nasal emission does not require surgical intervention; it is probably due to faulty learning and can usually be treated with speech therapy, if properly diagnosed.

2. *Vowel distortions secondary to hypernasality.*
   It is important for the clinician to differentiate between vowel distortions that may result from deviant articulatory placement and those that are deviations due to hypernasal resonance as the result of deficient velopharyngeal valving.

3. *Compensatory articulations.*
   Several types of compensatory articulations have been provided in Table 10.2. The clinician should differentiate between compensatory articulations that are used as substitutions and those that occur as coarticulations.

4. *Atypical backed articulation.*
   These articulations include back-velar substitutions for [l], [r], and [n]. The posterior shifts may result from attempting to capture airflow or use of the back of the tongue to help seal the velopharyngeal port. Such pro-

ductions should be analyzed to determine whether they are part of a phonological pattern of backing or whether they represent selective articulatory substitutions.

Clinical Implications: Therapeutics

Many children with cleft palates undergo palate repair by the age of 18 months. They remain free of compensatory sound production errors such as glottal for oral stops and pharyngeal for oral fricatives (Hall and Golding-Kushner, 1989). Other children require therapeutic intervention. To implement therapy with cleft palate clients, four overall goals should be kept in mind:

1. Improve the placement of consonant productions by promoting a more forward place of articulation.
2. Improve velopharyngeal valve function and decrease hypernasal resonance quality.
3. Modify compensatory articulations.
4. If developmental phonological errors exist, improve the child's phonological system (Van Demark and Hardin, 1990).

Improving the placement of consonant productions and modifying compensatory articulations are usually accomplished by direct work on place of articulation, that is, motor placement techniques. Glottal stops can easily be eliminated by using maneuvers that keep the vocal folds apart, such as gentle whispering, overaspiration, or the use of a sustained [h] (Golding-Kushner, 1995). Slight overaspiration by using a sustained [h] usually breaks the glottal pattern because it requires an open glottis. Voiceless oral stops are first introduced at the end of a prolonged [h]. In addition, the voiceless stop itself is overaspirated. If the word was *pie*, the production would sound similar to a prolonged [h] + [p] + *high*. Trost (1981) reports that teaching voiceless homorganic oral fricatives before establishing oral stops is a good tech-

nique for breaking up compensatory coarticulations. Nasal occlusion and release help to eliminate nasal snorting and to establish stops and fricatives. By occluding the nares, clients quickly learn to direct the airstream orally.

Sometimes, even after surgery, the velopharyngeal mechanism is only marginally adequate for articulatory function; hypernasality may still persist to varying degrees. If further surgery and/or prosthodontic intervention is not indicated, improving velopharyngeal valve function and decreasing hypernasal resonance quality might then become a treatment goal. There are several ways to improve velopharyngeal valve function. The velum has been massaged, as well as electrically stimulated, and various devices have been used to improve the effectiveness of these exercises (Starr, 1993). Behavioral approaches that provide feedback to clients are attempts to enhance their awareness and control of the velopharyngeal mechanism. Perceptual and acoustic feedback, visual feedback, and airflow and air pressure feedback have been offered with varying degrees of success (see Starr, 1993, for a review of these techniques). However, due to lack of clinical studies, outcome measures for these techniques remain unclear.

Decreasing hypernasal resonance may be another important therapy goal for cleft palate clients. Hypernasal resonance may occur in individuals with adequate and inadequate velopharyngeal competency. One such technique, increased mouth opening or orality (Boone and McFarlane, 1988; Waengler, 1981, Waengler and Bauman-Waengler, 1987b), will be described because of its overlap with previously mentioned articulatory principles.

Studies have shown (Waengler, 1981; Warren, 1979) that during sound articulation, varying degrees of velar activity occur. For example, stop-plosives require complete closure of the nasopharyngeal port for the necessary buildup of intraoral air pressure. Productions of [ɑ] or [w], on the other hand, do not demand the same degree of closure to prevent undue nasal resonance. Only during the production of stops and sounds with little articulatory possibility for oral air escape, sibilants and affricates, for example, is complete velopharyngeal closure necessary. With more "open" sounds, the same degree of closure is not required.

If "open" sounds require less velar activity to keep nasality effects from occurring, more open versions of the respective phoneme realizations should at least lessen, and possibly prevent, such consequences. Consider /i/ realizations as an example. They can be achieved in several ways, specifically with a more or less restricted oral passageway, without violating the boundaries of the phoneme's value. Under otherwise comparable conditions, orally more open productions will put less demand on proper velar function than the

orally more restricted ones and are, therefore, preferable for the purpose at hand.

Examples like this illustrate the clinical practicalities of the principle to be applied: The task is to train the hypernasal child to utilize systematically the widest oral-articulatory posture that doesn't interfere with the phoneme value the sound represents for the production of the sound in question (Waengler and Bauman-Waengler, 1987b). This might necessitate some preliminary practice in the form of relaxation exercises for lips, tongue, and, especially, jaw.

Many children with cleft palate, especially those with associated cognitive deficits and hearing impairments, are at risk for delays in speech-language development. Depending on kind and degree, developmental delays might or might not require therapeutic intervention. They should nevertheless always be kept therapeutically separate from the disorder-specific articulatory aberrations noted in cleft palate clients.

CLINICAL APPLICATION

Case Study JD

In the United States, the trend in recent years has been toward early closure of palatal clefts, typically between the ages of 6 and 18 months (Marsh and Lehman, 1988).

This case study is adapted from Albery and Russell (1990). JD was born with a cleft of the soft palate which was repaired relatively late at 2;6.

According to the authors, progression through the early speech stages with an open cleft had influenced his articulatory development. His deviant and restricted inventory is not, therefore, typical but does exemplify some of the compensatory articulation errors noted in Table 10.2.

JD's speech was highly unintelligible because the inventory restrictions caused the loss of numerous phonemic contrasts.

Phonetic Inventory:

[m], [n], [w], [j], [h]	Articulated in a regular manner in the prevocalic, intervocalic, and, where applicable, postvocalic word positions.
[ʔp], [ʔb]	A glottal component accompanied the bilabial productions in the prevocalic word positions.

Phonetic Inventory:

[p], [b], [t], [d], [k], [g],	→ ʔ	Stop-plosive productions (including [p] and [b] in intervocalic and
[f], [v], [ʃ], [ʒ], [θ], [ð]	→ ʔ	postvocalic positions), most fricatives, and affricates were realized as
[tʃ], [dʒ],	→ ʔ	glottal stops.
[s]	→ ħ	[s] was realized as a voiceless pharyngeal fricative [ħ] in all word positions.
[z]	→ ʕ	[z] was realized as a voiced pharyngeal fricative [ʕ] in all word positions.
[l]	→ ĩ	[l] was nasalized in the postvocalic word position.
[r]	→ w	[r] was realized as [w].

MENTAL DISABILITY

Definition and General Features

The various attempts to define mental disability reflect the different understanding of, and attitudes toward, the disorder at different times. At least nine different "official" definitions of mental retardation exist from 1921 to 1992. The 1992 definition by the American Association on Mental Retardation (AAMR), the successor organization of the former American Association for the Study of the Feebleminded and the American Association on Mental Deficiency, is no exception:

> *Mental retardation refers to substantial limitations in present functioning. It is characterized by significantly subaverage intellectual functioning, existing concurrently with related limitations in two or more of the following adaptive skill areas: communication, self-care, home living, social skills, community use, self-direction, health and safety, functional academics, leisure, and work. Mental retardation manifests before age 18. (AAMR, 1992, p. 5)*

In such a definition, three criteria stand out:

1. subaverage intellectual functioning
2. limitations in adaptive skills
3. manifestation before 18 years of age

Subaverage intellectual functioning refers in this definition to approximately two standard deviations below the mean on suitable standardized intelligence quotient tests, translating into a score of about 70 or below. *Adaptive skills* refers to functioning in two or more general areas of specified everyday living activities; limitations of such skills pertain essentially to restrictions in learning within the individual's own living circumstances. The manifestation of a mental disability before age 18 identifies such deficiencies as a developmental disorder beginning somewhere between the time of conception and official adulthood. This would eliminate individuals who in adulthood might show signs of dementia and demonstrate similar problems in adaptive behavior, for example.

The 1992 definition further states that an individual must show significant deficits in adaptive behavior relative to his or her own cultural group. This delineation is used to rule out linguistic and cultural differences that might limit the individual's functioning in a larger setting. Paul (1995) notes, "In the old days it sometimes happened that children were labeled retarded simply because they did not speak English as their first language and could not respond to testing or questions in the school language" (p. 114). By emphasizing adaptive behavior, these misdiagnoses are now, one hopes, eliminated.

Prevalence figures for this disorder depend, of course, on the definition of the disorder used. Because definitions changed in the past and will change in the future, these figures are notoriously unreliable. The President's Committee on Mental Retardation (1978) estimated the prevalence of this disorder to be about 3 percent of the population; however, other sources (Mercer, 1973; Tarjan, Wright, Eyman, and Keeran, 1973) support only a 1 percent prevalence.

For the first time in 1992, the AAMR definition eliminated severity classifications. When compared to former definitions, this amounts to a drastic change. However, many good reasons can be given for this change. Foremost, the widespread overrating of IQ scores and their possibly negative impact on aspects of care and education for mentally disabled individuals are arguments against this system. Nevertheless, classification according to severity is still practically very much a part of the general understanding of this disorder. Therefore, severity subgroups are delineated here for orientation purposes. The percentage of persons with mental disability in each of the classification categories is from the President's Committee on Mental Retardation (1978).

Classification	IQ score	Percentage of persons with a mental disability
mild	69 to 55	89%
moderate	54 to 40	6%
severe	39 to 25	3.5%
profound	below 25	1.5%

Specific associated problems may also impact the communicative behavior of this population. Both sensorineural and conductive hearing losses as well as abnormal middle ear function are prevalent in these individuals. Estimates of middle ear dysfunction range from 30 percent to 63 percent and seem to be especially high in individuals with severe retardation (Givens and Seidemann, 1977; Lloyd and Fulton, 1972). Nolan, McCartney, McArthur, and Rowson (1980) found that nearly half of the individuals with mental disabilities they tested had hearing impairments.

Articulatory/Phonological Characteristics

All subgroups of children with mental disabilities demonstrate a higher prevalence of speech problems. It has been estimated that 70 percent of these children have some form of speech production difficulty (Fristoe and Lloyd, 1979). Generally, their speech has been described as indistinct, slurred, and sluggish. They tend to lack articulatory precision and appropriate pauses and phrasing (Weiss, Gordon, and Lillywhite, 1987). The phonological characteristics of the population with mental disabilities can be summarized as follows (Shriberg and Widder, 1990):

1. Speech sound errors are more common than in the nondisabled population.
2. Deletion of consonants is the most frequent error.
3. Errors are typically inconsistent.
4. Patterns are similar to children who are not mentally disabled but demonstrate a functional delay.

In general, individuals with mental disabilities demonstrate the same phonological processes as nonretarded children but with a higher frequency of occurrence (Klink, Gerstman, Raphael, Schlanger, and Newsome, 1986; Moran, Money, and Leonard, 1984). The most common phonological processes are the reduction of consonant clusters and final consonant deletion (e.g., Bleile and Schwartz, 1984; Klink et al., 1986; Sommers, Patterson, and Wildgren, 1988). Variable use of these processes is also noted in this population. It has been hypothesized that individuals with mental disabilities may use these processes for other reasons than to simplify their speech.

For example, Shriberg and Widder (1990) suggest that consonant deletions may reflect cognitive processing constraints in the motor assembly stage of speech production.

Clinical Implications: Diagnostics

Individuals who are mentally disabled are a diverse group of people. Not only are individuals with mental disabilities quite different among themselves but also the boundaries between mentally disabled and what is considered to be norm are rather indistinct: "Mental retardation is on a continuum with normalcy" (Ingalls, 1978, p. 2). That is not to say that individuals with mental disabilities are not different from individuals who are considered to be normal; they are. For example, although the cognitive development of children with mental disabilities is said to be generally similar to that of nondisabled children, only slower (Owens, 1997), and cognitive skills have been proven to keep on growing through adulthood (Berry, Groenweg, Gibson, and Brown, 1984), organizational and recall problems, as well as difficulties in recognizing the significant feature of a given situation distinguish children with mental disabilities from their nondisabled peers (Das, Kirby, and Jarman, 1975; Meador, 1984).

With this group diversity in mind, assessment procedures will largely depend on the age of the individual and the level of speech and language functioning. Some individuals with mental disabilities will not have speech at all and alternative means of communication will need to be explored. For the very young child who is beginning to develop first words, an independent analysis can be used to examine the inventory of sounds the child is using. For older children and adults with more

> An independent analysis for children with emerging phonological systems is discussed in Chapter 6.

developed speech and language skills, the following assessment procedures could be used:

1. *Articulation test* to determine the consonant and vowel inventory. Phonological patterns can also be analyzed, as well as the intelligibility of the speech at the single-word level.

2. *Spontaneous speech sample* to determine the consonant and vowel inventory in conversational speech. Phonological patterns can be noted as well as the overall intelligibility in natural communicative situations. Differences in intelligibility between the spontaneous speech and the articulation test should be evaluated.

3. *Motor speech capabilities.* Speech structure and function should be assessed to determine the individual's motor capabilities.

4. *Hearing acuity and middle ear function.* Due to the large percentage of hearing losses and problems with middle ear function, it is important to have a complete understanding of the individual's current hearing realities.

5. *Language* should be assessed to determine the level of linguistic functioning.

6. *Assessment of the environment* in which the individual lives and works to determine communicative needs. One of the major roles of a clinician is to assess the communicative environment in which the individual resides. This should provide information about the circumstances demanding communication of some sort and how the client is currently communicating to express needs, wants, and desires.

Although the diagnostic assessment of the individual with mental disabilities is executed in a manner essentially similar to that used with nondisabled clients, specific factors need to be kept in mind. Individual differences such as age, level of cognitive functioning, level of speech and language functioning, and learning style will naturally alter the methods used.

Clinical Implications: Therapeutics

"Each child with mental retardation presents a unique pattern of communicative abilities and difficulties which must be identified as a result of a thorough individual assessment. There is, therefore, no intervention prescription for children with retardation" (Long and Long, 1994, p. 174). Some guiding principles for clinicians can nevertheless be suggested within an intervention framework. The following principles may be applicable to the treatment of articulatory/phonological disorders in the population with mental disabilities (Owens, 1997; Weiss, Gordon, and Lillywhite, 1987):

1. Use overlearning and repetition.
2. Train in the natural environment.
3. Begin as early as possible.
4. Follow developmental guidelines.
5. Concentrate more on overall intelligibility rather than on training individual sounds.

One could also add to this list:

6. Enlist the help of the client's caregivers.
7. Direct all therapeutic activities to communication training serving the daily routine.
8. All intervention efforts should be commensurate with the client's ability to grasp and attend to the respective tasks. This typically translates into short, repetitive, reinforced activities "meaningful to the situation and [resulting] in real consequences" (Owens, 1997, p. 495).

With very few exceptions, traditional motor approaches with these individuals have been of little value in the treatment of speech production problems (Sommers, 1969). Therefore, a sound-by-sound approach using placement techniques would probably not be a good choice. The cycles approach has been adapted for use with children with mental disabilities in classroom settings. In these cases, time allotments have been doubled for the children; thus, each phoneme or pattern is targeted for two hours rather than for sixty minutes (Hodson, 1989). A training period of three years or more may be required before substantial intelligibility gains are observed. Hodson (1989) summarizes by saying, "Mentally retarded children seem to be especially in need of a comprehensive, system-oriented phonological remediation approach because they lack the normal cognitive abilities requisite for integration of isolated phoneme parts" (p. 331).

Many of the treatment programs for children and adults with mental disabilities target the increase of overall functional language skills. Although intelligibility is an often noted problem with these individuals, there is very little information available on the treatment of the phonological systems. One possibility, developed by Swift and Rosin (1990), presents a remediation sequence for improving intelligibility of children with Down syndrome. Although this program was designed for a specific population of children, it could be adapted for other children with mental disabilities (in Swift and Rosin's study, the children were mildly and moderately retarded with little evidence of hypotonicity). The early and late linguistic stages of this program are more applicable to work on speech sound development.

During the early linguistic stage, single words and early two-word utterances are emphasized. In structured sound play, the clinician selects objects and toys that should elicit intended sounds. For example, if bilabial sounds were targeted, *ball, baby, bye-bye,* and *moo* could be selected. Drill work is then used to increase the target behavior, attention, and syllable sequencing. The authors also use other techniques, such as melodic speech, visual cues, cued speech, auditory bombardment, and an auditory training unit. Overlearned phrases associated with frequently occurring situations (scripts) are trained as well. In addition, augmentative communication is recognized as a valid option within the oral language intervention program.

During the late linguistic stage, drill work and the learning of scripts continue. In addition, repair strategies are now taught which may aid overall speech intelligibility. Repair strategies include a listener's request for clarification when the message is not understood, for example. Repair strategies from a speaker's point of view include repeating, rewording, and adaptations of the prosodic features (e.g., slowing the rate, adjusting phrasing, and using stress and inflection to enhance the meaning). Throughout the program, communication should be as functional as possible.

The decision to use an augmentative or alternative system for communication with individuals with mental disabilities should be based on the same criteria used with any client. If the cognitive and language comprehension levels allow it, alternative/augmentative communication devices can certainly increase the potential for successful communication. The general advice is to try speech therapy first—for one year at least—before nonspeech communicative means are introduced, even if all requirements for their use are met (Long and Long, 1994; Owens and House, 1984).

CLINICAL APPLICATION

Speech Goals and Activities for Facilitating the Development of Speech and Improving Intelligibility

The following goals and suggestions are offered by Miller (1988). Although they were proposed for Down syndrome children, they could be used with other children with mental disabilities who are in the beginning stages of speech and language development.

SPEECH GOALS FOR THE CHILD

1. *Increase the ability to respond to people and objects.* The more this skill can be promoted, the greater the opportunity for enhancing communication.
2. *Increase the frequency of vocal and verbal productions.* The more output, the more opportunity for modifying the quality of speech.
3. *Increase production of sounds and the variety of sounds made.* This includes not only the actual production of speech sounds but also speaking rate, loudness, and intonation changes. These variables will add to the intelligibility of the child.
4. *Making the transition from babbling behavior to using words* to represent objects and actions in the environment. It appears that children who are mentally disabled are trying to say words earlier than they are recognized by the caregivers in the children's environments. Their speech is often difficult to understand and the words they use are simply labels and not descriptive.

SUGGESTIONS FOR CAREGIVERS

1. Identify situations and activities throughout the day in which the child is most vocal. Make a list of these situations over a week or two, noting the situation, the length of time the situation continues, and how many times these situations occur during the day.
2. Document how much the child responds to people and things by looking, touching, or playing during a particular situation. Communication depends to a large degree upon responsiveness.
3. Try to increase the time the child spends in these communication-enhancing situations (noted in Number 1).
4. Introduce the children to music at an early age. Children frequently respond enthusiastically to this stimulation. The type of music will depend on the child.
5. Speech activities should be a natural part of the child's day. During ordinary caregiving tasks, talk to the child about the objects of the play and the activities. Introduce interactive games such as "pat-a-cake," "peek-a-boo," and "so big." While these activities promote vocalizations they also

develop responsiveness to turn taking and social interaction.

Based on a thorough assessment, the speech-language clinician can suggest sounds, sound patterns, and words that may be included in activities for the child's day. Suggestions offered in the child with an Emerging Phonological System section of Chapter 9 could also be incorporated here.

HEARING IMPAIRMENT

Definition and General Features

Hearing loss (or hearing impairment) is a generic term for any diminished ability in normal sound reception. The different etiologies that can result in hearing loss are only indirectly part of this definition. Commonly, hearing loss is described by type and degree of the particular auditory dysfunction (Northern and Downs, 1984). As far as the types of hearing impairment are concerned, conductive, sensorineural, and mixed dysfunctions are distinguished. The degree of hearing loss is categorized by reference to decibel (dB) levels, indicating the increase in intensity needed to make sound audible for the individual in question.

Conductive hearing loss refers to transmission problems affecting the travel of air-conducted sound waves from the external auditory canal to the inner ear. This affects the mechanical transfer of sound waves. A prominent medical condition causing conductive hearing loss is otitis media. **Sensorineural hearing loss** occurs as a consequence of damage to the sensory end organ, the cochlear hair cells, or the auditory nerve. In these cases, air-conduction and bone-conduction thresholds are typically comparable. Mumps, among other medical conditions, can cause a sensorineural auditory dysfunction. If both a conductive and a sensorineural loss can be established, a *mixed hearing loss* exists.

The different degrees of hearing loss indicate the severity of the problem according to the (approximate) threshold findings obtained. (*HL* stands for "hearing level.")

> To determine hearing loss, a three frequency average is typically used, which is the average for 500, 1,000, and 2,000 Hz in the better ear (Reed, 1994).

26 to 40 dB HL = mild hearing loss
41 to 55 dB HL = moderate hearing loss
56 to 70 dB HL = moderately severe hearing loss
71 to 95 dB HL = severe hearing loss
96+ dB HL = profound loss (Bess and McConnell, 1981)

Severity levels of hearing loss, determined by objective audiometric means, are not necessarily reliable indicators of speech-language function. Individuals deal differently with losses of hearing ability, especially within the context of communication. A loss of 50 dB HL bilaterally in two children, for example, can have a notably different influence on their verbal communication. Such different effects of an objectively established hearing loss can become especially important when dealing with children in various phases of their speech-language development. Even relatively mild auditory dysfunctions with relatively minor communicative consequences for adult speakers/listeners might have lasting detrimental developmental effects in children. Nevertheless, the diminished ability to receive sound for comprehension is normally identified by the degree of hearing loss.

Articulatory/Phonological Characteristics

Speech production in the hearing impaired is affected by the degree of hearing impairment and the frequencies involved. Generally, the greater the hearing loss, the more likely errors will extend from consonant and vowel productions to errors in stress, pitch, and voicing (Osberger and McGarr, 1982). Most of the literature describing the speech characteristics of hearing impaired individuals has examined children with severe to profound hearing losses. Little seems to be available about specific speech characteristics of children with less severe losses. Keeping this in mind, the following consonant, vowel, and prosodic feature differences have been noted in the speech of hearing impaired children.

Consonant production in hearing impaired children is generally characterized by deletions and substitutions. Both initial and final consonant deletions occur; however, final consonant deletions are far more prevalent (Abraham, 1989). Frequently occurring substitutions include (1) confusion of voiced and voiceless cognates, (2) substitution of stops for fricatives and liquids, and (3) confusion between oral and nasal consonants (Levitt and Stromberg, 1983). Studies with hard-of-hearing children have reported that consonants produced with the blade of the tongue ([t, d, s, z, ʃ, ʒ, tʃ, dʒ]) are more likely to be in error. The affricates are ranked as most difficult for both profoundly hearing impaired children and the hard-of-hearing (Markides, 1970; Smith, 1975). These findings are not, however, completely supported by an investigation by Abraham (1989). Based on the data obtained from thirteen severely and profoundly hearing impaired children, she found that there was a marked difference in the accuracy of production word-initially versus word-finally. All sounds demonstrated a lower percentage of accuracy word-finally. Although the affricates were below 50 percent accuracy, consonants with even lower percentages of accuracy included [z] and [ð].

Children with hearing impairments have been found to use at least partially rule-governed phonological systems (Abraham, 1989; Dodd, 1976). They use phonological processes similar to those of young normally developing children, although they use these processes more frequently. The overall intelligibility of speech is often reduced, particularly as linguistic complexity increases (Radziewicz and Antonellis, 1997).

Vowels tend to be neutralized; therefore, front and back vowels have a tendency to sound like central vowels (Ling, 1976). Other vowel errors include tense for lax (and lax for tense) substitutions, especially the front vowels [i] and [ɪ]. Due to poor control of timing, diphthongs are often produced as monophthongs and vice versa (Levitt and Stromberg, 1983).

Prosodic features can also be affected, although more difficulties are evidenced in profoundly impaired than in the hard-of-hearing population. Problems include reduced speech rate, slow articulatory transitions with frequent pauses, poor coordination of breathing with syntactic phrasing, use of duration to create stress patterns, and distorted resonance (Dunn and Newton, 1994).

Clinical Implications: Diagnostics

In addition to audiometric results, the speech-language diagnostician assessing the impact of impaired hearing on the articulatory/phonological status of a client needs a host of appraisal data before any diagnostic conclusion can be reached. These include cause, age of onset, and identification of the impairment; its etiology and type; and length of previous intervention efforts. Speech intelligibility measures as well as results of formal and informal testing for language skills should also be included in the assessment data. Finally, the client's and caregivers' attitudes toward the disorder and the need for intervention will give indications about the degree of motivation and possibly the impact of therapy.

Phonetic and phonological assessments need to be completed for the child with a hearing impairment. The following assessment procedures are outlined in Dunn and Newton (1994):

1. *Speech-motor assessment.* Used to rule out any gross neurological or anatomical limitations that might interfere with speech sound production.

2. *Syllable imitation.* Tests the coordination of the speech mechanism during nonmeaningful speech.

3. *Administration of the Phonetic Level Evaluation (PLE)* (Ling, 1976). This instrument evaluates suprasegmental and segmental skills through the imitation of nonsense syllables. The test provides a systematic, comprehensive hierarchy for the assessment of syllables with varied phonetic contexts. However, the PLE has specific shortcomings (see Dunn and Newton, 1994, pp. 130–132) and should not be used as the only evaluative measure for the hearing impaired child.

4. *Spontaneous speech sample.* Depending on the age and developmental level of the child, this could be either single words or continuous speech. Ideally, the speech sample should include both.

5. *Analysis of the segmental and suprasegmental characteristics of the spontaneous speech sample.* Segmental analysis should include those procedures outlined in this text in Chapter 7 (i.e., consonant and vowel inventory and distribution, syllable shape, and phonological pattern analysis). A suprasegmental analysis determines whether the child uses rate, pauses, stress, and intonational patterns appropriately. This can be done informally, with the clinician marking appropriate and inappropriate patterns. Dunn and Newton (1994) suggest a more formal measure developed at the National Technical Institute for the Deaf (Subtelny, 1980). This procedure provides rating scales for a variety of suprasegmental characteristics.

Clinical Implications: Therapeutics

With hearing impaired clients, the speech-language clinician's remedial task is mainly directed to the improvement of the client's speech intelligibility. "The term '**speech intelligibility**' may be defined generically as that aspect of oral speech-language output that allows a listener to understand what a speaker is saying" (Carney, 1994, p. 109). Such a task involves above all structured work on principal articulation errors and the selection of a suitable phonetic treatment program. Both of these objectives depend on two prerequisites (Dunn and Newton, 1994):

1. the improvement of the residual hearing by speech signal amplification and the methodical habituation of its application
2. the maximal utilization of the level of residual hearing for speech perception through systematic articulatory training

The first prerequisite presupposes wearing an individualized hearing aid at all times and, possibly, the use of auditory trainers during clinical sessions. In addition, it involves step-by-step procedures so that the client fully recognizes the speech-related benefits of the amplification. A primary responsibility of the speech-language clinician called to improve a client's intelligibility level is, therefore, to ensure constant proper amplification, not just during therapy, and to facilitate the client's adjustment to the new hearing situation.

The maximal utilization of the client's level of residual hearing poses another challenge. Hearing impaired children miss important information for the recognition of speech signals, which is the main reason for their lack of intelligibility. Essentially, they produce what they are able to hear, leaving out what they are unable to receive. In directing their attention systematically to specific oral/facial movements accompanying normal suprasegmental and segmental production, their residual hearing can be more effectively utilized which can, in turn, positively influence intelligibility. In connection with suitable amplification, these efforts should increase speech intelligibility, especially in respect to voice, suprasegmental realization, and vowel production, three especially conspicuous error areas of hearing impaired children.

However, the hearing impaired child will also need systematic training on the phonetic as well as the phonological level.

CLINICAL APPLICATION

Teaching Speech Sound Production to Individuals with Hearing Impairment

Several approaches have been implemented with hearing impaired individuals to teach speech sound production. Examples include the Auditory Global Approach (Calvert and Silverman, 1983) and multisensory approaches, prominent examples being Ling's program (1976) and Osberger's (1983) modification of the Ling approach. The multisensory approaches use a variety of sensory modalities to first achieve accurate imitative production at the syllabic level. When a certain level of accuracy is reached, instruction begins at the word level. These approaches train speech sound production; they do not provide hearing impaired children with a systematic means of developing their phonology.

Dunn and Newton (1994) suggest a program that simultaneously teaches phonetic and phonological skills. The training sequence is as follows:

1. *Establish a suprasegmental base.* This is initially achieved through coordination of pitch, duration, and intensity with babbling or vocal play. Once this suprasegmental base is established, it will carry over to the various other stages of treatment. Dunn and Newton

(1994) state in this context that "Clinicians' eagerness to work on consonants before a suprasegmental base is established may result in many of the disordered patterns characteristic of deaf speech" (p. 140).

2. *Teaching the segmental speech sounds.* This begins with basic vowel patterns. The patterns are first generated within any context the child can accurately produce, preferably a CV or VC syllable structure. Both Calvert and Silverman (1983) and Ling (1976) provide procedures and strategies for achieving a new sound with the hearing impaired population.

3. *Generalize a stable production by using different phonetic contexts and new syllable types.* Once a production is stable in one basic context, new contexts are selected. Productions move from various other syllable types to monosyllabic words and, finally, to two-syllable words. With one- and two-syllable words, the child is responsible only for accurate production of the target sound. For example, if the target sound is [b] and the selected word is *boat,* [bo] would be considered an accurate production. Two-syllable words begin with those containing reduplicated syllables such as *bye-bye* or *booboo.* In this phase, acceptable speech sound production is applied to meaningful words. In addition, prosodic variation is practiced with these words.

MOTOR SPEECH DISORDERS: ACQUIRED APRAXIA OF SPEECH

Definition and General Features

The general term *apraxia* refers to a disorder in the execution of purposeful movements; reflexive or automatic motor actions remain largely intact. For example, as soon as an otherwise reflexive action is intended—upon request, for example, or by one's own volition—gross execution difficulties occur. *Acquired apraxia of speech,* therefore, is the impaired volitional production of articulation and prosody (Kent and Rosenbek, 1983). These articulatory and prosodic aberrations do not result from muscle weakness or slowness but from impairment to the central nervous system's programming of oral movements. Apraxia of speech represents an inability to program and sequence articulatory requirements for volitional speech (Darley, Aronson, and Brown, 1975; Johns and Darley, 1970). Thus, **apraxia of speech** is a disorder of expressive communication as a result of brain damage affecting the normal realization of speech sounds, sound sequences, and prosodic features representing speech. Auditory comprehension, in principle, remains intact (Darley et al., 1975).

Damage to two central nervous system areas is held responsible for the communication disorder found in apraxia of speech. The most common cause is injury to the dominant side of the brain's frontal lobe, more specifically its posterior inferolateral regions, otherwise known as *Broca's area*. However, lesions to several cortical and subcortical areas might be involved as well, specifically those of the supplemental motor cortex and the basal ganglia (Dworkin, 1991).

Apraxia of speech should be separated from the dysarthrias, another motor speech disorder that affects verbal expression. The following guidelines are given for differentiation between the two (Darley et al., 1975; LaPointe and Wertz, 1974; Shipley and McAfee, 1992; Wertz, LaPointe, and Rosenbek, 1984):

Apraxia of speech	Dysarthria
Absence of any muscular weakness, paralytic condition, or discoordination.	Presence of muscular weakness. Change in muscular tone secondary to neurologic involvement.
Speech process of articulation is primarily affected.	All processes for speech are affected: respiration, phonation, resonation, and articulation.
Speech errors result from disruption of the central nervous system's programming of oral movements.	Speech errors result from disruption of the central and peripheral nervous system's control of muscular movements.
Inconsistent articulatory errors.	Consistent, predictable articulatory errors.

Apraxia of speech differs from the aphasias by the language involvement of the latter. Such a differentiation appears quite clear as long as a comparison is made between apraxic speakers, on the one hand, and those afflicted with Wernicke's or sensory aphasia, on the other. A valid distinction between apraxic speakers and those with Broca's, that is, expressive or motor aphasia, is far less obvious and has triggered an ongoing discussion of long standing (Martin, 1974; Noll, 1983). Both apraxic speakers and Broca's aphasics have little, if any, language involvement and somewhat common problems with verbal output (Benson, 1979; Luria and Hutton, 1977). Of course, statements like these depend largely on the definition of the term *language involvement*. When the syntactic realization of grammatical rules is taken into account, individuals with Broca's aphasia are dysgrammatic; apraxics are not. Thus, although some vagueness between the terms *Broca's aphasia* and *apraxia of speech* certainly remains, one can generally summarize that

Aphasia is a language disorder caused by injury to the dominant hemisphere responsible for processing the language code. Apraxia is a motor speech disorder resulting from damage

to neural circuits of the dominant hemisphere responsible for programming speech movements. (Marquardt, 1982, p. 3)

Apraxia of speech can, of course, co-occur with aphasia and does so frequently (Metter, 1985).

Apraxia of speech should also be distinguished from oral (nonverbal) apraxia. **Oral (nonverbal) apraxia** is a disturbance of the planning and execution of volitional *nonspeech* movements of oral structures, that is, those movements not representing speech production. For example, if a client is asked to lick his lips, he might blow instead (Johns, 1985). The same client might be perfectly able to drink some juice, swallow the sip, and lick a drop off his lips without any problem (Meitus and Weinberg, 1983). Upon request, though, he cannot perform the same motor action; attempts will probably result in a series of laborious, bizarre trials. As might be expected, clients with apraxia of speech often suffer from oral (nonverbal) apraxia as well.

Articulatory/Phonological Characteristics

The following characteristics of apraxia of speech have been noted (Bauman and Waengler, 1977; Darley, 1978; Darley et al., 1975; Deal and Darley, 1972; Johns and Darley, 1970; LaPointe and Johns, 1975; Shankweiler and Harris, 1966; Waengler and Bauman-Waengler, 1980, 1987a; Wertz, LaPointe, and Rosenbek, 1984):

1. *Effortful, trial-and-error groping of articulatory movements and attempts at self-correction.* This may result in equalization of syllabic stress patterns, slow rate of speech, and other prosodic alterations.
2. *Prosodic disturbances.*
3. *Difficulty initiating utterances.*
4. *Articulatory inconsistency on repeated production of the same utterance.* However, is-

lands of clear, well-articulated speech exist.
5. *Sound substitution errors predominate.* Additions and prolongations also occur; distortions and omissions are less frequent.
6. *Sound or syllable transpositions may occur.*
7. *Occasionally, articulatory errors are complications rather than simplifications.* A consonant cluster may be substituted for a single consonant.
8. *Errors are typically phonetically related to one another.* Substitutions, for example, may be related in place or manner of articulation to the intended sound.
9. *More errors occur on consonants that require more precise articulatory adjustments,* for example, fricatives and affricates.
10. *Number of errors and articulatory struggle increase as the word increases in length.*
11. *Speech comprehension and word recognition abilities are often far better than speech production abilities.*
12. *Clients recognize their errors.* This may cause numerous retrials or self-correction attempts.
13. *Under otherwise comparable conditions, more sound production errors occur in stressed than in unstressed syllables.*

Clinical Implications: Diagnostics

A diagnosis of apraxia of speech may not have been made before a clinician sees the client. Therefore, the following areas should be included in a thorough evaluation of a client with suspected apraxia of speech (Haynes and Pindzola, 1998):

1. aphasia test
2. intelligence, cognitive, and memory tests, as needed
3. apraxia battery
4. speech-motor mechanism examination
5. articulation test
6. spontaneous speech sample

For the purposes at hand, this diagnostic section will concentrate on those testing procedures that involve only aspects of articulation and phonology, that is, on numbers 3 through 6 of the above-mentioned categories.

CLINICAL APPLICATION

Formal and Informal Tests for Apraxia of Speech in Adults

Test of oral and limb apraxia	DeRenzi, Pieczuro, and Vignolo, 1966
Oral apraxia test	Darley, Aronson, and Brown, 1975
Test of verbal, oral, and limb apraxia	Rosenbek and Wertz, 1976
Test of oral and limb apraxia	Helm-Estabrooks, 1996
Dworkin-Culatta Oral Mechanism Examination	Dworkin and Culatta, 1980
Apraxia Battery for Adults	Dabul, 1979
Oral movement battery	Moore, Rosenbek, and LaPointe, 1976
Tests of integrity and consistency of phoneme production	Johns and Darley, 1970
Motor Speech Evaluation	Wertz, LaPointe, and Rosenbek, 1984

Some of these tests can be used to evaluate the presence of oral and limb apraxia as well as specific characteristics of apraxia of speech. Others will give the clinician information about the client's abilities to sequence words of varying length and complexity.

The speech-motor assessment examines the structure and function of the articulators. While the function of the articulators is often assessed with one of the apraxia batteries, the oral-mechanism examination can also be used to determine the presence of oral (nonverbal) apraxia. If the structure is intact but commands eliciting nonverbal movements such as "pucker your lips" or "stick out your tongue" result in laborious, bizarre movements, oral apraxia may be suspected.

Both the articulation test and the spontaneous speech sample should answer the following questions:

- Does the client have difficulty initiating utterances? Does this difficulty have a pattern? For example, is it better with words or sentences? Does the content of the message play a role?
- Are there any islands of well-articulated speech? These are usually automatic-reactive responses such as the days of the week or "I can't say that"; however, are there others?
- Which sound errors occur? Evaluate the differences between one-word articulation tests and spontaneous speech. Also note the errors that occur as the complexity of the word or utterance increases. Furthermore, register substitutions, additions, prolongations, transpositions, distortions, and omissions.
- Do sound errors have a pattern? Errors are typically related to the target sound. A place-manner-voice analysis could demonstrate which patterns are occurring. Observations should include ascertaining difficulties with fricatives, affricates, and consonant clusters, all typical problems for the individual with apraxia of speech.
- Which prosodic aberrations occur? Stress realizations (stressed versus unstressed syl-

lables), intonation, rate of speech, and pausing should be observed and analyzed.

Clinical Implications: Therapeutics

In apraxia of speech, the client's ability to program and sequence articulatory requirements for volitional speech is impaired. This impairment ranges from mild to severe, with each client demonstrating a different clinical picture. Some may have difficulty only in sequencing certain multisyllabic words or with specific clusters; others may have extreme problems sequencing a simple CV word. Obviously, such varying degrees of impairment will influence the selection of therapeutic measures. In addition, certain aspects of motor production affect the error patterns of apraxic speakers (Wertz et al., 1984). These general guidelines can be utilized when structuring therapy:

1. *Articulatory accuracy is better for meaningful than for nonmeaningful utterances.* Therefore, avoid nonsense syllables; all treatment stimuli should be meaningful.

2. *Errors increase as words increase in length.* Determine the level at which the client demonstrates accurate production most of the time, then build on that level. For example, if the assessment reveals that the client can produce CV, CVC, and VC words fairly accurately, start with this level of functioning and slowly build to CVCV structures or "easier" two-syllable words.

3. *Errors increase as the distance between successive points of articulation increases.* Evaluate your word material. Organize it so that this factor is taken into consideration. If you are working on consonant clusters, [st] should be easier than [sk]. If you are structuring words, *toilet* should be easier than *shopping*.

4. *Errors increase on consonants that require more precise articulatory adjustments.* Fricatives, affricates, and consonant clusters are extremely difficult for some apraxics. Begin with

other sound classes until more volitional control is achieved.

Darley et al. (1975) advocate the *phonetic placement approach* to help the client relearn the positioning of the articulators for the standard realization of speech sounds. Cognition, sensory perception, and neuromuscular action are (by definition) essentially unimpaired. Therefore, the positioning of the articulators necessary for the realization of the sound in question should be relatively easy to achieve.

The *sound modification method* presupposes the presence of some regular sound realizations. Applying the knowledge of phonetic sound production features, the clinician attempts to derive the target sound out of elements of another sound the client can realize in a regular manner. For example, assume that a client with generally acceptable [d] sounds demonstrates difficulty with [t], especially when initiating a stressed syllable. The client may actually need to be instructed only that the main phonetic differences between [d] and [t] pertain to voicing and lenis versus fortis production—organ, place, and manner of articulation are in both cases directly comparable. Thus, any whispered [d] will automatically result in a weak [t], which a slightly increased production effort will normalize. The client will not have to learn [t] productions "from scratch." The sound modification method might prove to be beneficial for individual clients.

MOTOR SPEECH DISORDERS: THE DYSARTHRIAS

Definition and General Features

The word *articulation* has its origin in the Greek root *arthr-*, referring to the jointed connection between the many different parts of the speaking process. *Dys-arthr-ia,* therefore, literally means "disordered articulation." To be sure, in this context, "articulation" is to be

---

CLINICAL APPLICATION

Apraxia of Speech: A Phonological Disorder?

According to popular contemporary definitions that subsume articulation difficulties under the category of phonological disorders (e.g., Elbert, 1997), apraxia of speech would be labelled a phonological disorder. The treatment for apraxia of speech has historically been phonetically based, that is, followed traditional articulation principles. However, taking the apraxics' relatively preserved language, cognitive, and perceptual skills into account, a remediation program based on phonological principles could offer some additional advantages.

1. Articulatory accuracy is, as a rule, better for meaningful than for nonmeaningful utterances. A minimal pair approach, for example, would speak directly to this issue by focusing on meaningful and meaning-differentiating communication.
2. Many of the minimal pair approaches are based on communicative breakdown. For example, the child actually means *key* but says *tea* and, therefore, receives the wrong picture card. Apraxic clients are very aware of errors and communicative breakdowns that occur when production accuracy fails. Therefore, this method could in some cases be more motivating than imitating nonsense syllables.

Generally, though, a minimal pair approach falls short for the communicative needs of the apraxic individual. There are just not very many minimal pairs that are used contrastively in everyday communicative situations. Nevertheless, for certain clients, adding phonemic to phonetic principles of treatment might be beneficial. Phonetic principles such as awareness of the articulatory complexity of the utterance, the consonants it contains, and the helpful or hindering coarticulation features could be easily combined with meaningful, communicatively contrasting situations.

---

understood in the broadest possible sense, that is, as signifying all articulated movements that result in speech. The technical term *dysarthria,* on the other hand, denotes a rather explicit group of articulation disorders, namely, those caused by neurogenic abnor-malities, more specifically by the impairment of a single portion or several portions of the (central and/or peripheral) nervous system that control and coordinate speech. **Dysarthrias** are neuromuscular speech disorders (Marquardt, 1982).

Dysarthrias have many different causes. Accident-induced trauma, tumors, cerebrovascular accidents (strokes), congenital conditions, and infectious and degenerative neurogenetic diseases are prominent among them. All of these events can bring about more or less pronounced paralytic conditions and coordination impairments of the voluntary musculature required for speech production. The result: dysarthrias.

Articulatory/Phonological Characteristics

It is customary to classify the dysarthrias according to the locus of the damage and its neuropathic consequences into five main types:

1. spastic dysarthria
2. ataxic dysarthria
3. hypokinetic dysarthria
4. hyperkinetic dysarthria
5. flaccid dysarthria

In addition, any simultaneous occurrence of characteristics of several types is labelled:

6. mixed dysarthria

Every main type has its cluster of speech impairing phonetic-articulatory production features (Darley et al., 1975; Dworkin, 1991; Wertz, 1985). They are summarized in Table 10.3.

Summaries like these are helpful, but any division of dysarthric characteristics into just five subtypes suggests more group uniformity than is actually the case. Although some within-group similarities can probably serve as general guidelines, several across-group fea-

TABLE 10.3 Summary of Features of the Various Types of Dysarthria

TYPES	FEATURES

Spastic Dysarthria

(Resulting from upper motor neuron system disorders. Example: Pseudobulbar palsy.)

Respiration:	Low respiratory frequency with shallow inspiration and lack of expiratory control.
Phonation:	Strained, harsh, low-pitch voice; reduced pitch and loudness ranges.
Resonation:	Hypernasality; nasal air emission.
Articulation:	Slow, labored, imprecise phoneme realization, especially of consonants.

Ataxic Dysarthria

(Resulting from cerebellar lesions. Example: Cerebellar ataxia.)

Respiration:	Shallow inspiration and lack of expiratory control. Rapid, irregular, forced breathing patterns.
Phonation:	Forced, hoarse-breathy, trembling voice. Generally reduced (but sometimes excessive) use of pitch and loudness.
Resonation:	Normal.
Articulation:	Slow, imprecise phoneme realization, especially of consonants. Sound prolongations. Irregular pausing between words, syllables, and sounds.

Hypokinetic Dysarthria

(Resulting from disorders of the extrapyramidal system. Example: Parkinsonism.)

Respiration:	Frequent respirations with shallow inspiratory phases and lack of expiratory control.
Phonation:	Harsh, tremorous voice; reduced pitch and loudness levels.
Resonation:	Normal.
Articulation:	Fluctuating imprecise articulation. Articulatory bursts. Low intelligibility.

Hyperkinetic Dysarthria

(Resulting from disorders of the extrapyramidal system. Examples: Athetosis, chorea.)

Respiration:	Frequent respirations with shallow inspirations and incomplete expirations; lack of respiratory control.
Phonation:	Strained, tremorous voice. Uncontrolled but generally reduced ranges in the expressive use of pitch and loudness.
Resonation:	Alternating hypernasality.
Articulation:	Variable imprecision of phoneme, especially consonant, realization.

Flaccid Dysarthria

(Resulting from lower motor neuron system disorders. Example: Bulbar palsy.)

Respiration:	Shallow, audible inspirations. Uneven, incomplete expirations. Low respiratory frequency; low expiratory air pressure.
Phonation:	Breathy, hoarse voice lacking expressive pitch and loudness variation.
Resonation:	Marked hypernasality with nasal air emission.
Articulation:	Slow, imprecise phoneme realization, especially of consonants.

Source: Summarized from Darley et al. (1975); Dworkin (1991); and Waengler and Bauman-Waengler (1987a).

tures overlap considerably, "thus challenging the usefulness of group classifications" (Dworkin, 1991, p. 6). Several of the deficiencies mentioned belong in some measure simply to the clinical picture of most dysarthrias. These include:

Respiration: Irregular, generally shallow breathing patterns might suddenly become interrupted by some deep breaths; rapid inspiration, incomplete expiration phases; waste of expiratory air during speaking; lack of respiratory support.

Phonation: Strained voice; deviations from suitable loudness levels (either too loud or too soft) and voice quality (either too harsh or too "breathy," aphonic).

Resonation: Hypernasality and nasal air emission as consequence of incomplete velopharyngeal closure, distorting all speech sounds with the exception of nasals.

Articulation: Labored, indistinct sound articulation, especially of consonants, resulting in distortions or substitutions. Consonant errors might affect whole sound classes; stops, for example, might be realized as homorganic fricatives. Also, second and third elements of consonant clusters might be deleted; rate of speech usually slower than normal (bradylalia), but bursts of fast speech (tachylalia) might occur as well; qualitative and quantitative misrepresentations of vowels.

Prosody: Narrow range of intonational configurations ("monopitch"); (often greatly) reduced variety of expressive loudness levels ("monoloudness"); this generally reduced range of prosodic elements is sometimes interrupted by exaggerated stress and intonation patterns (Darley et al., 1975; Dworkin,

1991; Waengler and Bauman-Waengler, 1987a).

The physiological basis for all of these characteristics is a striking imbalance in the constant and subtle changes between phases of (relative) muscular tension and relaxation leading to normal speech events. The delicate synergism between the interaction of individual muscles and whole muscle groups to produce speech is in all cases of dysarthria disturbed. Instead, a disproportionate influence of agonistic and antagonistic forces determines dysarthric speech motor activity, distorting its normally smooth flow into effortful, poorly controlled speech production.

Common characteristics such as these exist across and within the main groups of dysarthrias. However, individual clients medically diagnosed with a specific type of dysarthria often show significant deviations from the noted group features. These individual differences are especially important within the assessment and intervention process. The speech-language clinician will always need to find out the specific deviations from norm each individual client displays.

Clinical Implications: Diagnostics

Most dysarthric clients are referred to us by physicians or medical institutions. As a rule, an official diagnosis has already been established, usually down to the subtype the client belongs to medically—spastic dysarthria, for example. What, then, remains for speech-language pathologists to assess and evaluate? Actually, quite a bit.

Even in the appraisal section of our assessment process, we need to go far beyond the initial (mainly medical) information available to us. As mentioned earlier, dysarthric subtype characteristics are somewhat vague and indeterminate and, therefore constitute little more than a point of departure for any appropriate collection of clinical data. They are both helpful and insufficient for our purposes. They are helpul because they indicate what to suspect and what to look for. They are insufficient because individual cases more often than not show considerable deviations from average, book-based descriptions. That is why *all* dysarthric symptoms contributing to abnormal voice and speech production need to be appraised as precisely as possible.

One possible aid to precise appraisal is the use of instrumentation. There is certainly no scarcity of instruments available to be used to objectify the data. The problem does not lie in a lack of suitable instrumentation but in their proper application to the task at hand. Many clinicians are not trained well enough in instrumentation to feel comfortable with its proper use or do not have easy access to instrumentation. Another reason for the rare use of instruments in a clinical setting is a time concern: Clinicians feel too pressed for time to engage in the utilization of instruments in order to make their appraisal data more objective and verifiable.

A second way to make the appraisal of dysarthric clients more comparable, reliable, and precise is the use of a suitable protocol. Such a protocol might look like that found in Figure 10.1.

CLINICAL APPLICATION

Protocols for the Appraisal of the Speech Characteristics of Clients with Dysarthria

Frenchay Dysarthria Assessment	Enderby, 1980, 1983
Dysarthria Examination Battery	Drummond, 1993
Point-Place System	Rosenbek and LaPointe, 1985
Motor Speech Evaluation	Wertz, LaPointe, and Rosenbek, 1984
Assessments of Intelligibility of Dysarthric Speech	Yorkston and Beukelman, 1981

Some of these assessment instruments give profiles for the various diagnostic categories, whereas others provide severity ratings.

After having identified kind and severity of the dysarthric disturbances within the main subsystems contributing to speech, the clinician is now ready to interpret and evaluate them in their totality, that is, to draw a composite picture of the problem at hand—diagnosis in the narrow sense of the term. Diagnoses lead directly into therapy planning. They form the very basis for the professional selection of appropriate intervention measures.

Clinical Implications: Therapeutics

The speech-language clinician's main therapeutic goal is the improvement of the dysarthric client's intelligibility. Because the established deficits are caused by central and/or peripheral nervous system damage, this is done primarily by searching for, and training, compensatory measures. The diagnostic results should provide the necessary information

FIGURE 10.1 Protocol for Assessing Respiration, Phonation, Resonation, and Articulation of Dysarthric Speech

1. Rate the degree of normal, near normal, or abnormal behavior on a scale from 1 to 5 by marking the double line at the judged value.

	normal		→		abnormal
	1	2	3	4	5

Respiration
Silent breathing
Speech breathing
  Inspiration
  Expiration
  Breath support
  Shouting
  Shortness of breath

Resonation
Nasality
Quality of prolonged vowels
  Constant   check one   [   ]
  Intermittent   [   ]

Phonation
Voice
Pitch
Volume

Lips
Appearance in resting position
Lip protrusion
Movement during speaking

Jaw
Appearance in resting position
Movement during speaking

Tongue
Appearance in resting position
Protrusion
Elevating tip of tongue
Lowering tip of tongue
Lateral movements
During speaking
Strength

Articulation
Vowels
  Quality
  Duration
Consonants
Clusters

Prosody
Stress
Intonation
Tempo
Rhythm

2. Itemize the most salient characteristic in each of the categories with a rating of 3 or more.

3. Repeat the rating process at least one more time on a different day.

about the kind and degree of shortcomings in the various subsystems constituting normal speech production (i.e., respiration, phonation, resonation, and articulation). This information becomes the basis for therapy planning.

Most therapy plans are based on the principle of treating disordered facets of the subsystems contributing to speech thoroughly and methodically (Dworkin, 1991; Johns, 1985; Rosenbek and LaPointe, 1985; Yorkston, Beukelman, and Bell, 1988). Because speech results from cumulative effects of secondary physiological functions, the primary functions of structures in which speech is rooted have to be considered as well. Thus, speech breathing has to evolve out of systematically modified breathing patterns for vital silent breathing; articulation out of natural conditions of lip, tongue, and jaw movements; the voicing/unvoicing of sound segments and suitable intonation patterning out of previously normalized voice production. In this way, an elaborate system of suitable exercises is created and diligently practiced. If aspects of different subsystems need to be combined—as in the case of respiratory preconditions for specific voice effects such as changes in pitch, loudness, quality and quantity, for example—matters can quickly become complicated. Superior planning and tenacity as well as flexibility during the implementation of the program are prerequisite ingredients for the successful treatment of practically all dysarthric clients. A general guideline for this task pertains to the observance of certain sequences. For example, postural adjustments precede every specific measure; respiratory and resonatory dysfunctions have to be addressed before phonatory, articulatory, and prosodic ones (Dworkin, 1991).

The following general treatment goals are summarized by Rosenbek and LaPointe (1985):

1. *Help the person to become a productive patient.* Clinician and client have agreed on the necessity and value of treatment, what is to be accomplished, and the treatment procedures.
2. *Modify abnormalities of posture, tone, and strength.*
3. *Modify respiration.*
4. *Modify phonation.*
5. *Modify resonation.*
6. *Modify articulation.*
7. *Modify prosody.*
8. *If indicated, provide alternative or augmentative modes of communication.*

The ordering of these goals does not imply a certain progression with one exception: The patient must accept an active role in treatment before changes in speech are possible. Exercises for each of these treatment goals are listed in Rosenbek and LaPointe (1985).

Dworkin (1991) provides a procedure based on a specific order of speech subsystems. The first-order subsystems consist of resonation and respiration; the second order is phonation; and the third order consists of articulation and prosody. First-order subsystems are treated first; second-order subsystems second, and third-order subsystems are last in the treatment sequence. Inhibition and facilitation techniques will probably need to precede the specific subsystem treatments. Inhibition techniques are implemented for increased tone and any associated weakness and paresis, hyperactive reflexes, hyperkinesia, and hypersensitivity. On the other hand, facilitation techniques are introduced to improve functioning of any of the following abnormal features: decreased tone and any associated weakness and paresis, hypoactive reflexes, and hyposensitivity.

The following general treatment objectives are provided by Dworkin (1991):

1. Promote adequate orofacial postures.

2. Promote integration of orofacial reflexes.
3. Improve orofacial muscle tone and strength.
4. Improve range, speed, timing, and coordination of orofacial muscle activities.

These general goals must be seen in light of the treatment hierarchy that includes first-, second-, and third-order subsystems. Detailed exercises for each of the subsystems are included in Dworkin (1991).

CLINICAL APPLICATION

Resources for Treatment of the Adult Client with Dysarthria

The following selected references are given to aid the clinician in the treatment of adult clients with dysarthria:

Berry, W. R. (1983). *Clinical dysarthria.* San Diego: College-Hill.

Darley, F. L., Aronson, A. E., & Brown, J. R. (1975). *Motor speech disorders.* Philadelphia: W. B. Saunders.

Duffy, J. R. (1995). *Motor speech disorders: Substrates, differential diagnosis, and management.* St. Louis: Mosby Year Book.

Dworkin, J. P. (1991). *Motor speech disorders: A treatment guide.* St. Louis: Mosby Year Book.

Farber, S. D. (1982). Neurorehabilitation: A multisensory approach. Philadelphia: W. B. Saunders.

Johns, D. F. (Ed.). (1985). *Clinical management of neurogenic communicative disorders* (2nd ed.). Boston: Little, Brown.

McNeil, M. R., Rosenbek, J. C., & Aronson, A. E. (Eds.). (1984). *The dysarthrias: Physiology-acoustics-perception-management.* San Diego: College-Hill.

Moore, C., Yorkston, K., & Beukelman, D. (Eds.). (1991). *Dysarthria and apraxia of speech: Perspectives on management.* Baltimore: Paul H. Brooks.

SUMMARY

There are several communication disorders with articulatory/phonological deficits as one of their central characteristics. This chapter provided an overview of the most prominent among them. First, the childhood disorders developmental apraxia of speech, cerebral palsy, clefting, mental disability, and hearing impairment have been reviewed. Acquired communication disorders with articulatory deficits commonly occurring in adults were then represented by apraxia of speech and the dysarthrias. Each of these disorders has been defined and general characteristics have been listed. Such an outline served as a foundation for the subsequent discussion of specific articulatory and phonological problems which are found in these populations. Assessment principles for the respective speech problems noted have been pointed out followed by selected therapeutic measures for the treatment of individuals within the seven populations.

For each of the disorders mentioned, an impressive list of specialized literature exists. References have been given throughout the chapter to guide interested students and practitioners to more in-depth information. Each disorder represents a complex entity including many important variables and involving several groups of professionals. This chapter briefly summarized basic considerations of articulatory and phonological features and their clinical intervention.

GLOSSARY

acoustic phonetics   The study of the transmission properties of speech.

addental [s]   A frequent s-sound distortion marked by too close an approximation of the organ of articulation and the place of articulation causing the resulting s-sounds to lose its regular stridency, giving a "dull" or "flat" sound impression.

affricate   Manner of articulation marked by a homorganic release of a stop with the auditory effect of a stop + fricative sequence, e.g., [ʧ].

affrication   The replacement of fricatives by homorganic affricates. Example: [ʧu] for "shoe."

age appropriate   In accordance with developmental norm values of a given age.

allophonic variation   The phonetic realization of a phoneme; also called phonetic variation. *See:* speech sounds.

alveolar   Alveolar ridge of upper (frontal) teeth as place of articulation for consonant production, e.g., [t].

alveolarization   The change of nonalveolar sounds, mostly interdentals and labio-dentals, into alveolar sounds.

anticipatory assimilation   *See:* Regressive assimilation.

apical   Tip of the tongue as organ of articulation for consonant production, e.g., [θ].

apico-alveolar   Referring to the organ of articulation (apex of the tongue) and the place of articulation (alveolar ridge) for sound production.

appraisal   Beginning phase of the assessment process. The collection of data to be interpreted and evaluated in the diagnostic phase.

apraxia of speech   A disorder of expressive communication as a result of brain damage affecting the normal realization of speech sounds, sound sequences, and prosodic features representing speech (Darley et al., 1975).

approximant   A speech sound marked by the approximation of an organ of articulation toward a place of articulation not resulting in an audible friction noise, e.g., [r].

articulation   The totality of motor processes involved in the planning and execution of smooth sequences of highly overlapping gestures that result in speech.

articulation disorder   Refers to difficulties with the motor production aspects of speech, or an inability to produce certain speech sounds that results in aberrations in their form when compared to regular pronunciation. Articulation disorders are phonetic in nature. *See:* phonological disorder.

articulators   Anatomical structures utilized to generate speech sounds: Organs and places of articulation.

articulatory backing   A compensatory measure of cleft palate children to produce speech sounds more posteriorly in the oral cavity than is normally the case (Trost, 1981).

articulatory phonetics   Deals with the production features of speech sounds, their categorization and classification according to specific production parameters.

aspirate   Referring to [h] as a speech sound consisting of an audible puff of breath.

assessment   Clinical evaluation of a client's disorder.

assimilation   Adaptive articulatory changes by which one speech sound becomes similar, sometimes identical, to a neighboring sound segment.

assimilatory process   Describes changes in which a sound becomes similar to, or is influenced by, a neighboring sound of an utterance.

association lines   Indicators for connections between autosegments on different tiers.

auditory phonetics   The study of speech (sound) perception.

autosegmental phonology   One of the nonlinear phonologies proposing to factor out changes within the boundary of a segment by putting them onto another "tier."

avoidance factor   The avoidance of words that do not contain sounds within a child's inventory.

bifid uvula   A uvula medially divided into two portions, a split uvula (uvula bifida).

binary system   A system using a plus (+) and minus (–) system to signal the presence (+) or absence (–) of certain features.

bunched "r" Referring to the "bunched" corpus of the tongue during an r-sound production.

canonical babbling Collective term for the reduplicated and nonreduplicated babbling stages.

categorical perception The tendency of listeners to perceive speech sounds varied along a continuum according to the phonemic categories of their native language.

cerebral palsy (CP) A nonprogressive disorder of motor control caused by damage to the developing brain during pre-, peri-, or early postnatal periods.

checked syllable *See:* closed syllable.

chronological mismatch Persistence of early phonological processes together with processes characteristic of later stages of phonological development.

citation articulation test Examines speech sound articulation in selected isolated words.

citing A single-word test response, e. g., the naming of a picture.

clefting A division of a continuous structure by a cleavage, a split prominently caused by a failure of the palate to fuse during fetal development.

close Referring to the relative closeness between the dorsum of the tongue and the roof of the mouth during vowel production, e.g., [u] (when compared to [ʊ]).

closed syllable A syllable that has a coda, e.g., *stop*; a checked syllable.

coalescence *See:* total assimilation.

coarticulation The concept that the articulators are continually moving into position for other segments over a stretch of speech.

coda All the sound segments of a syllable following its peak.

cognate Referring to the similarity between two sounds, e.g., [u] and [ʊ] are both u-type vowels.

communication augmentation Any approach designed to support, enhance, or augment the communication of individuals who cannot use speech in all situations.

complete assimilation *See:* total assimilation.

comprehensive evaluation A series of activities and tests that allow a more detailed and complete collection of data than do screenings.

conductive hearing loss Refers to transmission problems affecting the travel of air-conducted sound waves from the external auditory canal to the inner ear.

consonant A speech sound with a significant constriction within the vocal tract, mainly in the oral and pharyngeal cavities, foremost along the sagittal midline of the oral cavity.

contact assimilation Also contiguous assimilation. An assimilatory process modifying immediately adjacent sounds.

contiguous assimilation *See:* contact assimilation.

contoid Nonphonemic consonantlike sound production.

coronal Pertaining to the corona of the tongue as organ of articulation, i.e., its frontal and lateral edges forming a near three-quarter circle. Example: [d].

coronal place node In feature geometry, refers to articulation of both the tongue tip and the tongue blade segments.

cuing techniques Visual and/or tactile cues used to help the child articulate certain sounds or sound sequences.

deaffrication The realization of affricates as homorganic fricatives. Example: [ʃiz] for "cheese."

denasalization The replacement of nasals by homorganic stops. Example: [dud] for "noon."

dental Upper teeth as place of articulation for consonant production, e.g., [f].

dentalization Nonstandard articulatory variation in the production of nondental consonants: Using the dental place of articulation for a nondental consonant, e.g., [s̪] for [s].

derhotacization Loss of r-coloring during the production of [r] and rhotacized central vowels.

derivational morpheme Any grammatically significant addition to the word stem by affixes (prefixes, infixes, suffixes).

developmental apraxia of speech (DAS) Refers to children who evidence a lack of motor control of the oral mechanism for speech production that is not attributable to other problems of muscular control (Hall, Jordan, and Robin, 1993).

developmental verbal dyspraxia (DVD) *See:* developmental apraxia of speech (DAS).

diacritics Marks added to sound transcription symbols in order to give them a particular phonetic value.

diagnosis The end result of studying and interpreting of data collected during appraisal.

dialect   A language variation spoken by the members of a particular regional, cultural, or social community.

diphthong   A vowel in which there is a change in quality during its duration.

distinctive features   Phonetic constituents that distinguish between phonemes.

distribution of speech sounds   Refers to where the norm and aberrant articulations occurred within a word.

dorsal place node   In feature geometry, refers to those segments (vowels and consonants) articulated with the dorsum of the tongue.

dorsum   Surface area of the tongue.

duration symbols   Diacritics to mark the length of speech sounds.

dysarthrias   Neuromuscular speech disorders.

emerging phonology   The time span during childhood in which conventional words begin to appear as a means of communication.

epenthesis   A syllable structure process marked by the insertion of a sound segment into a word, mostly (but not always) a schwa insertion between two consonants, e.g., [pəliz] for "please."

facilitating context   Phonetic aspects of neighboring speech sounds able to support sound features to be acquired.

feature geometry   A group of nonlinear phonological theories which have adopted the tiered representation of features used in autosegmental phonology. Feature geometry attempts to explain why some features are affected by assimilation processes (known as "spreading" or "linking" features) while others are affected by neutralization or deletion processes (known as "delinking").

final consonant deletion   A syllable structure process by which a CVC syllable is by the omission of the final consonant converted into a CV syllable. The omission of a syllable-arresting consonant.

first word   An entity of relatively stable phonetic form that is produced consistently by the child in a particular context and is recognizably related to the adultlike word form of a particular language.

fortis   Refers to relatively more articulatory effort among consonant cognates. Most voiceless sounds are fortis.

fricative   A manner of articulation characterized by an audible friction noise established by forcing expiratory air through a constricted passage in the oral cavity. Example: [f]. Extensive constrictions cause the hissing noise of sibilants, a subcategory of fricatives. Examples: [s], [ʃ].

fronting   A substitution process marked by the "fronting" of organ and place of articulation for palatal sounds into the coronal-alveolar region (palatal fronting) or the change of velar consonants into either palatal or alveolar consonants (velar fronting). Example: t/k substitution.

generative phonology   The application of principles of generative (or transformational) grammar to phonology.

glide   Manner of articulation, a shifting movement of the articulators from a narrower to a wider consonantal constriction, e.g., [w]; also called semivowel, sonorant.

gliding   A substitution process characterized by the replacement of liquids with glides.

gliding of liquids/fricatives   The replacement of liquids or fricatives by glides. Example: [wɛd] for "red."

glossing   Repeating with normal pronunciation what the client has just said for easier identification later.

groping behavior   An ongoing series of movements of the articulators in an attempt to find the desired articulatory position.

harmony process   *See:* assimilation process.

hearing loss   A generic term for any diminished ability in normal sound reception.

holophrastic period   The span of time during which the child uses one word to indicate a complete idea.

idiosyncratic (or unusual) error patterns   Error patterns not (or infrequently) seen in the normal speech development of children.

idiosyncratic processes   Phonological processes found only in the speech of individual children with disordered phonology.

independent analysis   Takes only the client's productions into account, they are not compared to the adult norm model.

individual sound approach   Traditional or motor approach referring to the treatment of individual speech sounds in sequence. *See:*

motor approach. *See:* Traditional approach. *See:* Single-sound approach.

intelligibility Refers to a judgment made by a clinician based on how much of an utterance can be understood.

interdental "s" A frequent s-sound distortion marked by the visibility of the tongue tip between the upper and lower incisors. Interdental s-productions sound very much like [θ] and [ð], respectively.

intervocalic Consonants or consonant clusters occurring between two vowels, typically at the juncture of two syllables.

inventory of speech sounds A list of speech sounds that the client can articulate within normal limits.

item learning The acquisition of word forms as unanalyzed units, as productional wholes.

jargon stage Characterized by strings of babbled utterances that are modulated primarily by intonation, rhythm, and pausing.

juncture symbols Diacritics to mark juncture phenomena within an utterance, e.g., a + nice man versus an + ice man.

labial Organ of articulation (lower lip), place of articulation (upper lip), e.g., [m] (bilabial).

labial assimilation The change of a nonlabial into a labial sound under the influence of a neighboring labial sound.

labialization Consonant productions with lip rounding, e.g., [s̪up] for [sup]. Equivalent to rounding of (unrounded) vowels.

labial place node In feature geometry, designates the lip articulation of the rounded vowels and the consonants /w/, /p/, /b/, /m/, /f/, /v/, and possibly /r/ in General American English.

laryngeal node In feature geometry, designates the glottal characteristics of the segment.

lateral Manner of articulation in which a midline closure within the oral cavity lets the expiratory airstream pass laterally into the cheeks, e.g., [l]; together with the rhotics collectively referred to as liquids.

lateral "s" A nonstandard s-sound production characterized by (uni- or bilateral) air flow during /s/ realizations. The result is an unusual, openly conspicuous "slurping" noise component.

lax Referring to a lesser degree of muscular activity during vowel production, e.g., [ɪ] (when contrasted to [i]).

lenis Refers to comparatively less articulatory effort among consonant cognates. Most voiced sounds are lenis.

limitation Occurs when differences between the child's and the adult's system become limited to only specific sounds, sound classes, or sound sequences.

linear phonologies Phonological theories characterized by an assumption that all meaning-distinguishing sound segments are serially arranged.

linkage condition Any condition governing the association of units on each tier.

lip symbols Diacritics to mark rounding or unrounding of the lips during normally unrounded or rounded consonant realizations, e.g., [tʷɪn] = labialized, rounded [t].

liquid Group term for the consonant categories laterals, and rhotics; different from the glides since liquids lack an audible articulatory movement. Together with the glides and nasals (as well as all vowels), the liquids fall under the cover term sonorants.

liquid assimilation The articulatory influence of a liquid on a neighboring nonliquid sound.

manner of articulation The type of constriction the organ and place of articulation produce for the realization of a particular consonant.

manner of articulation features Specify in generative phonology the way organ and place of articulation cooperate to produce sound classes, signalling differences between stops and fricatives, for example.

markedness (Of phonemes) refers to sounds that are relatively more difficult to produce and are found less frequently in languages.

mediodorsal Central portion of the tongue as organ of articulation for consonant production, e.g., [j].

mediopalatal Central portion of hard palate as place of articulation for consonant production, e.g., [j].

metalinguistic awareness The ability to think about and reflect on the nature of language and how it functions.

metaphonology Involves the child's conscious awareness of the sounds within that particular language.

metaphon therapy A therapy approach marked by the systematic training of phonological awareness, especially the awareness of sound properties.

metathesis The transposition of sounds within an utterance.

metrical phonology One of the nonlinear phonologies emphasizing stress by building metrical trees which reflect the syntactic structure of an utterance.

micrognathia Referring to an unusually small mandible.

minimal pair Words that differ in only one phoneme value among their sound constituents, e.g., *book* versus *cook*.

minimal pair contrast therapy The therapeutic use of pairs of words that differ by one phoneme only.

monophthong A vowel that remains qualitatively the same throughout its entire production; a pure vowel.

morphophonemic function The role of phonemes to signal grammatical units. For example: /s/ is a phoneme of the English language, as demonstrable by the minimal pair "sick" versus "thick." However, /s/ also signals plurality, "book" versus "books," a morphological function.

morphophonology The study of the different allomorphs of the morpheme and the rules governing their use.

motor approach Referring to the treatment of individual sounds based on the placement of the articulators for normal speech sound production. *See:* individual sound approach, single-sound approach, traditional approach.

motor-based problem A phonetic disorder characterized by misarticulations seen as disruptions at a relatively peripheral level of the articulatory process involving inadequate motor learning.

multilinear phonologies *See:* nonlinear phonologies.

multiple sound approach Attempts to therapeutically influence several error sounds simultaneously.

nasal Manner of articulation for consonants produced with the velum lowered so that the expiratory air can pass freely through the nasal cavity, e.g., [m].

nasal assimilation The articulatory influence of a nasal on a neighboring nonnasal sound.

nasality symbols Diacritics to mark passing/nonpassing of expiratory air through the nasal cavity. Only nonnasal sounds can be nasalized, only nasals denasalized.

nasal "s" Irregular s-productions marked by nasal air flow caused by organic or functional deficiencies of velar movement resulting in incomplete nasal-pharyngeal closure.

natural class Phonemes that share one or more features and usually have similar patterns within a language system (Grunwell, 1987). *See:* naturalness.

naturalness (Of phonemes) designates the sound aspects, (1) the relative simplicity of a sound production and (2) its high frequency of occurrence in languages.

natural phonology A theory that incorporates features of naturalness theories and was specifically designed to explain the development of the child's phonological system.

natural process A process common in the speech development of children across languages.

near minimal pairs Pairs of words that differ by more than one phoneme; the vowel preceding or following the target sound remains constant in both words.

noncontiguous assimilation *See:* remote assimilation.

nonlinear phonologies A group of phonological theories understanding segments as governed by more complex linguistic dimensions.

nonphonemic diphthong A diphthong that can be realized in its initial vowel-like portion without a change in word meaning, i.e., [heᴵ] or [he] for "hay."

nonreduplicated babbling Demonstrates variation of both consonants and vowels from syllable to syllable. Also called variegated babbling.

obstruents Consonants characterized by a complete or narrow constriction between the articulators hindering the expiratory airstream; includes the stops, the fricatives, and the affricatives.

offglide The end portion of a diphthong, e.g., [ɪ] in [eᴵ].

onglide The beginning portion of a diphthong, e.g., [e] in [eᴵ].

onset Consists of all sound segments of a syllable prior to its peak.

open Referring to the relative open space between the dorsum of the tongue and the roof of the mouth during vowel production, e.g., [ʊ] (when contrasted to [u]).

open syllable   A syllable that does not contain a coda, e.g., *do;* an unchecked syllable.

oral (nonverbal) apraxia   A disturbance of the planning and execution of volitional *non-speech* movements of the oral structures.

oral stops   Manner of articulation with obstruction of the oral cavity by free nasal passage of the airstream, e.g., nasals.

ordering   Occurs when substitutions that appeared unordered and random become more organized.

organ of articulation   The part within the vocal tract that actually moves to achieve the articulatory result; the active articulator.

palatal   Hard palate as place of articulation for consonant production.

palatalization   Irregular articulatory variation in the production of consonants. Using the palate as place of articulation for nonpalatal consonants.

palatal "s"   Irregular s-production characterized by a palatal (rather than alveolar or predorsal) approximation of the organ of articulation toward the place of articulation. The result is an auditory impression of a voiceless j-sound, transcribed as [ç].

partial assimilation   Assimilatory influence of one sound segment on another by which only parts of the phonetic characteristics of the influencing sound are imposed on the influenced sound resulting in a higher degree of similarity between the respective sound segments.

peak   The most prominent, acoustically most intense part of a syllable; usually a vowel.

perceptual constancy   The ability to identify the same sound across different speakers, pitches, and other changing environmental conditions.

perseverative assimilation   *See:* progressive assimilation.

persisting normal processes   The use of certain phonological processes beyond their typical age limits.

phoneme   The smallest linguistic unit that is able, when combined with other such units, to establish word meanings and distinguish between them; exemplified by minimal pairs, e.g., *seek* versus *peak.*

phonemic diphthong   A diphthong that cannot be produced in only its initial vowel-like por-

tion without a change in word meaning, i.e., [mas] versus [maᵘs].

phonemic error   The consistent replacement of one (American English) phoneme with another.

phonemic inventory   The repertoire of phonemes used contrastively by an individual.

phonemic problem   Any misarticulation based on difficulties with the language-specific linguistic function of speech sounds, their phoneme values.

phonetically consistent form   *See:* proto-word, quasi-word, vocable.

phonetic approaches   Each error sound is treated individually, one after the other. Also referred to as traditional or motor approach.

phonetic context   The segmental, suprasegmental, and phonotactic environment in which a given speech sound occurs.

phonetic inventory   The repertoire of speech sounds for a particular client, including all his or her characteristic production features.

phonetic placement method   The clinician instructs the client how to position the articulators in order to produce a norm production.

phonetic problem   Any misarticulation based on phonetic production difficulties.

phonetics   The study of speech emphasizing the description and classification of speech sounds according to their production, transmission, and perceptual features.

phonetic variability   Refers to the unstable pronunciations of the child's first fifty words.

phonetic variation   The phonetic realization of a phoneme; also called allophonic variation.

phonological development   Refers to the acquisition of speech sound form and function within the language system.

phonological disorder   Refers to an impaired system of phonemes and phoneme patterns within the context of spoken language. Exemplified by the improper use of speech sounds to signify linguistic meaning within a language. Phonological disorders are phonemic in nature. *See:* articulation disorder.

phonological idiom   Refers to accurate sound productions that are later replaced by inaccurate ones. Also called regression.

phonological process   "A mental operation that applies in speech to substitute for a class of sounds or sound sequences presenting a common difficulty to the speech capacity of the individual (Stampe, 1979, p. 1).

phonological rules Used to demonstrate the relationship between the underlying (phonological) and the surface (phonetic) forms. In generative phonological analysis, also formalized statements about the patterns of sound substitutions and deletions.

phonology The description of the systems and patterns of phonemes that occur in a language. Phonologists analyze the language-specific distinctive phonemes and the rules that describe the set of changes that result when these phonemes occur in different relationships with other phonemes.

phonotactics The description of the allowed combinations of phonemes in a particular language.

place node In feature geometry, groups together all the different places of articulation.

place of articulation The area within the vocal tract that remains motionless during consonant articulation, that is, the passive articulator; the part that the organ of articulation approaches or contacts directly.

plosive Manner of articulation resulting from a previous complete occlusion at some point of the vocal tract; the sudden release phase of a stop.

postalveolar Posterior portion of the alveolar ridge as place of articulation.

postdorsal Posterior portion of the tongue as organ of articulation for consonant production, e.g., [k].

postpalatal Posterior portion of hard palate as place of articulation for consonant production.

postvocalic Consonants or consonant clusters following a vowel, typically occurring at the end of a word or utterance.

predorsal Anterior portion of the dorsum as organ of articulation for consonant production, e.g., predorsal [z] realization.

predorsal-alveolar Referring to the organ of articulation (predorsal portion of the tongue) and the place of articulation (alveolar ridge) for the production of speech sounds.

prelinguistic development Refers to all vocalizations prior to the first actual words.

prepalatal Anterior portion of hard palate as place of articulation for consonant production, e.g., [ʒ].

presystematic stage The stage in the phonological development of children when contrastive word units (rather than contrastive sounds of phoneme value) are acquired.

prevocalic Consonants or consonant clusters preceding a vowel, typically occurring at the beginning of a word or utterance.

progressive assimilation The assimilatory influence of a preceding sound on a following sound segment. Also called perseverative assimilation.

prosodic features Larger linguistic units, elements that occur across segments, influencing what we say.

proto-word Vocalizations used consistently by a child in particular contexts but without a recognizable adult model. Also called vocables, phonetically consistent forms, and quasi-words.

quasi-word *See:* phonetically consistent form, proto-word, vocable.

raised tongue position Too high a tongue position for the production of the vowel in question.

reduplicated babbling Marked by similar strings of consonant-vowel productions.

reduplication A syllable structure process since the syllable in question is "simplified" by a mere repetition of the first, e.g., [baba] for "bottle."

regression *See:* phonological idiom.

regressive assimilation The change of a sound's phonetic production characteristics under the influence of a following consonant, e.g., [ɪʃi] for "is she." Also called anticipatory assimilation.

remote assimilation Assimilatory process modifying a speech sound separated by at least one other segment, especially when both the influencing and the influenced sounds belong to two different syllables. Also called noncontiguous assimilation.

retroflexed Produced with the tip of the tongue "curled back," e.g., one form of standard [r] production.

retroflexed "r" Referring to the tip of the tongue curled upward and back during a specific type of [r]-production.

rhotic Manner of articulation characterized by r-coloring.

rhyme Cover term for nucleus (vowel) and coda (the arrest of the syllable).

root node   In feature geometry, links the segment to the prosodic tiers.

salience factor   A child's active selection in early word productions of words containing sounds that are important or remarkable (salient) to the child.

screening   Activities or tests that identify individuals for further evaluation.

segmental   Referring to the discrete, sequentially arranged speech segments, to vowels and consonants.

semivowels   The sonorants, especially the glides among them, as productionally characterized by an articulatory movement from a sagittally more constricted to a sagittally more open oral cavity.

sensorineural hearing loss   Occurs as a consequence of damage to the sensory end organ, the cochlear hair cells, or the auditory nerve.

sequencing errors   Disruptions in the production of the correct ordering of speech sounds or syllables

sibilant   A fricative sound characterized by a sharper sound due to the presence of high-frequency components. Example: [s], [ʃ].

silent posturing   Refers to the positioning of the articulators for a specific articulation without sound production.

skeletal (or CV) tier   A representation of a syllable and its hierarchically related components onset and rhyme.

sonorant consonants   Consonants produced with a relatively open expiratory passageway; include the nasals, glides, and liquids.

sound modification method   Based on deriving the target sound from a phonetically similar sound that the client can accurately produce. Also called derivation method.

speech intelligibility   "That aspect of oral speech-language output that allows a listener to understand what a speaker is saying" (Carney, 1994, p. 109).

speech sounds   Represent physical sound realities; end products of articulatory motor processes.

speech sound development   Refers primarily to the gradual articulatory mastery of speech sound forms within a given language.

stimulability testing   Testing the client's ability to produce a misarticulated sound in an ap-propriate manner when "stimulated" by the clinician to do so.

stop   Manner of articulation resulting from a complete occlusion at some point of the vocal tract brought about by the cooperation of an (active) organ of articulation and a (passive) place of articulation; the buildup of expiratory airstream pressure behind this closure, e.g., [p].

stopping   A substitution process. The substitution of stops for homorganic fricatives or the omission of the fricative portion of affricates.

stress markers   Diacritics to indicate different levels of syllable prominence in an utterance.

strident [s]   An irregular s-production named after the auditory impression it creates, i.e., a shrill, irritating, often whistlelike sound component.

substitution   The replacement of one sound/phoneme with another.

substitution process   Describes those sound changes in which one sound class is replaced by another.

suppression   Refers to the abolishment of one or more phonological processes as children move from the innate speech patterns to the adult norm production.

suprasegmentals   Intonation, stress, juncture, tempo, and rhythm as speech characteristics "added to" its segmental (speech sound) components.

syllabification   1. The division of a (spoken or written) word into syllables.   2. The shifting of the syllable nucleus from a vowel to the following consonant, [bʌtən] → [bʌtn̩].

syllable arresting sounds   *See:* Coda.

syllable constraint   Refers to any restriction or limitations established in the production of syllable shapes.

syllable nucleus   The "core" of a syllable carrying its highest intensity and prosodic features, typically a vowel.

syllable releasing sounds   *See:* onset.

syllable shape   Refers to the structure of the syllables within a word.

syllable shape reduction   The reduction of a syllable shape usually by the deletion of one of its consonant members.

syllable structure process   Describes those sound changes that affect the structure of the syllable.

system   An orderly combination of parts forming a complex unity.

systematic sound preference   Pertains to the use of a single phonetic realization for several different phonemes.

system learning   The acquisition of phonemic principles that apply to the phonological system in question.

tense   Referring to a higher degree of muscular activity during vowel production, e.g., [i] (when compared to [ɪ]).

tiers   Separable and independent levels that represent a sequence of gestures or a unified set of acoustic features.

tone unit   An organizational unit imposed on prosodic data.

tongue symbols   Diacritics to describe deviations from normal tongue placement for speech sound realizations, e.g., [d̪il] = dentalized [d].

tongue thrust   Refers to excessive anterior tongue movement during swallowing and a more anterior tongue position during rest.

tongue thrust swallow   Referring to excessive anterior tongue movement during swallowing and a more anterior tongue position during rest. *See:* tongue thrust.

total assimilation   The assimilatory influence of a sound segment on another by which all the phonetic properties of the influenced sound are changed into the sound category of the influencing sound. Also called complete assimilation.

traditional-motor approaches   *See:* phonetic approaches.

trill   The sound produced by the vibratory action of an organ of articulation tapping rapidly against a place of articulation.

unchecked syllable   *See:* open syllable.

underlying form   A purely theoretical concept that is thought to represent a mental reality behind the way people use language.

unrounding   Spreading of the lips during sound production, e.g., [i] (when compared to [ɪ]).

unstressed syllable deletion   A syllable structure process (also called weak syllable deletion) marked by the omission of the unstressed syllable of a multisyllable word.

variable use of processes   Processes operating on one target sound in a certain context that are in other contexts already suppressed or different processes operating on the same target phoneme.

variegated babbling   *See:* nonreduplicated babbling.

velar   Soft palate as place of articulation for consonant production, e.g., [g] in [gup].

velar assimilation   The change of a nonvelar sound into a velar one under the influence of a neighboring velar sound.

velar harmony   A (regressive) assimilation process in which a postdorsal-velar stop-plosive causes a preceding coronal-alveolar stop-plosive to change its organ and place of articulation, e,g., [gag] for [dag].

velarization   The change of a nonvelar consonant into a velar one under the influence of a neighboring velar sound. Example: [gag] for "dog."

vocable   *See:* phonetically consistent form, proto-word, quasi-word.

vocalization (vowelization)   The replacement of syllabic liquids and nasals, foremost [l], [r], and [n], by vowels. Example: [lædə] for "ladder."

vocoid   Nonphonemic vowel-like sound production.

voice symbols   Diacritics to mark the voicing of an unvoiced or the unvoicing of a voiced consonant.

voicing   The presence or absence of simultaneous vibration of the vocal cords resulting in voiced or voiceless consonants.

vowel   A speech sound that is formed without significant constriction of the oral and pharyngeal cavities, especially along the sagittal midline of the oral cavity; normally serving as syllable nucleus.

vowelization   The replacement of syllabic liquids and nasals, foremost [l], [r], and [n], by vowels. Example: [lædʊ] for "ladder."

weak syllable deletion   A syllable structure process (also called unstressed syllable deletion) marked by the omission of the unstressed syllable of a multisyllable word.

Abercrombie, D. (1967). *Elements of general phonetics*. Chicago: Aldine.

Abkarian, G. G., & Dworkin, J. P. (1993). Treating severe motor speech disorders: Give speech a chance. *Journal of Medical Speech-Language Pathology, 1,* 258–287.

Abraham, S. (1989). Using a phonological framework to describe speech errors of orally trained, hearing-impaired school-agers. *Journal of Speech and Hearing Disorders, 54,* 600–609.

Air, D. H., Wood, A. S., & Neils, J. R. (1989). Considerations for organic disorders. In N. Creaghead, P. W. Newman, & W. Secord (Eds.), *Assessment and remediation of articulatory and phonological disorders* (2nd ed.) (pp. 265–301). New York: Macmillan.

Albert, M., Sparks, R., & Helm, N. (1973). Melodic intonation therapy for aphasia. *Archives of Neurology, 29,* 130–131.

Albery, E., & Russell, J. (1990). Cleft palate and orofacial abnormalities. In P. Grunwell (Ed.), *Developmental speech disorders* (pp. 63–82). New York: Churchill Livingstone.

American Association on Mental Retardation. (1992). *Mental retardation: Definition, classification, and systems of support* (9th ed.). Washington, DC: Author.

American Cleft Palate-Craniofacial Association and Cleft Palate Foundation. (1997). *About cleft lip and cleft palate*. Chapel Hill, NC: Author.

American Speech-Language-Hearing Association. (1985). Guidelines for identification audiometry. *ASHA, 27,* 49–52.

American Speech-Language-Hearing Association. (1989). Report of the ad hoc committee on labial-lingual posturing function. *ASHA, 31,* pp. 92–94.

American Speech-Language-Hearing Association. (1990). Guidelines for screening for hearing impairments and middle ear disorders. *ASHA, 32* (Suppl. 2), 17–24.

American Speech-Language-Hearing Association. (1991). The role of the speech-language pathologist in management of oral myofunctional disorders. *ASHA, 33* (Suppl. 5), 7.

American Speech-Language-Hearing Association Ad Hoc Committee on Communication Processes and Nonspeaking Persons. (1980). Nonspeech communication: A position paper. *ASHA, 22,* 267–272.

American Speech-Language-Hearing Association Audiologic Assessment Panel 1996. (1997). *Guidelines for audiologic screening*. Rockville, MD: Author.

Anderson, P. (1941). *The relationship of normal and defective articulation of the consonant [s] in various phonetic contexts to auditory discrimination between normal and defective [s] productions among children from kindergarten through fourth grade*. Master's thesis, State University of Iowa, Iowa City.

Andrews, N., & Fey, M. E. (1986). Analysis of the speech of phonologically impaired children in two sampling conditions. *Language, Speech, and Hearing Services in Schools, 17,* 187–198.

Aram, D. M. (1984). Preface. In W. H. Perkins & J. L. Northern (Eds.), *Seminars in speech and language*. New York: Thieme-Stratton.

Aram, D. M., & Glasson, C. (1979). *Developmental apraxia of speech*. Paper presented at the annual meeting of the American Speech-Language-Hearing Association, Atlanta, GA.

Aram, D. M., & Nation, J. E. (1982). *Child language disorders*. St. Louis, MO: C. V. Mosby.

Archangeli, D. (1988). Aspects of underspecification theory. *Phonology, 5,* 183–207.

Archangeli, D., & Pulleyblank, D. (1994). *Grounded phonology*. Cambridge, MA: MIT Press.

Arlt, P. B., & Goodban, M. T. (1976). A comparative study of articulatory acquisition as based on a study of 240 normals, aged three to six. *Language, Speech, and Hearing Services in Schools, 7,* 173–180.

Arnold, G. E. (1943). Die nasalen Sigmatismen. *Archives für Ohren-, Hals- und Nasenheilkunde, 153,* 57.

Arnold. G. E. (1954). Nasal sigmatisms. *Talk, 35,* 2.

Atkinson-King, K. (1973). Children's acquisition of phonological stress contrasts. *UCLA Working Papers in Phonetics, 25,* 184–191.

Aungst, L., & Frick, J. (1964). Auditory discrimination ability and consistency of articulation of /r/. *Journal of Speech and Hearing Disorders, 29,* 76–85.

Baker, R. D., & Ryan, B. P. (1971). *Programmed conditioning for articulation.* Monterey, CA: Monterey Learning Systems.

Ball, M. J., & Kent, R. D. (1997). *The new phonologies. Developments in clinical linguistics.* San Diego, CA: Singular.

Bally, S. J. (1996). Communication strategies for adults with hearing loss. In M. J. Moseley & S. J. Balley (Eds.), *Communication therapy. An integrated approach to aural rehabilitation with deaf and hard of hearing adolescents and adults.* Washington, DC: Gallaudet University Press.

Bankson, N. W., & Bernthal, J. E. (1990). *Bankson-Bernthal test of phonology.* Chicago: Riverside Press.

Bankson, N. W., & Bernthal, J. E. (1998a). Analysis and interpretation of assessment data. In J. E. Bernthal & N. W. Bankson, *Articulation and phonological disorders* (4th ed.) (pp. 270–298). Boston: Allyn & Bacon.

Bankson, N. W., & Bernthal, J. E. (1998b). Phonological assessment procedures. In J. E. Bernthal & N. W. Bankson, *Articulation and phonological disorders* (4th ed.) (pp. 233–269). Boston: Allyn & Bacon.

Bankson, N. W., & Bernthal, J. E. (1998c). Remediation concepts, principles, and methodologies. In J. E. Bernthal & N. W. Bankson, *Articulation and phonological disorders* (4th ed.) (pp. 299–377). Boston: Allyn & Bacon.

Bardach, J., & Morris, H. L. (Eds.). (1990). *Multidisciplinary management of cleft lip and palate.* Philadelphia: W. B. Saunders.

Barlow, S., & Farley, G. (1989). Neurophysiology of speech. In D. P. Kuehn, M. L. Lemme, & J. M. Baumgartner, (Eds.), *Neural bases of speech, hearing, and language* (pp. 146–200). Boston: Little, Brown.

Barton, D. P. (1976). *The role of perception in the acquisition of speech.* Unpublished doctoral dissertation, University of London.

Barton, D. P. (1980). Phonemic perception in children. In G. Yeni-Komshian, J. Kavanagh, & C. A. Ferguson (Eds.), *Child phonology: Volume 2. Perception,* (pp. 97–116). New York: Academic Press.

Bashir, A. S., Grahamjones, F., & Bostwick, R. Y. (1984). A touch-cue method of therapy for developmental verbal apraxia. In W. H. Perkins & J. L. Northern (Eds.), *Seminars in Speech and Language* (pp. 127–137). New York: Thieme-Stratton.

Baudouin de Courtenay, J. (1895). Versuch einer Theory phonetischer Alternationen: Ein Capitel aus der Psychophonetik. Translation in E. Stankiewicz (Ed.), *Selected writings of Baudouin de Courtenay.* Bloomington: Indiana University Press.

Bauer, H. R. (1988). The ethologic model of phonetic development: I. *Clinical Linguistics and Phonetics, 2,* 347–380.

Bauer, H. R., & Robb, M. P. (1989). *Phonetic development between infancy and toddlerhood: The phonetic product estimator.* Paper presented at the national convention of the American Speech-Language-Hearing Association, St. Louis.

Bauman, J. A., & Waengler, H.-H. (1977). Measurements of sound durations in the speech of apraxic adults. *Hamburger Phonetische Beiträge,* Monograph 23. Hamburg: H. Buske Verlag.

Bauman-Waengler, J. A. (1987). Experimental-phonetic analysis of duration in the speech of Parkinson's patients. *Beiträge zur Phonetik und Linguistik, 52, Festschrift H.-H. Waengler.* Hamburg: Helmut Buske Verlag.

Bauman-Waengler, J. A. (1991). Phonological processes in three groups of preschool children: A longitudinal study. *Proceedings from the XII International Congress of Phonetic Sciences, Aix-en-Provence, 3,* 354–357.

Bauman-Waengler, J. A. (1993a). *Dialect versus disorder: Articulation errors in African American preschool children.* Presentation at the state convention of the Pennsylvania Speech-Language-Hearing Association, Harrisburg, PA.

Bauman-Waengler, J. A. (1993b). *Language testing of African American children: Assessing assessment instruments.* Seminar presented at the state convention of the Pennsylvania Speech-Language-Hearing Association, Harrisburg, PA.

Bauman-Waengler, J. A. (1994a). Normal phonological development. In R. Lowe, *Phonology: Assessment and intervention applications in speech pathology* (pp. 35–72). Baltimore: Williams & Wilkins.

Bauman-Waengler, J. A. (1994b). *Phonetic-phonological features in the speech of African American preschoolers.* Paper presented at the national convention of the American Speech-Language-Hearing Association, New Orleans, LA.

Bauman-Waengler, J. A. (1995). *Articulatory differences between two groups of African American preschoolers*. Paper presented at the national convention of the Canadian Association of Speech-Language Pathologists and Audiologists, Ottawa, Canada.

Bauman-Waengler, J. A. (1996). *Problems in assessing African American children with phonological disorders*. Seminar presented at the national convention of the Black American Speech-Language-Hearing Association, Milwaukee, WI.

Bauman-Waengler, J. A., & Waengler, H.-H. (1980). Sound duration: Comparison between performances of subjects with central nervous disorders and normal speakers. *Proc. XVIII. Congress of the International Association of Logopedics and Phoniatrics, I*, 67–72.

Bauman-Waengler, J. A., & Waengler, H.-H. (1988). *Phonological process analysis in three groups of preschool children*. Paper presented at the national convention of the American Speech-Language-Hearing Association, Boston.

Bauman-Waengler, J. A., & Waengler, H.-H. (1990). *Individual variation in phonologically disordered preschoolers: A longitudinal study*. Paper presented at the national convention of the American Speech-Language-Hearing Association, Seattle.

Beebe, H. (1957). Dyslalia in a pair of twin girls. *Folia Phoniatrica, 9*, 91–95.

Bell, A. M. (1867). *Visible speech: The science of universal alphabetics*. London: Simpkin, Marshall.

Benson, D. F. (1979). Aphasia rehabilitation. *Archives of Neurology, 36*, 187–189.

Bernhardt, B. (1990). *Application of nonlinear phonological theory to intervention with six phonologically disordered children*. Unpublished Ph.D. dissertation. University of British Columbia.

Bernhardt, B. (1992a). The application of nonlinear phonological theory to intervention with one phonologically disordered child. *Clinical Linguistics and Phonetics, 6*, 283–316.

Bernhardt, B. (1992b). Developmental implications of nonlinear phonological theory. *Clinical Linguistics and Phonetics, 6*, 259–281.

Bernhardt, B. (1994). The prosodic tier and phonological disorders. In M. Yavaş (Ed.), *First and second language phonology* (pp. 149–172). San Diego, CA: Singular.

Bernhardt, B., & Gilbert, J. (1992). Applying linguistic theory to speech-language pathology: The case for nonlinear phonology. *Clinical Linguistics and Phonetics, 6*, 123–145.

Bernhardt, B., & Stemberger, J. P. (1998). *Handbook of phonological development from the perspective of constraint-based nonlinear phonology*. San Diego, CA: Academic Press.

Bernhardt, B., & Stoel-Gammon, C. (1994). Nonlinear phonology: Introduction and clinical application: Tutorial. *Journal of Speech and Hearing Research, 37*, 123–143.

Bernthal, J. E., & Bankson, N. W. (1998). *Articulation and phonological disorders* (4th ed.). Boston: Allyn & Bacon.

Berry, P., Groenweg, G., Gibson, D., & Brown, R. (1984). Mental development of adults with Down syndrome. *American Journal of Mental Deficiency, 89*, 252–256.

Bertoncini, J., Morais, J., Bijeljac-Babic, R., McAdams, S., Peretz, I., & Mehler, J. (1989). Dichotic perception and laterality in neonates. *Brain and Language, 37*, 591–605.

Bess, F., & McConnell, F. (1981). *Audiology, education and the hearing impaired child*. St. Louis, MO: Mosby.

Best, S., Bigge, J., & Sirvis, B. (1994). Physical and health impairments. In N. Haring, L. McCormick, & T. Haring (Eds.), *Exceptional children and youth: An introduction to special education* (pp. 300–341). New York: Merrill.

Beukelman, D. R., Yorkston, K. M., & Dowden, P. A. (1985). *Communication augmentation: A casebook of clinical management*. San Diego, CA: College-Hill Press.

Bigge, J. (1991). *Teaching individuals with physical and multiple disabilities* (3rd ed.). New York: Merrill.

Bird, J., & Bishop, D. V. (1992). Perception and awareness of phonemes in phonologically impaired children. *European Journal of Disorders of Communication, 27*, 289–311.

Bird, J., Bishop, D. V., & Freeman, N. H. (1995). Phonological awareness and literacy development in children with expressive phonological impairments. *Journal of Speech and Hearing Research, 38*, 446–462.

Birnholz, J. C., & Benacerraf, B. R. (1983). The development of human fetal hearing. *Science, 222*, 516–518.

Bishop, D. (1994). Grammatical errors in specific language impairment: Competence or performance limitations. *Applied Psycholinguistics, 15*, 507–550.

Bishop, D., & Adams, C. (1990). A prospective study of the relationship between specific language impairment, phonological disorders and reading retardation. *Journal of Child Psychology and Psychiatry, 31,* 1027–1050.

Bishop, D., & Edmundson, A. (1987). Language-impaired four year olds: Distinguishing transient from persistent impairment. *Journal of Speech and Hearing Disorders, 52,* 156–173.

Bishop, D., & Robson, J. (1989). Unimpaired short-term memory and rhyme judgement in congenitally speechless individuals: Implications for the notion of "articulatory coding." *Quarterly Journal of Experimental Psychology, 41A,* 123–140.

Blache, S. (1978). *The acquisition of distinctive features.* Baltimore: University Park Press.

Blache, S. (1982). Minimal word-pairs and distinctive feature training. In M. A. Crary & D. Ingram (Eds.), *Phonological intervention: Concepts and procedures* (pp. 61–96). San Diego, CA: College-Hill Press.

Blache, S. (1989). A distinctive feature approach. In N. Creaghead, P. Newman, & W. Secord (Eds.), *Assessment and remediation of articulatory and phonological disorders* (2nd ed.) (pp. 361–382). New York: Macmillan.

Blache, S., Parsons, C., & Humphreys, J. (1981). A minimal-word-pair model for teaching the linguistic significance of distinctive feature properties. *Journal of Speech and Hearing Disorders, 46,* 291–296.

Blakeley, R. W. (1977). *Test for apraxia of speech and oral apraxia—Children's battery.* Rochester, MN: Mayo Clinic.

Blakeley, R. W. (1980). *Screening test for developmental apraxia of speech.* Tigard, OR: C. C. Publications.

Bleile, K., & Schwarz, I. (1984). Three perspectives on the speech of children with Down's syndrome. *Journal of Communication Disorders, 17,* 87–94.

Blockcolsky, V., Frazer, J., & Frazer, D. (1987). *40,000 selected words.* Tucson, AZ: Communication Skill Builders.

Bloom, L. (1973). *One word at a time: The use of single word utterances before syntax.* The Hague: Mouton.

Blumstein, S. (1973). *A phonological investigation of aphasic speech.* The Hague: Mouton.

Bobath, B. (1967). The very early treatment of cerebral palsy. *Developmental Medicine and Childhood Neurology, 9,* 373–390.

Bobath, K., & Bobath, B. (1972). Cerebral palsy, Part II: The neurodevelopmental approach to treatment. In P. H. Pearson & C. E. Williams (Eds.), *Physical therapy services in the developmental disabilities* (pp. 114–185). Springfield, IL: Charles C. Thomas.

Bonvillian, J., Raeburn, V., & Horan, E. (1979). Talking to children—the effect of rate, intonation and length on children's sentence imitation. *Journal of Child Language, 6,* 459–467.

Boone, D. R., & McFarlane, S. C. (1988). *The voice and voice therapy.* Englewood Cliffs, NJ: Prentice-Hall.

Boothroyd, A. (1988). Perception of speech pattern contrasts from auditory presentation of voice fundamental frequency. *Ear and Hearing, 9,* 313–321.

Bosma, J. F. (1975). Anatomic and physiologic development of the speech apparatus. In E. L. Eagles (Ed.), *Human communication and its disorders* (Vol. 3) (pp. 469–481). New York: Raven Press.

Boysson-Bardies, B., de, & Vihman, M. (1991). Adaptation to language. *Language, 67,* 297–339.

Bradley, D. P. (1989). A systematic multiple-phoneme approach. In. N. A. Creaghead, P. W. Newman, & A. Secord (Eds.), *Assessment and remediation of articulatory and phonological disorders* (2nd ed.) (pp. 305–322). Columbus, OH: Merrill.

Brady, S. (1986). Short-term memory, phonological processing and reading ability. *Annals of Dyslexia, 36,* 138–153.

Brady, S., & Fowler, A. E. (1988). Phonological precursors to reading acquisition. In R. L. Masland & M. W. Masland (Eds.), *Preschool prevention of reading failure* (pp. 204–215). Parkton, MD: York Press.

Briere, E. (1966). An investigation of phonological interference. *Language, 42,* 768–796.

Broen, P. A., & Moller, K. T. (1993). Early phonological development and the child with cleft palate. In K. T. Moller & C. D. Starr (Eds.), *Cleft palate. Interdisciplinary issues and treatment* (p. 219–249). Austin, TX: PRO-ED.

Brogan, W. J., & Woodings, T. L. (1976). A decline in the incidence of cleft lip and palate deformities in humans. *Clinics in Plastic Surgery, 3,* 647.

Bronstein, A. J. (1960). *The pronunciation of American English. An introduction to phonetics.* New York: Appleton-Century-Crofts.

Bross, R. (1992). An application of structual linguistics to intelligibility measurements of impaired speakers of English. In R. D. Kent (Ed.), *Intelligibility in speech disorders: Theory, measurement, and management* (pp. 35–65). Amsterdam: John Benjamins.

Brown, R. (1973). *A first language: The early stages.* Cambridge, MA: Harvard University Press.

Bruner, J. (1975). The ontogenesis of speech acts. *Journal of Child Language, 2,* 1–19.

Bryen, D., Goldman, A., & Quinlisk-Gill, S. (1988). Sign language with students with severe/profound mental retardation: How effective is it? *Education and Training in Mental Retardation, 23,* 129–137.

Butcher, A. (1990). The uses and abuses of phonological assessment. *Child Language Teaching and Therapy, 6,* 262–276.

Bzoch, K. (1979). Measurement and assessment of categorical aspects of cleft palate speech. In K. R. Bzoch (Ed.), *Communicative disorders related to cleft lip and palate* (2nd ed.) (pp. 161–191). Boston: Little, Brown.

Bzoch, K. (1997). Clinical assessment, evaluation, and management of 11 categorical aspects of cleft palate speech disorders. In K. R. Bzoch (Ed.), *Communication disorders related to cleft lip and palate* (4th ed.) (pp. 261–311). Austin, TX: PRO-ED.

Calvert, D. R., & Silverman, S. R. (1983). *Speech and deafness: A text for learning and teaching* (rev. ed.). Washington, DC: Alexander Graham Bell Association for the Deaf.

Camp, B., Burgess, D., Morgan, L., & Zerbe, G. (1987). A longitudinal study of infant vocalizations in the first year. *Journal of Pediatric Psychology, 12,* 321–331.

Campbell, T., & Shriberg, L. (1982). Associations among pragmatic functions, linguistic stress, and natural phonological processes in speech-delayed children. *Journal of Speech and Hearing Research, 25,* 547–553.

Capute, A. J. (1974). Developmental disabilities: An overview. *Dental Clinics of North America, 18,* 557–577.

Carney, A. E. (1994). Understanding speech intelligibility in the hearing impaired. In K. G. Butler (Ed.), *Hearing impairment and language disorders* (pp. 109–121). Gaithersburg, MD: Aspen.

Carney, E. (1979). Inappropriate abstraction in speech assessment procedures. *British Journal of Disorders of Communication, 14,* 123–135.

Carrell, J., & Tiffany, W. R. (1960). *Phonetics: Theory and application to speech improvement.* New York: McGraw-Hill.

Carterette, E., & Jones, M. (1974). *Informal speech: Alphabetic and phonemic texts with statistical analyses and tables.* Berkeley: University of California Press.

Carver, C. M. (1987). Dialects. In S. Flexner & L. C. Hauck (Eds.), *The Random House dictionary of the English language* (2nd ed.) (pp. xxv–xxvi). New York: Random House.

Chaney, C. (1992). Language development, metalinguistic skills and print awareness in 3 year old children. *Applied Psycholinguistics, 13,* 485–514.

Chapman, K. L. (1993). Phonological processes in children with cleft palate. *Cleft Palate-Craniofacial Journal, 30,* 64–71.

Chapman, K. L., & Hardin, M. A. (1992). Phonetic and phonologic skills of two year olds with cleft palate. *Cleft Palate-Craniofacial Journal, 29,* 435–443.

Chapman, R. S., & Miller, J. (1980). Analyzing language and communication in the child. In R. Schiefelbusch (Ed.), *Nonspeech language and communication: Analysis and intervention* (pp. 159–196). Baltimore: University Park Press.

Chappell, G. E. (1973). Childhood verbal apraxia and its treatment. *Journal of Speech and Hearing Disorders, 38,* 362–368.

Chen, H. P., & Irwin, O. C. (1946). Infant speech: Vowel and consonant types. *Journal of Speech Disorders, 11,* 27–29.

Cheng, L. L. (1991). *Assessing Asian language performance: Guidelines for evaluating limited-English proficient students* (2nd ed.). Oceanside, CA: Academic Communication Associates.

Cheng, L. L. (1993). Asian-American cultures. In D. Battle (Ed.), *Communication disorders in multicultural populations* (pp. 38–77). Boston: Andover Medical.

Cheng, L. L. (1994). Asian/Pacific students and the learning of English. In J. Bernthal & N. Bankson (Eds.), *Child phonology: Characteristics, assessment, and intervention with special populations* (pp. 255–274). New York: Thieme.

Chin, S. B., & Dinnsen, D. A. (1991). Feature geometry in disordered phonologies. *Clinical Linguistics and Phonetics, 5,* 329–337.

Chomsky, C. (1971). *Linguistic development in children from 6 to 10.* Office of Education: Final Report.

Chomsky, N. (1957) *Syntactic structures.* The Hague: Mouton.

Chomsky, N. (1967). Some general properties of phonological rules. *Language, 43,* 102–128.

Chomsky, N. (1982). *Lectures on government and binding.* New York: Foris.

Chomsky, N. (1988). *Language and problems of knowledge.* Cambridge, MA: MIT Press.

Chomsky, N., & Halle, M. (1968). *The sound pattern of English.* New York: Harper & Row.

Christensen, M., & Hanson, M. (1981). An investigation of the efficacy of oral myofunctional therapy as a precursor to articulation therapy for pre-first-grade children. *Journal of Speech and Hearing Disorders, 46,* 160–165.

Christian, D., Wolfram, W., & Nube, N. (1988). *Variation and change in geographically isolated communities: Appalachian English and Ozark English.* Tuscaloosa, AL: University of Alabama Press.

Clark, M. C., & Goldstein, B. (1996). *Analysis of vowel error patterns in children with phonological disorders.* Paper presented at the annual convention of the American Speech-Language-Hearing Association, Seattle, WA.

Clarke-Klein, S., & Hodson, B. (1995). A phonologically based analysis of misspellings by third graders with disordered-phonology histories. *Journal of Speech and Hearing Research, 38,* 839–849.

Clements, G. (1985). The geometry of phonological features. *Phonology Yearbook, 2,* 225–252.

Cohen, J., & Diehl, C. (1963). Relation of speech sound discrimination ability to articulation-type speech defects. *Journal of Speech and Hearing Disorders, 28,* 187–190.

Cole, R. A., & Perfetti, C. A. (1980). Listening for mispronunciations in a children's story: the use of context by children and adults. *Journal of Verbal Learning and Verbal Behavior, 19,* 297–315.

Compton, A. J. (1970). Generative studies of children's phonological disorders. *Journal of Speech and Hearing Disorders, 35,* 315–339.

Compton, A. J. (1975). Generative studies of children's phonological disorders: A strategy for therapy. In S. Singh (Ed.), *Measurement procedures in speech, hearing, and language* (pp. 55–90). Baltimore: University Park Press.

Compton, A. J. (1976). Generative studies of children's phonological disorders: Clinical ramifications. In D. Morehead & A. Morehead (Eds.), *Normal and deficient child language* (pp. 61–96). Baltimore: University Park Press.

Conly, U., Bauman-Waengler, J. A., & Waengler, H.-H. (1989). *Aberrant phonology in Japanese learners of American-English: Assessment and Intervention.* Paper presented at the American Speech-Language-Hearing Association national convention, New Orleans, LA.

Connolly, J. H. (1986). Intelligibility: A linguistic view. *British Journal of Disorders of Communication, 21,* 371–376.

Conti-Ramsden, G., & Jones, M. (1997). Verb use in specific language impairment. *Journal of Speech and Hearing Research, 40,* 1298–1313.

Cooper, E. (1985). The method of meaningful contrasts. In P. Newman, N. Creaghead, & W. Secord (Eds.), *Assessment and remediation of articulatory and phonological disorders* (pp. 369–382). Columbus, OH: Merrill.

Copenhagen Conference. (1925). Association Phonétique Internationale, Copenhagen, Denmark.

Cornett, R. (1972). *Cued speech parent training and follow-up program.* Final report. Washington, DC: Bureau of Education for the Handicapped, DHEW, 96.

Costello, J. (1975). Articulation instruction based on distinctive features theory. *Language, Speech, and Hearing Services in Schools, 6,* 61–71.

Crary, M. A. (1983). Phonological process analysis from spontaneous speech: The influence of sample size. *Journal of Communication Disorders, 16,* 133–141.

Crary, M. A. (1984). Phonological characteristics of developmental verbal dyspraxia. In W. H. Perkins & J. L. Northern (Eds.), *Seminars in speech and language* (pp. 71–83). New York: Thieme-Stratton.

Crary, M. A. (1993). *Developmental motor speech disorders.* San Diego, CA: Singular.

Crary, M. A., & Comeau, S. (1981). Phonologically based assessment and intervention in spastic cerebral palsy: A case analysis. *South African Journal of Communication Disorders, 28,* 31–36.

Creaghead, N., & Newman, P. (1989). Articulatory phonetics and phonology. In N. Creaghead, P. Newman, & W. Secord (Eds.), *Assessment and remediation of articulatory and phonological disorders* (2nd ed.) (pp. 9–32). New York: Macmillan.

Creaghead, N. A., Newman, P. W., & Secord, W. A. (Eds.). (1989). *Assessment and remediation of articulatory and phonological disorders* (2nd ed.). New York: Macmillan.

Cruttenden, A. (1981). Item-learning and system-learning. *Journal of Psycholinguistic Research, 10,* 79–88.

Cruttenden, A. (1985). Intonation comprehension in 10-year-olds. *Journal of Child Language, 12,* 643–661.

Crystal, D. (1981). *Clinical linguistics.* New York: Springer-Verlag.

Crystal, D. (1986). Prosodic development. In P. Fletcher & M. Garman (Eds.), *Language acquisition* (2nd ed.) (pp. 174–197). Cambridge: Cambridge University Press.

Crystal, D. (1987). *The Cambridge encyclopedia of language.* Cambridge: Cambridge University Press.

Culatta, R., Page, J. L., & Wilson, L. (1987). *Speech rates of normally communicative children.* Paper presented at the annual convention of the American Speech-Language-Hearing Association, New Orleans, LA.

Culp, D. M. (1989). Developmental apraxia and augmentative or alternative communication— A case study. In International Society for Augmentative and Alternative Communication, *AAC Augmentative and Alternative Communication* (pp. 27–34). Baltimore: Williams & Wilkins.

Dabul, B. (1979). *Apraxia battery for adults.* Tigard, OR: C. C. Publications.

Dalbor, J. (1980). *Spanish pronunciation: Theory and practice: An introductory manual of Spanish phonology and drill* (2nd ed.). New York: Holt, Rinehart and Winston.

Dalston, R. (1997). The use of nasometry in the assessment and remediation of velopharyngeal inadequacy. In K. R. Bzoch (Ed.), *Communication disorders related to cleft lip and palate* (4th ed.) (pp. 331–346). Austin, TX: PRO-ED.

Dalston, R., Warren, D., & Dalston, E. (1991). Use of nasometry as a diagnostic tool for identifying patients with velopharyngeal impairment. *Cleft Palate-Craniofacial Journal, 28,* 184–189.

Darley, F. (1978). Differential diagnosis of acquired motor speech disorders. In F. Darley & D. C. Spriestersbach (Eds.), *Diagnostic methods in speech pathology* (2nd ed.) (pp. 492–513). New York: Harper & Row.

Darley, F. (Ed.). (1979). *Evaluation and appraisal in speech and language disorders.* Reading, MA: Addison-Wesley.

Darley, F. (1984). Apraxia of speech: A neurogenic articulation disorder. In H. Winitz (Ed.), *Treating articulation disorders: For clinicians by clinicians* (pp. 289–305). Baltimore: University Park Press.

Darley, F. (1991). A philosophy of appraisal and diagnosis. In F. Darley & D. Spriestersbach (Eds.), *Diagnostic methods in speech pathology* (2nd ed.) (pp. 1–23). New York: Harper & Row.

Darley, F. L., Aronson, A. E., & Brown, J. R. (1975). *Motor speech disorders.* Philadelphia: W. B. Saunders.

Das, J., Kirby, J., & Jarman, R. (1975). Simultaneous and successive synthesis: An alternative model for cognitive abilities. *Psychological Bulletin, 82,* 87–103.

Davis, B., Marquardt, T. P., & Sussman, H. M. (1985). *Developmental apraxia of speech: Case study.* Paper presented at the annual meeting of the American Speech-Language-Hearing Association, Washington, DC.

Davis, B. L., & MacNeilage, P. F. (1990). Acquisition of correct vowel production: A quantitative case study. *Journal of Speech and Hearing Research, 33,* 16–27.

Davis, L. F. (1987). Respiration and phonation in cerebral palsy: A developmental model. *Seminars in Speech and Language, 8,* 101–106.

Deal, J., & Darley, F. (1972). The influence of linguistic and situational variables on phonemic accuracy in apraxia of speech. *Journal of Speech and Hearing Research, 15,* 639–653.

Dean, E., Howell, J., Hill, A., & Waters, D. (1990). *Metaphon resource pack.* Windsor, UK: NFER Nelson.

DeCasper, A., & Fifer, W. P. (1980). On human bonding: Newborns prefer their mothers' voices. *Science, 208,* 1174–1176.

Delack, J. B., & Fowlow, P. J. (1978). The ontogenesis of differential vocalization: Development of prosodic contrastivity during the first year of life. In N. Waterson & C. Snow (Eds.), *The development of communication* (pp. 93–110). New York: John Wiley.

Denes, P. B., & Pinson, E. N. (1963). *The speech chain: The physics and biology of spoken language.* Garden City, NY: Anchor Press/Doubleday.

Denes, P. B., & Pinson, E. N. (1973). *The speech chain.* Garden City, NY: Anchor Press.

DeRenzi, E., Pieczuro, A., & Vignolo, L. A. (1966). Oral apraxia and aphasia. *Cortex, 2,* 50–73.

Dewey, G. (1923). *Relative frequency of English speech sounds.* Cambridge, MA: Harvard University Press.

DiCarlo, L. M. (1974). Communication therapy for problems associated with cerebral palsy. In S. Dickson (Ed.), *Communication disorders: Remedial principles and practices* (2nd ed.) (pp. 358–397). Glenview, IL: Scott, Foresman.

Dickson, S. (1962). Differences between children who spontaneously outgrow and children who retain functional articulation errors. *Journal of Speech and Hearing Research, 5,* 263–271.

Diedrich, W. (1983). Stimulability and articulation disorders. In J. Locke (Ed.), *Assessing and treating phonological disorders: Current approaches. Seminars in Speech and Language, 4.* New York: Thieme-Stratton.

Dillow, K. A., Dzienkowski, R. C., Smith, K. K., & Yucha, C. B. (1996). Cerebral palsy: A comprehensive review. *The Nurse Practitioner, 21,* 45–61.

Dinnsen, D. A. (1984). Methods and empirical issues in analyzing functional misarticulations. In M. Elbert, D. A. Dinnsen, & G. Weismer (Eds.), *Phonological theory and the misarticulating child, ASHA Monograph No. 22* (pp. 1–4). Rockville, MD: ASHA.

Dinnsen, D. A. (1996). Context-sensitive underspecification and the acquisition of phonemic contrasts. *Journal of Child Language, 23,* 57–79.

Dinnsen, D. A. (1997). Nonsegmental phonologies. In M. J. Ball & R. D. Kent (Eds.), *The new phonologies* (pp. 77–125). San Diego, CA: Singular.

Dinnsen, D. A., & Chin, S. B. (1993). Individual differences in phonological disorders and implications for a theory of acquisition. In F. R. Eckman (Ed.), *Confluence: Linguistics, L2 acquisition, and speech pathology* (pp. 137–152). Amsterdam: John Benjamins.

Dinnsen, D. A., & Elbert, M. (1984). On the relationship between phonology and learning. In M. Elbert, D. Dinnsen, & G. Weismer (Eds.),

Phonological theory and the misarticulating child, ASHA Monograph, 22 (pp. 59–68). Rockville, MD: ASHA.

Dodd, B. (1976). The phonological systems of deaf children. *Journal of Speech and Hearing Disorders, 41,* 185–198.

Dodd, B., & Iacano, T. (1989). Phonological disorders in children: Changes in phonological process use during treatment. *British Journal of Disorders of Communication, 24,* 333–351.

Donegan, P. J., & Stampe, D. (1979).The study of natural phonology. In D. A. Dinnsen (Ed.), *Current approaches to phonological theory* (pp. 126–173). Bloomington, IN: Indiana University Press.

Dore, J. (1975). Holophrases, speech acts and language universals. *Journal of Child Language, 3,* 22–39.

Dore, J., Franklin, M. B., Miller, R. T., & Ramer, A. L. (1976). Transitional phenomena in early language acquisition. *Journal of Child Language, 3,* 13–29.

Doszak, A. L., McNeil, M. R., & Jancosek, E. (1981). *Efficacy of melodic intonation therapy with developmental apraxia of speech.* Paper presented at the national convention of the American Speech-Language-Hearing Association, Los Angeles.

Drummond, S. S. (1993). *Dysarthria examination battery.* Austin, TX: PRO-ED.

DuBois, E., & Bernthal, J. E. (1978). A comparison of three methods for obtaining articulatory responses. *Journal of Speech and Hearing Disorders, 43,* 295–305.

Duffy, J. R. (1995). *Motor speech disorders. Substrates, differential diagnosis, and management.* St. Louis, MO: Mosby Year Book.

Dunn, C., & Newton, L. (1994). A comprehensive model for speech development in hearing-impaired children. In K. G. Butler (Ed.), *Hearing impairment and language disorders* (pp. 122–143). *Topics in language disorders series.* Gaithersburg, MD: Aspen.

Dunn, L. M., Dunn, L., Whetton, C., & Pintilie, D. (1982). *British picture vocabulary scales.* Windsor: NFER Nelson.

Dworkin, J. P. (1991). *Motor speech disorders: A treatment guide.* St. Louis, MO: Mosby Year Book.

Dworkin, J. P., & Culatta, R. A. (1980). *Dworkin-Culatta oral mechanism examination.* Nicholasville, KY: Edgewood Press.

Edwards, H. T. (1997). *Applied phonetics: The sounds of American English* (2nd ed.). San Diego, CA: Singular.

Edwards, M. (1973). Developmental verbal dyspraxia. *British Journal of Disorders of Communication, 8,* 64–70.

Edwards, M. L. (1992). Clinical forum: Phonological assessment and treatment. In support of phonological processes. *Language, Speech, and Hearing Services in Schools, 23,* 233–240.

Eilers, R. E. (1980). Infant speech perception: History and mystery. In G. Yeni-Komshian, J. Kavanagh, & C. A. Ferguson (Eds.), *Child phonology: Volume 2. Perception* (pp. 23–39). New York: Academic Press.

Eimas, P. D., Siqueland, E. R., Jusczyk, P., & Vigorito, J. (1971). Speech perception in infants. *Science, 171,* 303–306.

Eisenson, J. (1972). *Aphasia in children* (pp. 189–202). New York: Harper & Row.

Elbers, L. (1982). Operating principles in repetitive babbling: A cognitive approach. *Cognition, 12,* 45–63.

Elbert, M. (1992). Clinical forum: Phonological assessment and treatment. Consideration of error types: A response to Fey. *Language, Speech, and Hearing Services in Schools, 23,* 241–246.

Elbert, M. (1997). From articulation to phonology: The challenge of change. In B. W. Hodson & M. L. Edwards (Eds.), *Perspectives in applied phonology* (pp. 43–60). Gaithersburg, MD: Aspen.

Elbert, M., Dinnsen, D., & Powell, T. (1984). On the prediction of phonologic generalization learning patterns. *Journal of Speech and Hearing Disorders, 49,* 309–317.

Elbert, M., & Gierut, J. (1986). *Handbook of clinical phonology: Approaches to assessment and treatment.* San Diego, CA: College-Hill Press.

Elliott, L. L. (1979). Performance of children aged 9–17 years on a test of speech intelligibility in noise using sentence material with controlled word predictability. *Journal of the Acoustical Society of America, 66,* 651–653.

Elliott, L. L., Connors, S., Kille, E., Levin, S., Ball, K., & Katz, D. (1979). Children's understanding of monosyllabic nouns in quiet and in noise. *Journal of the Acoustical Society of America, 66,* 12–21.

Emerick, L. L., & Haynes, W. O. (1986). *Diagnosis and evaluation in speech pathology* (3rd. ed.). Englewood Cliffs, NJ: Prentice-Hall.

Enderby, P. (1980). Frenchay dysarthria assessment. *British Journal of Disorders of Communication, 15,* 165–173.

Enderby, P. (1983). The standardized assessment of dysarthria is possible. In W. R. Berry (Ed.), *Clinical dysarthria* (pp. 109–119). San Diego, CA: College-Hill Press.

Erenberg, G. (1984). Cerebral palsy. Current understanding of a complex problem. *Postgraduate Medicine, 75,* 87–93.

Estrem, T., & Broen, P. A. (1989). Early speech productions of children with cleft palate. *Journal of Speech and Hearing Research, 32,* 12–23.

Eyer, J., & Leonard, L. (1994). Learning past tense morphology with specific language impairment: A case study. *Child Language Teaching and Therapy, 10,* 127–138.

Faircloth, M. A., & Faircloth, S. R. (1970). An analysis of the articulatory behavior of a speech-defective child in connected speech and in isolated-word responses. *Journal of Speech and Hearing Disorders, 35,* 51–61.

Faircloth, S. R., & Faircloth, M. A. (1973). *Phonetic science: A program of instruction.* Englewood Cliffs, NJ: Prentice-Hall.

Farmer, A., & Lencione, R. (1977). An extraneous vocal behavior in cerebral palsied speakers. *British Journal of Communication Disorders, 12,* 109–118.

Farwell, C. B. (1976). Some strategies in the early production of fricatives. *Papers and Reports on Child Language Development, 12,* 97–104.

Fasold, R., & Wolfram, W. (1975). Some linguistic features of Negro dialect. In P. Stoller (Ed.), *Black American English* (pp. 49–87). New York: Deli.

Fawcus, R. (1971). Features of a psychological and physiological study of articulatory performance. *British Journal of Disorders of Communication, 6,* 99–106.

Ferguson, C. A. (1976). Learning to pronounce: The earliest stages of phonological development in the child. In F. D. Minifie & L. L. Floyd (Eds.), *Communicative and cognitive abilities: Early behavioral assessment* (pp. 273–297). Baltimore: University Park Press.

Ferguson, C. A., & Farwell, C. (1975). Words and sounds in early language acquisition: English initial consonants in the first fifty words. *Language, 51,* 419–439.

Ferguson, C. A., & Garnica, O. (1975). Theories of phonological development. In E. Lenneberg & E. Lenneberg (Eds.), *Foundation of language development* (Vol. 1) (pp. 153–180). New York: Academic Press.

Fernald, A., Taeschner, T., Dunn, J., Papousek, M., Boysson-Bardies, B., de, & Fukui, I. (1989). A cross-language study of prosodic modification in mother's and father's speech to preverbal infants. *Journal of Child Language, 16,* 477–503.

Ferrier, E., & Davis, M. (1973). A lexical approach to the remediation of final sound omissions. *Journal of Speech and Hearing Disorders, 38,* 126–131.

Ferry, P. C., Hall, S. M., & Hicks, J. L. (1975). "Dilapidated" speech: Developmental verbal dyspraxia. *Developmental Medicine and Child Neurology, 17,* 749–756.

Fey, M. E. (1992). Clinical forum: Phonological assessment and treatment. Articulation and phonology: Inextricable constructs in speech pathology. *Language, Speech, and Hearing Services in Schools, 23,* 225–232. (Reprinted from *Human Communication Canada, 1985, 9,* 7–16.)

Fey, M. E., Cleave, P., Ravida, I., Long, S., Dejmal, A., & Easton, D. (1994). Effects of grammar facilitation on the phonological performance of children with speech and language impairments. *Journal of Speech and Hearing Research, 37,* 594–607.

Firth, J. R. (1948). Sounds and prosodies. *Transactions of the Philological Society.* Oxford: Blackwell.

Fisher, H. B., & Logemann, J. A. (1971). *The Fisher-Logemann test of articulation competence.* Boston: Houghton Mifflin.

Fisichelli, R. M. (1950). *An experimental study of the prelinguistic speech development of institutionalized infants.* Unpublished doctoral dissertation, Fordham University.

Fleming, K. (1971). Guidelines for choosing appropriate phonetic contexts for speech-sound recognition and production practice. *Journal of Speech and Hearing Disorders, 36,* 356–367.

Fletcher, P., & Peters, J. (1984). Characterizing language impairment in children: An exploratory study. *Language Testing, 1,* 33–49.

Fletcher, S. G. (1970). Theory and instrumentation for quantitative measurement of nasality. *Cleft Palate Journal, 7,* 601–609.

Fletcher, S. G. (1992). *Articulation. A physiological approach.* San Diego, CA: Singular.

Fletcher, S. G., Casteel, R., & Bradley, D. (1961). Tongue-thrust swallow, speech articulation, and age. *Journal of Speech and Hearing Disorders, 26,* 201–208.

Fletcher, S. G., & Newman, D. G. (1991). /s/ and /ʃ/ as a function of lingua-palatal contact place and sibilant groove width. *Journal of the Acoustical Society of America, 89,* 850–858.

Flexner, S. B. (Ed.). (1987). *The Random House dictionary of the English language.* (2nd ed.). New York: Random House.

Fokes, J. (1982). Problems confronting the theorist and practitioner in child phonology. In M. Crary & D. Ingram (Eds.), *Phonological intervention: Concepts and procedures* (pp. 13–34). San Diego, CA: College-Hill Press.

Foster, D., Riley, K., & Parker, F. (1985). Some problems in the clinical application of phonological theory. *Journal of Speech and Hearing Disorders, 50,* 294–297.

Fourcin, A. J. (1978). Acoustic patterns and speech acquisition. In N. Waterson & C. Snow (Eds.), *Development of communication* (pp. 47–72). New York: John Wiley.

Fox, B., & Routh, D. K. (1975). Analyzing spoken language into words, syllables, and phonemes: A developmental study. *Journal of Psycholinguistic Research, 4,* 331–342.

French, A. (1988). What shall we do with 'medial' sounds? *British Journal of Disorders of Communication, 23,* 41–50.

French, A. (1989). The systematic acquisition of word forms by a child during the first-fifty-word stage. *Journal of Child Language, 16,* 69–90.

French, N., Carter, C., & Koenig, W. (1930). The words and sounds of telephone conversations. *Bell System Technical Journal, 9,* 290–324.

Fristoe, M., & Lloyd, L. (1979). Nonspeech communication. In N. R. Ellis (Ed.), *Handbook of mental deficiency, psychological theory and research* (2nd ed.) (pp. 401–430). Hillsdale, NJ: Erlbaum Associates.

Froeschels, E. (1952). *Dysarthric speech: Speech in cerebral palsy.* Magnolia, MA: Expression Co.

Fudala, J., & Reynolds, W. (1994). *Arizona articulation proficiency scale* (2nd ed.). Los Angeles: Western Psychological Services.

Garnica, O. (1973). The development of phonemic speech perception. In T. Moore (Ed.), *Cognitive development and the acquisition of language* (pp. 215–222). New York: Academic Press.

Gesell, A., & Thompson, H. (1934). *Infant behavior: Its genesis and growth*. New York: McGraw-Hill.

Gierut, J. (1985). *On the relationship between phonological knowledge and generalization learning in misarticulating children*. Bloomington: Indiana University Linguistics Club.

Gierut, J. (1989). Maximal opposition approach to phonological treatment. *Journal of Speech and Hearing Disorders, 54,* 9–19.

Gierut, J. (1990). Differential learning of phonological oppositions. *Journal of Speech and Hearing Research, 33,* 540–549.

Gierut, J. (1991). Homonymy in phonological change. *Clinical Linguistics and Phonetics, 5,* 119–137.

Gierut, J. (1992). The conditions and course of clinically induced phonological change. *Journal of Speech and Hearing Research, 35,* 1049–1063.

Gierut, J., & Neumann, H. (1992). Teaching and learning /θ/: A nonconfound. *Clinical Linguistics and Phonetics, 6,* 191–200.

Gilbert, J. H., & Purves, B. A. (1977). Temporal constraints on consonant clusters in child speech production. *Journal of Child Language, 4,* 417–32.

Giles, S. B. (1971). *A study of articulatory characteristics of /l/ allophones in English*. Unpublished doctoral dissertation, University of Iowa.

Givens, G., & Seidemann, M. (1977). Middle ear measurements in a difficult to test mentally retarded population. *Mental Retardation, 15,* 40–42.

Gleitman, L., Gleitman, H., & Shipley, E. (1972). The emergence of the child as a grammarian. *Cognition, 1,* 137–164.

Goguillot, L. (1889). Comment on fait parler les sounds-muets. Paris: G. Masson.

Golding-Kushner, K. J. (1995). Treatment of articulation and resonance disorders associated with cleft palate and VPI. In R. J. Shprintzen & J. Bardach (Eds.), *Cleft palate speech management. A multidisciplinary approach* (pp. 327–351). St. Louis, MO: Mosby Year Book.

Goldman, R., & Fristoe, M. (1986). *Goldman-Fristoe test of articulation* (2nd ed.). Circle Pines, MN: American Guidance Service.

Goldman, R., Fristoe, M., & Woodcock, R. (1970). *Goldman-Fristoe-Woodcock test of auditory discrimination*. Circle Pines, MN: American Guidance Service.

Goldsmith, J. A. (1976). *Autosegmental phonology*. Bloomington, IN: Indiana University Linguistics Club.

Goldsmith, J. A. (1990). *Autosegmental and metrical phonology*. Cambridge, MA: Basil Blackwell.

Goldstein, B. (1995). Spanish phonological development. In H. Kayser (Ed.), *Bilingual speech-language pathology: An Hispanic focus* (pp. 17–38). San Diego, CA: Singular.

Gordon-Brannan, M. (1994). Assessing intelligibility: Children's expressive phonologies. In K. Butler & B. Hodson (Eds.), *Topics in Language Disorders, 14,* 17–25.

Goswami, U., & Bryant, P. E. (1990). *Phonological skills and learning to read*. Hillsdale, NJ: Lawrence Erlbaum.

Greenlee, M. (1974). Interacting processes in the child's acquisition of stop-liquid clusters. *Papers and Reports on Child Language Development* (Stanford University), *7,* 85–100.

Grunwell, P. (1975). The phonological analysis of articulation disorders. *British Journal of Disorders of Communication, 10,* 31–42.

Grunwell, P. (1981). The development of phonology: A descriptive profile. *First Language, 2,* 161–191.

Grunwell, P. (1985a). *Phonological assessment of child speech*. San Diego, CA: College-Hill Press.

Grunwell, P. (1985b). Forum: Phonetic and phonological features. Comment on the terms "phonetics" and "phonology" as applied in the investigation of speech disorders. *British Journal of Disorders of Communication, 20,* 165–170.

Grunwell, P. (1986). Aspects of phonological development in later childhood. In K. Durkin (Ed.), *Language development in the school years* (pp. 34–56). London: Croom Helm.

Grunwell, P. (1987). *Clinical phonology* (2nd ed.). Baltimore: Williams & Wilkins.

Grunwell, P. (Ed.). (1990). *Developmental speech disorders: Clinical issues and practical implications*. New York: Churchill Livingstone.

Grunwell, P. (1997). Developmental phonological disability: Order in disorder. In B. W. Hodson & M. L. Edwards (Eds.), *Perspectives in applied phonology* (pp. 61–104). Gaithersburg, MD: Aspen.

Gutzmann, A. (1895). *Die Gesundheitspflege der Sprache*. Breslau: F. Hirt.

Gutzmann, H. (1912). *Sprachheilkunde: Vorlesungen über die Störungen der Sprache mit besondere Berücksichtigung der Therapie*. Berlin: Kornfeld.

Guyette, T. W., & Diedrich, W. M. (1981). A critical review of developmental apraxia of speech. In N. J. Lass (Ed.), *Speech and language: Advances in basic research and practice* (Vol. 5) (pp. 1–49). New York: Academic Press.

Haas, W. (1963). Phonological analysis of a case of dyslalia. *Journal of Speech and Hearing Disorders, 28*, 239–246.

Haelsig, P. C., & Madison, C. L. (1986). A study of phonological processes exhibited by 3-, 4-, and 5-year-old children. *Language, Speech, and Hearing Services in Schools, 17*, 107–114.

Hakes, D. T. (1982). The development of metalinguistic abilities: What develops. In S. Kuczaj (Ed.), *Language development* (Vol. II) (pp. 163–210). Hillsdale, NJ: Lawrence Erlbaum.

Hall, C., & Golding-Kushner, K. J. (1989). *Long-term follow-up of 500 patients after palate repair performed prior to 18 months of age.* Presented at the Sixth International Congress on Cleft Palate and Related Craniofacial Anomalies, Israel.

Hall, M. (1938). Auditory factors in functional articulatory speech defects. *Journal of Experimental Education, 7*, 110–132.

Hall, P. K. (1989). The occurrence of developmental apraxia of speech in a mild articulation disorder: A case study. *Journal of Communication Disorders, 22*, 265–276.

Hall, P. K., Hardy, J. C., & LaVelle, W. E. (1990). A child with signs of developmental apraxia of speech with whom a palatal lift prosthesis was used to manage palatal dysfunction. *Journal of Speech and Hearing Disorders, 55*, 454–460.

Hall, P. K., Jordan, L. S., & Robin, D. A. (1993). *Developmental apraxia of speech: Theory and clinical practice.* Austin, TX: PRO-ED.

Hall, P. K., Robin, D. A., & Jordan, L. S. (1986). *The presence of word-retrieval deficits in developmental verbal apraxia.* Paper presented at the annual meeting of the American Speech-Language-Hearing Association, Detroit, MI.

Halle, M. (1962). Phonology in generative grammar. *Word, 18*, 54–72.

Halle, M., & Stevens, K. (1979). Some reflections on the theoretical basis of phonetics. In B. Lindblom, S. Ohman, & G. Fant (Eds.), *Frontiers of speech communication research* (pp. 335–349). London: Academic Press.

Hallé, P. A., Boysson-Bardies, B., de, & Vihman, M. (1991). Beginnings of prosodic organization: Intonation and duration patterns of disyllables produced by Japanese and French infants. *Language and Speech, 34*, 299–318.

Halliday, M. A. (1975). *Learning how to mean: Explorations in the development of language.* New York: Elsevier.

Hanson, M. L. (1988). Orofacial myofunctional therapy: Guidelines for assessment and treatment. *International Journal of Orofacial Myology, 14*, 27–32.

Hanson, M. L. (1994). Oral myofunctional disorders and articulatory patterns. In J. E. Bernthal & N. W. Bankson (Eds.), *Child phonology: Characteristics, assessment, and intervention with special populations* (pp. 29–53). New York: Thieme.

Hanson, M. L., & Barrett, R. H. (1988). *Fundamentals of orofacial myology.* Springfield, IL: Charles C. Thomas.

Hardcastle, W. J., Morgan-Barry, R. A., & Clark, C. J. (1987). Articulatory and voicing characteristics of adult dysarthric and verbal dyspraxic speakers: An instrumental study. *British Journal of Disorders of Communication, 20*, 249–270.

Hardy, J. C. (1983). *Cerebral palsy.* Englewood Cliffs, NJ: Prentice-Hall.

Hardy, J. C. (1994). Cerebral palsy. In W. A. Secord, G. H. Shames, & E. Wiig (Eds.), *Human communication disorders: An introduction* (4th ed.) (pp. 562–604). New York: Merrill.

Hare, G. (1983). Development at 2 years. In J. V. Irwin & S. P. Wong (Eds.), *Phonological development in children: 18–72 months* (pp. 55–85). Carbondale, IL: Southern Illinois University Press.

Hargrove, P. (1982). Misarticulated vowels: A case study. *Language, Speech, and Hearing Services in Schools, 13*, 86–95.

Harkins, C. S., Berlin, A., Harding, R., Longacre, J., & Snodgrass, R. (1960). Report of the nomenclature committee. *Cleft Palate Bulletin, 10*, 11.

Harkins, C. S., Berlin, A., Harding, R., Longacre, J., & Snodgrass, R. (1962). A classification of cleft lip and palate. *Plastic and Reconstructive Surgery, 29*, 31.

Harlan, N. T. (1984). Treatment approach for a young child evidencing developmental verbal apraxia. *Australian Journal of Human Communication Disorders, 12*, 121–127.

Hawkins, S. (1979). Temporal coordination of consonants in the speech of children: Further data. *Journal of Phonetics, 13*, 235–267.

Haynes, S. (1985). Developmental apraxia of speech: Symptoms and treatment. In D. F. Johns (Ed.), *Clinical management of neurogenic communication disorders* (2nd ed.) (pp. 259–266). Boston: Little, Brown.

Haynes, W., & Moran, M. (1989). A cross-sectional developmental study of final consonant production in Southern Black children from preschool through third grade. *Language, Speech, and Hearing Services in Schools, 20,* 400–406.

Haynes, W. O., & Pindzola, R. H. (1998). *Diagnosis and evaluation in speech pathology* (5th ed.). Boston: Allyn & Bacon.

Haynes, W. O., Pindzola, R. H., & Emerick, L. L. (1992). *Diagnosis and evaluation in speech pathology* (4th ed.). Englewood Cliffs, NJ: Prentice-Hall.

Healy, T. J., & Madison, C. L. (1987). Articulation error migration: A comparison of single word and connected speech samples. *Journal of Communicaton Disorders, 20,* 129–136.

Heffner, R-M. S. (1975). *General phonetics.* Madison, WI: University of Wisconsin Press.

Helfrich-Miller, K. R. (1984). Melodic intonation therapy with developmentally apraxic children. In W. H. Perkins & J. L. Northern (Eds.), *Seminars in speech and language* (pp. 119–125). New York: Thieme-Stratton.

Helm-Estabrooks, N. (1996). *Test of oral and limb apraxia (TOLA).* Chicago: Applied Symbols.

Hickman, L. A., (1997). *The apraxia profile.* San Antonio, TX: Psychological Corporation.

Hilton, L. (1984). Treatment of deviant phonological systems: Tongue thrust. In W. Perkins (Ed.), *Phonological-articulatory disorders* (pp. 47–54). New York: Thieme-Stratton.

Hodson, B. W. (1984). Facilitating phonological development in children with severe speech disorders. In H. Winitz (Ed.), *Treating articulation disorders. For clinicians by clinicians* (pp. 75–89). Baltimore: University Park Press.

Hodson, B. W. (1986). *The assessment of phonological processes—revised.* Danville, IL: Interstate.

Hodson, B. W. (1989). Phonological remediation: A cycles approach. In N. A. Creaghead, P. W. Newman, & W. A. Secord (Eds.), *Assessment and remediation of articulatory and phonological disorders* (2nd ed.) (pp. 323–333). New York: Macmillan.

Hodson, B. W. (1992). Clinical forum: Phonological assessment and treatment, applied phonology: Constructs, contributions, and issues. *Language, Speech, and Hearing Services in Schools, 23,* 247–253.

Hodson, B. W. (1994). Helping individuals become intelligible, literate, and articulate: The role of phonology. *Topics in Language Disorders, 14(2),* 1–16.

Hodson, B. W., & Paden, E. P. (1981). Phonological processes which characterize unintelligible and intelligible speech in early childhood. *Journal of Speech and Hearing Disorders, 46,* 369–373.

Hodson, B. W., & Paden, E. P. (1983). *Targeting intelligible speech: A phonological approach to remediation.* San Diego, CA: College-Hill Press.

Hodson, B. W., & Paden, E. P. (1991). *Targeting intelligible speech: A phonological approach to remediation* (2nd ed.). San Diego, CA: College-Hill Press.

Hoek, D., Ingram, D., & Gibson, D. (1986). Some possible causes of children's early word extensions. *Journal of Child Language, 13,* 477–494.

Hoffman, P. (1990). Spelling, phonology, and the speech-language pathologist: A whole language perspective. *Language, Speech, and Hearing Services in Schools, 21,* 238–243.

Hoffman, P., Norris, J., & Monjure, J. (1990). Comparison of process targeting and whole language treatments for phonologically delayed preschool children. *Language, Speech, and Hearing Services in Schools, 21,* 102–109.

Hoffman, P., Schuckers, G., & Daniloff, R. (1989). *Children's phonetic disorders: Theory and treatment.* Boston: Little, Brown.

Hogg, R., & McCully, C. B. (1989). *Metrical phonology: A course book.* Cambridge: Cambridge University Press.

Holmgren, K., Lindblom, B., Aurelius, G., Jalling, B., & Zetterstrom, R. (1986). On the phonetics of infant vocalization. In B. Lindblom & R. Zetterstrom (Eds.), *Precursors of early speech* (pp. 51–63). New York: Stockton Press.

Hornby, P. A., & Hass, W. A. (1970). Use of contrastive stress by preschool children. *Journal of Speech and Hearing Research, 13,* 395–399.

Howell, J. (1989). *The metalinguistic awareness of phonologically disordered and normally developing children: A comparative study.* Unpublished doctoral dissertation, University of Newcastle Upon Tyne, Great Britain.

Howell, J., & Dean, E. (1991). *Treating phonological disorders in children: Metaphon-theory to practice.* San Diego, CA: Singular.

Howell, J., & Dean, E. (1994). *Treating phonological disorders in children: Metaphon-theory to practice* (2nd ed.). London: Whurr.

Hulme, C., & Snowling, M. (1992). Deficits in output phonology: An explanation of reading failure? *Cognitive Neuropsychology, 9,* 47–72.

Hutchinson, B. B., Hanson, M. L., & Mecham, M. J. (Eds.). (1979). *Diagnostic handbook of speech pathology.* Baltimore: Williams & Wilkins.

Hyman, L. (1975). *Phonology: Theory and analysis.* New York: Holt, Rinehart & Winston.

Ianucci, D., & Dodd, D. (1980). The development of some aspects of quantifier negation. *Papers & Reports on Child Language Development, 19,* 88–94.

Iglesias, A., & Anderson, N. (1995). Dialectal variations. In J. E. Bernthal & N. W. Bankson (Eds.), *Articulation and phonological disorders* (3rd ed.) (pp. 147–161). Boston: Allyn & Bacon.

Iglesias, A., & Goldstein, B. (1998). Language and dialectal variations. In J. Bernthal & N. Bankson, *Articulation and phonological disorders* (4th ed.) (pp. 148–171). Boston: Allyn & Bacon.

Ingalls, R. P. (1978). *Mental retardation: The changing outlook.* New York: John Wiley & Sons.

Ingram, D. (1974). Phonological rules in young children. *Journal of Child Language, 1,* 49–64.

Ingram, D. (1976). *Phonological disability in children.* New York: Elsevier.

Ingram, D. (1979). Phonological development: Production. In P. Fletcher & M. Garman (Eds.), *Language acquisition* (2nd ed.) (pp. 223–239). Cambridge: Cambridge University Press.

Ingram, D. (1981). *Procedures for the phonological analysis of children's language.* Baltimore: University Park Press.

Ingram, D. (1989a). *First language acquisition: Method, description, and explanation.* Cambridge: Cambridge University Press.

Ingram, D. (1989b). *Phonological disability in children: Studies in disorders of communication* (2nd ed.). London: Cole & Whurr.

Ingram, D., Christensen, L., Veach, S., & Webster, B. (1980). The acquisition of word-initial fricatives and affricates in English by children between 2 and 6 years. In G. H. Yeni-Komshian, J. F. Kavanagh, & C. A. Ferguson (Eds.), *Child phonology: Vol. I. Production* (pp. 169–192). New York: Academic Press.

Ingram, T. T. S. (1966). The neurology of cerebral palsy. *Archives of Diseases of Childhood, 41,* 337–357.

Ingram, T. T. S., & Barn, J. (1961). A description and classification of common speech disorders associated with cerebral palsy. *Cerebral Palsy Bulletin, 3,* 57–69.

International Phonetic Alphabet (revised 1993, updated 1996). *Association Phonétique Internationale.* Victoria, BC (University of Victoria), Canada.

Irwin, J. V., & Wong, S. P. (Eds.). (1983). *Phonological development in children 18 to 72 months.* Carbondale, IL: Southern Illinois University Press.

Irwin, O. C. (1945). Reliability of infant speech sound data. *Journal of Speech Disorders, 10,* 227–235.

Irwin, O. C. (1946). Infant speech: Equations for consonant-vowel ratios. *Journal of Speech Disorders, 11,* 177–180.

Irwin, O. C. (1947a). Infant speech: Consonantal sounds according to place of articulation. *Journal of Speech and Hearing Disorders, 12,* 397–401.

Irwin, O. C. (1947b). Infant speech: Consonant sounds according to manner of articulation. *Journal of Speech and Hearing Disorders, 12,* 402–404.

Irwin, O. C. (1948). Infant speech: Development of vowel sounds. *Journal of Speech and Hearing Disorders, 13,* 31–34.

Irwin, O. C. (1951). Infant speech: Consonantal position. *Journal of Speech and Hearing Disorders, 16,* 159–161.

Irwin, O. C. (1965). *Speech and hearing therapy.* Pittsburgh, PA: Stanwix House.

Irwin, O. C., & Chen, H. P. (1946). Infant speech: Vowel and consonant frequency. *Journal of Speech and Hearing Disorders, 11,* 123–125.

Ivimey, G. P. (1975). The development of English morphology: An acquisition model. *Language and Speech, 18,* 120–144.

Jackson, M. R., & Hall, P. K. (1987). *A longitudinal study of articulation characteristics in developmental verbal apraxia.* Paper presented at the annual meeting of the American Speech-Language-Hearing Association, New Orleans, LA.

Jacobson, J., Boersma, D., Fields, R., & Olson, K. (1983). Paralinguistic features of adult speech to infants and small children. *Child Development, 54,* 436–442.

Jaffe, M. (1989). Feeding at-risk infants and toddlers. *Topics in Language Disorders, 10(1),* 13–25.

Jaffe, M. B. (1984). Neurological impairment of speech production: Assessment and treatment. In A. Holland & J. M. Costello (Eds.), *Handbook of speech and language disorders* (pp.157–186). San Diego, CA: College-Hill Press.

Jakobson, R. (1949). On the identification of phonemic entities. *Travaux du Cercle Linguistique de Prague, 5*, 205–213.

Jakobson, R. (1962). Zur Struktur des Phonems (pp. 280–310). *Selected Writings I. Vol. 1, Phonological studies*. The Hague: Mouton.

Jakobson, R. (1968). *Child language, aphasia and phonological universals*. The Hague: Mouton. (Original work published 1942)

Jakobson, R., Fant, G., & Halle, M. (1952). *Preliminaries to speech analysis: The distinctive features and their correlates*. Cambridge, MA: MIT Press.

Jakobson, R., & Halle, M. (1956). *Fundamentals of language*. The Hague: Mouton.

Jakobson, R., & Halle, M. (1971). *Fundamentals of language* (2nd ed.). The Hague: Mouton.

Jakobson, R., & Lotz, J. (1949). Notes on the French phonemic pattern. In *R. Jakobson's Selected Writings I* (1962, pp. 426–434). The Hague: Mouton.

Jensen, T. S., Boggild-Andersen, B., Schmidt, J., Ankerhus, J., & Hansen, E. (1988). Perinatal risk factors and first-year vocalizations: Influence on preschool language and motor performance. *Developmental Medicine and Child Neurology, 30*, 153–161.

Jespersen, O. (1889). *The articulation of speech sounds*. Marburg: Elwert Verlag.

Jespersen, O. (1913). *Lehrbuch der Phonetik*. Leipzig: Teubner.

Johns, D. F. (1985). *Clinical management of neurogenic communication disorders*. Boston: Little, Brown.

Johns, D. F., & Darley, F. L. (1970). Phonemic variability in apraxia of speech. *Journal of Speech and Hearing Research, 13*, 556–583.

Johnston, J. (1982). Interpreting the Leiter IQ: Performance profiles of young normal and language-disordered children. *Journal of Speech and Hearing Research, 25*, 291–296.

Johnston, J., & Schery, T. (1976). The use of grammatical morphemes by children with communication disorders. In D. Morehead & A. Morehead (Eds.), *Normal and deficient child language* (pp. 239–258). Baltimore: University Park Press.

Jones, C. L., & Lorman, J. S. (1986). *Apraxia: A guide for the patient and family*. Stow, OH: Interactive Therapeutics.

Jones, D. (1938). Concrete and abstract sounds. *Proceedings of the 3rd International Congress of Phonetic Sciences*. Ghent: Belgium.

Jones, D. (1950). *The phoneme: Its nature and use*. Cambridge: Heffer.

Jordan, L. S. (1988). *Gestures for cuing phonemes in verbal apraxia: A case study*. Paper presented at the annual meeting of the American Speech-Language-Hearing Association, Boston, MA.

Jordan, L. S. (1991). *Treating apraxia of speech*. Paper presented at the Midwest Aphasiology Conference, Iowa City, IA.

Jusczyk, P. W. (1992). Developing phonological categories from the speech signal. In C. A. Ferguson, L. Menn, & C. Stoel-Gammon (Eds.), *Phonological development: Models, research, implications* (pp. 17–64). Parkton, MD: York Press.

Kagan, J. (1971). *Change and continuity in infancy*. New York: Wiley.

Kamhi, A. G. (1992). Clinical forum: Phonological assessment and treatment. The need for a broad-based model of phonological disorders. *Language, Speech, and Hearing Services in Schools, 23*, 261–268.

Kamhi, A. G., Friemoth-Lee, R., & Nelson, L. (1985). Word, syllable and sound awareness in language disordered children. *Journal of Speech and Hearing Disorders, 50*, 207–212.

Kamhi, A. G., Minor, J. S., & Mauer, D. (1990). Content analysis and intratest performance profiles on the Columbia and the TONI. *Journal of Speech and Hearing Research, 33*, 375–379.

Kantner, C., & West, R. (1960). *Phonetics* (rev. ed.). New York: Harper & Brothers.

Kay Elemetrics Corporation (1988). *Instruction manual for the nasometer, Model 6200*. Pine Brooks, NJ: Author.

Kenney, K. W., & Prather, E. M. (1986). Articulation development in preschool children: Consistency of productions. *Journal of Speech and Hearing Research, 29*, 29–36.

Kent, R. (1982). Contextual facilitation of correct sound production. *Language, Speech, and Hearing Services in Schools, 13*, 66–76.

Kent, R. D. (1997). *The speech sciences*. San Diego, CA: Singular.

Kent, R. D. (1998). Normal aspects of articulation. In J. E. Bernthal & N. W. Bankson, *Articulation and phonological disorders* (4th ed.) (pp. 1–62). Boston: Allyn & Bacon.

Kent, R. D., & Bauer, H. R. (1985). Vocalizations of one-year-olds. *Journal of Child Language, 13*, 491–526.

Kent, R. D., Miolo, G., & Bloedel, S. (1994). The intelligibility of children's speech: A review of evaluation procedures. *American Journal of Speech-Language Pathology, 3(2),* 81–95.

Kent, R. D., & Murray, A. D. (1982). Acoustic features of infant vocalic utterances at 3, 6, and 9 months. *Journal of the Acoustical Society of America, 72,* 353–365.

Kent, R. D., & Netsell, R. (1978). Articulatory abnormalities in athetoid cerebral palsy. *Journal of Speech and Hearing Disorders, 43,* 353–373.

Kent, R. D., & Rosenbek, J. C. (1982). Prosodic disturbance and neurologic lesion. *Brain and Language, 15,* 259–291.

Kent, R. D., & Rosenbek, J. C. (1983). Acoustic patterns in apraxia of speech. *Journal of Speech and Hearing Disorders, 26,* 231–248.

Kercher, M. B., & Bauman-Waengler, J. (1992). *Performances of Black English speaking children on standardized language tests.* Presentation at the national convention of the American Speech-Language-Hearing Association, San Antonio, TX.

Kertesz, A. (1980). *Western aphasia battery.* London, Ontario: University of Western Ontario.

Khan, L. (1988). *Vowel remediation: A case study.* Paper presented at the American Speech-Language-Hearing Association Convention, Boston, MA.

Khan, L., & James, S. (1983). Grammatical morpheme development in three language disordered children. *Journal of Childhood Communication Disorders, 6,* 85–100.

Khan, L., & Lewis, N. (1986). *Khan-Lewis phonological analysis.* Circle Pines, MN: American Guidance Service.

King, G., & Fletcher, P. (1993). Grammatical problems in school-age children with specific language impairment. *Clinical Linguistics and Phonetics, 7,* 339–352.

Kiparsky, P. (1982). From cyclic phonology to lexical phonology. In H. van der Hulst & H. Smith (Eds.), *The structure of phonological representations* (Vol. II, pp. 131–176). Dordrecht: Foris.

Kiparsky, P., & Menn, L. (1977). On the acquisition of phonology. In J. Macnamara (Ed.), *Language learning and thought* (pp. 47–78). New York: Academic Press.

Kitamura, H. (1991). Evidence for cleft palate as a postfusion phenomenon. *Cleft Palate Journal, 28,* 195–211.

Klein, E. (1995). *Clinical phonology: Assessment and treatment of articulation disorders in children and adults.* San Diego, CA: Singular.

Klein, H. B. (1984). Procedure for maximizing phonological information from single-word responses. *Language, Speech, and Hearing Services in Schools, 15,* 267–274.

Klich, R. J., Ireland, J. V., & Weidner, W. E. (1979). Articulatory and phonological aspects of consonant substitutions in apraxia of speech. *Cortex, 15,* 451–470.

Klick, S. L. (1985). Adapted cueing technique for use in treatment of dyspraxia. *Language, Speech, and Hearing Services in Schools, 16,* 256–259.

Klink, M., Gerstman, L., Raphael, L., Schlanger, B., & Newsome, L. (1986). Phonological process usage by young EMR children and nonretarded preschool children. *American Journal of Mental Deficiency, 91,* 190–195.

Kramer, J. (1939). *Der Sigmatismus, seine Bedingungen und seine Behandlung.* Solothurn: St. Antonius-Verlag.

Krauss, T., & Galloway, H. (1982). Melodic intonation therapy with language delayed apraxic children. *Journal of Music Therapy, 19,* 102–113.

Krech, H. (1969). *Die Behandlung gestörter s-Laute.* Berlin: VEB Verlag Volk und Gesundheit.

Kronvall, E., & Diehl, C. (1954). The relationship of auditory discrimination to articulatory defects of children with no known organic impairment. *Journal of Speech and Hearing Disorders, 19,* 335–338.

Kruszewski, N. (1881). *Über Lautabwechslung.* Kasan': Universitätsbuchdruckerei.

Kudrjavcev, T., Schoenberg, B. S., Kurland, L. T., & Groover, R. V. (1983). Cerebral palsy—trends in incidence and changes in concurrent mortality: Rochester, MN, 1950–1976. *Neurology, 33,* 1433–1438.

Kuhl, P. K. (1980). Perceptual constancy for speech sound categories in early infancy. In G. Yeni-Komshian, J. Kavanagh, & C. A. Ferguson (Eds.), *Child phonology: Volume 2. Perception* (pp. 41–66). New York: Academic Press.

Kuhl, P. K. (1987). Perception of speech and sound in early infancy. In P. Salapatek & L. Cohen (Eds.), *Handbook of infant perception: Volume 2. From perception to cognition* (pp. 275–382). New York: Academic Press.

Kussmaul, A. (1885). Die Störungen der Sprache. In H. V. Ziemsson (Ed.), *Handbuch der Speciellen*

Pathologie und Therapie: Volume 12 (pp. 1–299). Leipzig: F. C. W. Vogel.

Ladefoged, P. (1971). *Preliminaries to linguistic phonetics.* Chicago: University of Chicago Press.

Ladefoged, P. (1982). *A course in phonetics* (2nd ed.). New York: Harcourt Brace Jovanovich.

Ladefoged, P. (1993). *A course in phonetics* (3rd ed.). New York: Harcourt Brace Jovanovich.

Lahey, M. (1988). *Language disorders and language development.* New York: Macmillan.

Lahey, M., & Bloom, L. (1977). Planning a first lexicon: Which words to teach first. *Journal of Speech and Hearing Disorders, 42,* 340–350.

Lapko, L., & Bankson, N. (1975). Relationship between auditory discrimination, articulation stimulability and consistency of misarticulation. *Perceptual and Motor Skills, 40,* 171–177.

LaPointe, L. L., & Johns, D. F. (1975). Some phonemic characteristics in apraxia of speech. *Journal of Communication Disorders, 8,* 259–269.

LaPointe, L. L., & Wertz, R. T. (1974). Oral-movement abilities and articulatory characteristics of brain-injured adults. *Perceptual Motor Skills, 39,* 39–43.

LaVoi, G. W. (1986). *A comparative analysis of selected variables in apraxic and nonapraxic children.* Paper presented at the annual meeting of the American Speech-Language-Hearing Association, Detroit, MI.

Lecanuet, J.-P., Granier-Deferre, C., & Bushnel, M.-C. (1989). Differential fetal auditory reactiveness as a function of stimulus characteristics and state. *Seminars in Perinatology, 13,* 421–429.

Lee, L., Koenigsknecht, R., & Mulhern, S. (1975). *Interactive language development teaching.* Evanston, IL: Northwestern University Press.

Lehiste, I. (1970). *Suprasegmentals.* Cambridge: Massachusetts Institute of Technology.

Leinonen-Davis, E. (1988). Assessing the functional adequacy of children's phonological systems. *Clinical Linguistics and Phonetics, 2,* 257–270.

Leonard, L. (1988). Lexical development and processing in specific language impairment. In R. Schiefelbusch & L. Lloyd (Eds.), *Language perspectives: Acquisition, retardation, and intervention* (2nd ed.) (pp. 69–87). Austin, TX: PRO-ED.

Leonard, L. (1994). Some problems facing accounts of morphological deficits in children with specific language impairments. In R. Watkins & M. Rice (Eds.), *Specific language impairments in children* (pp. 91–106). Baltimore: Brookes.

Leonard, L., & Brown, B. (1984). Nature and boundaries of phonologic categories: A case study of an unusual phonologic pattern in a language-impaired child. *Journal of Speech and Hearing Disorders, 49,* 419–428.

Leonard, L., & Leonard, J. (1985). The contribution of phonetic context to an unusual phonological pattern: A case study. *Language, Speech, and Hearing Services in Schools, 16,* 110–118.

Leonard, L., & McGregor, K. (1991). Unusual phonological patterns and their underlying representations: A case study. *Journal of Child Language, 18,* 261–271.

Leonard, L., McGregor, K., & Allen, G. (1992). Grammatical morphology and speech perception in children with specific language impairment. *Journal of Speech and Hearing Research, 35,* 1076–1085.

Leonard, L., Newhoff, M., & Mesalam, L. (1980). Individual differences in early child phonology. *Applied Psycholinguistics, 1,* 7–30.

Leonard, L., Schwartz, R., Folger, M., Newhoff, M., & Wilcox, M. (1979). Children's imitations of lexical items. *Child Development, 50,* 19–27.

Leonard, L., Schwartz, R., Morris, B., & Chapman, K. (1981). Factors influencing early lexical acquisition: Lexical orientation and phonological composition. *Child Development, 52,* 882–887.

Leopold, W. F. (1947). *Speech development of a bilingual child: A linguist's record.* Evanston, IL: Northwestern University Press.

Leopold, W. F. (1948). Semantic learning in infant language. *Word: Journal of the Linguistic Circle of New York, 4,* 173–180.

Lepschy, G. C. (1970). *A survey of structural linguistics.* London: Faber and Faber.

Levitt, H., & Stromberg, H. (1983). Segmental characteristics of the speech of hearing-impaired children: Factors affecting intelligibility. In I. Hochberg, H. Levitt, & M. J. Osberger (Eds.), *Speech of the hearing impaired: Research, training, and personnel preparation* (pp. 53–73). Baltimore: University Park Press.

Liberman, I. Y., & Shankweiler, D. (1985). Phonology and the problems of learning to read and write. *Topical Issues: Remedial and Special Education, 6,* 8–17.

Liberman, I. Y., Shankweiler, D., Fisher, W., & Carter, B. (1974). Reading and the awareness of linguistic segments. *Journal of Experimental Child Psychology, 18,* 201–212.

Liberman, I. Y., Shankweiler, D., Liberman, A. M., Fowler, C., & Fischer, F. W. (1977). Phonetic segmentation and recording in the beginning reader. In A. S. Reber & H. Scarborough (Eds.), *Toward a psychology of reading.* Hillsdale, NJ: Lawrence Erlbaum.

Liberman, M. (1975). *The intonational system of English.* Doctoral dissertation, Massachusetts Institute of Technology, Cambridge, MA.

Liberman, M., & Prince, A. (1977). On stress and linguistic rhythm. *Linguistic Inquiry, 8,* 249–336.

Ling, D. (1976). *Speech and the hearing-impaired child: Theory and practice.* Washington, DC: Alexander Graham Bell Association for the Deaf.

Lipsitt, L. (1966). Learning processes of human newborns. *Merrill-Palmer Quarterly, 12,* 45–71.

Lloyd, L., & Fulton, R. (1972). Audiology's contribution to communications programming with the retarded. In J. McLean, D. Yoder, & R. Schiefelbusch (Eds.), *Language intervention with the retarded: Developmental strategies* (pp. 111–129). Baltimore: University Park Press.

Local, J. (1983). How many vowels in a vowel? *Journal of Child Language, 10,* 449–453.

Locke, J. L. (1980a). Mechanisms of phonological development in children: Maintenance, learning, and loss. *Papers from the Sixteenth Regional Meeting of the Chicago Linguistic Society.* Chicago: Chicago Linguistic Society.

Locke, J. L. (1980b). The inference of speech perception in the phonologically disordered child, part I: A rationale, some criteria, the conventional tests. *Journal of Speech and Hearing Disorders, 45,* 431–434.

Locke, J. L. (1980c). The inference of speech perception in the phonologically disordered child, part II: Some clinically novel procedures, their use, some findings. *Journal of Speech and Hearing Disorders, 45,* 435–468.

Locke, J. L. (1983). *Phonological acquisition and change.* New York: Academic Press.

Locke, J. L. (1990). Structure and stimulation in the ontogeny of spoken language. *Developmental Psychobiology, 23,* 621–643.

Locke, J. L., Bleile, K., Fey, M., & Folkins, J. (1996). *Does the distinction between articulation and phonology have clinical significance?* Paper presented at the National Convention of the American Speech-Language-Hearing Association, Seattle, WA.

Lohr, F. E. (1978). The nonverbal apraxic child: Definition, evaluation, and therapy. *Western Michigan University Journal of Speech, Language, and Hearing, 12,* 71–82.

Long, S. H., & Long, S. T. (1994). Language and children with mental retardation. In V. R. Reed, *An introduction to children with language disorders* (2nd ed.) (pp. 153–191). New York: Merrill.

Lorentz, J. P. (1976). An analysis of some deviant phonological rules of English. In D. M. Morehead & A. E. Morehead (Eds.), *Normal and deficient child language* (pp. 29–59). Baltimore: University Park Press.

Love, R. J. (1992). *Childhood motor speech disability.* Boston: Allyn & Bacon.

Love, R. J., & Fitzgerald, M. (1984). Is the diagnosis of developmental apraxia of speech valid? *Australian Journal of Human Communication Disorders, 12,* 71–82.

Lowe, R. J. (1986). *Assessment link between phonology and articulation: ALPHA.* Moline, IL: LinguiSystems.

Lowe, R. J. (1994). *Phonology: Assessment and intervention applications in speech pathology.* Baltimore: Williams & Wilkins.

Lowe, R. J. (1996). *Assessment link between phonology and articulation: ALPHA* (rev. ed.). Mifflinville, PA: Speech and Language Resources.

Lowe, R. J., Knutson, P., & Monson, M. (1985). Incidence of fronting in preschool children. *Language, Speech, and Hearing Services in Schools, 16,* 119–123.

Lowe, R. J., Mount-Weitz, J., & Schmidt, C. (1992). *Activities for the remediation of phonological disorders.* DeKalb: Janelle.

Luchsinger, R., & Arnold, G. E. (1965). *Voice-speech-language. Clinical communicology: Its physiology and pathology.* Belmont, CA: Wadsworth.

Lund, N. J., & Duchan, J. F. (1992). *Assessing children's language in naturalistic contexts* (3rd ed.). Englewood Cliffs, NJ: Prentice-Hall.

Lundberg, I. (1988). Preschool prevention of reading failure: Does training in phonological awareness work? In R. L. Masland & M. W. Masland (Eds.), *Preschool prevention of reading failure* (pp. 163–176). Parkton, MD: York Press.

Lundberg, I., Olofsson, A., & Wall, S. (1980). Reading and spelling skills in the first school years predicted from phonemic awareness skills in kindergarten. *Scandinavian Journal of Psychology, 21,* 159–173.

Luria, A. R., & Hutton, J. T. (1977). A modern assessment of the basic forms of aphasia. *Brain and Language, 4,* 129–151.

Lynch, J. I. (1986). Langugage of cleft infants: Lessening the risk of delay through programming. In B. J. McWilliams (Ed.), *Current methods of assessing and treating children with cleft palates* (pp. 255–268). Seminars in Speech and Language, Vol. 7.

Mader, J. (1954). The relative frequency occurrence of English consonant sounds in words in the speech of children in grades one, two, and three. *Speech Monographs, 21,* 294–300.

Magnusson, E. (1983). The phonology of language disordered children: Production, perception and awareness. *Travaux de l'Institut de Linguistique de Lund XVIII.* Lund: CWK Gleerup.

Magnusson, E. (1991). Metalinguistic awareness in phonologically disordered children. In M. Yavaş (Ed.), *Phonological disorders in children: Theory, research and practice* (pp. 87–120). London: Routledge.

Magnusson, E., & Naucler, K. (1987). Language disordered and normally speaking children's development of spoken and written language: Preliminary results from a longitudinal study. *RUVL 16,* Uppsala University: Department of Linguistics.

Malikouti-Drachman, A., & Drachman, G. (1975). The acquisition of stress in Modern Greek. *Salzburger Beiträge zur Linguistik, 2,* 277–289.

Marcos, H. (1987). Communicative function of pitch range and pitch direction in infants. *Journal of Child Language, 14,* 255–268.

Marion, M. J., Sussman, H. M., & Marquardt, T. P. (1993). The perception and production of rhyme in normal and developmentally apraxic children. *Journal of Communication Disorders, 26,* 129–160.

Markides, A. (1970). The speech of deaf and partially-hearing children with special reference to factors affecting intelligibility. *British Journal of Disorders of Communication, 5,* 126–140.

Marquardt, T. P. (1982). *Acquired neurogenic disorders.* Englewood Cliffs, NJ: Prentice-Hall.

Marquardt, T. P., Reinhart, J. B., & Peterson, H. A. (1979). Markedness analysis of phonemic sub-stitution errors in apraxia of speech. *Journal of Communication Disorders, 12,* 481–494.

Marquardt, T. P., & Sussman, H. M. (1991). Developmental apraxia of speech: Theory and practice. In D. Vogel & M. P. Cannito (Eds.), *Treating disordered speech motor control* (pp. 341–390). Austin, TX: PRO-ED.

Marsh, J. L., & Lehman, J. A. (1988). *Cleft care in 1986: An ACPA survey* [abstract]. American Cleft Palate–Craniofacial Annual Meeting, Williamsburg, VA.

Martin, A. D. (1974). Some objections to the term apraxia of speech. *Journal of Speech and Hearing Disorders, 39,* 53–64.

Martinet, A. (1960). *Elements de linguistique général I.* [Elements of general linguistics I]. Paris: Armand Colin.

Mase, D. (1946). Etiology of articulatory speech defects. *Teacher's College Contribution to Education, no. 921.* New York: Columbia University.

Matheny, N., & Panagos, J. (1978). Comparing the effects of articulation and syntax programs on syntax and articulation improvement. *Language, Speech, and Hearing Services in Schools, 9,* 57–61.

McCabe, R. B., & Bradley, D. P. (1975). Systematic multiple phonemic approach to articulation therapy. *Acta Symbolica, 6,* 1–18.

McCarthy, J. (1988). Feature geometry and dependency: A review. *Phonetica, 43,* 84–108.

McCarthy, J., & Prince, A. (1993). *Prosodic morphology I: Constraint interaction and satisfaction.* Unpublished manuscript. Amherst, MA: University of Massachusetts.

McDonald, E. T. (1964). *A deep test of articulation—picture form.* Pittsburgh, PA: Stanwix.

McMahon, K., Hodson, B., & Allen, E. (1983). Phonological analysis of cerebral palsied children's utterances. *Journal of Childhood Communication Disorders, 7,* 28–35.

McNeil, M. R., Rosenbek, J. C., & Aronson, A. E. (1984). *The dysarthrias: Physiology, acoustics, perception, management.* San Diego, CA: College-Hill Press.

McReynolds, L. V., & Bennett, S. (1972). Distinctive feature generalization in articulation training. *Journal of Speech and Hearing Disorders, 37,* 462–470.

McReynolds, L. V., & Elbert, M. (1981). Criteria for phonological process analysis. *Journal of Speech and Hearing Disorders, 46,* 197–204.

McReynolds, L. V., & Engmann, D. (1975). *Distinctive feature analysis of misarticulations*. Baltimore: University Park Press.

McReynolds, L. V., Engmann, D., & Dimmitt, K. (1974). Markedness theory and articulation errors. *Journal of Speech and Hearing Disorders, 39*, 93–103.

Meador, D. (1984). Effects of color on visual discrimination of geometric symbols by severely and profoundly mentally retarded individuals. *American Journal on Mental Deficiency, 89*, 275–286.

Mehler, J., Jusczyk, P., Lambertz, G., Halsted, N., Bertoncini, J., & Amiel-Tison, C. (1988). A precursor of language acquisition in young infants. *Cognition, 29*, 143–178.

Mehrabian, A. (1970). Measures of vocabulary and grammatical skills for children up to age six. *Developmental Psychology, 2*, 439–446.

Meitus, I. J., & Weinberg, B. (1983). *Diagnosis in speech-language pathology*. Baltimore: University Park Press.

Menn, L. (1971). Phonotactic rules in beginning speech. *Lingua, 26*, 225–251.

Menn, L. (1976). *Pattern, control and contrast in beginning speech: A case study in the development of word form and word function*. Unpublished doctoral dissertation, University of Illinois, Urbana-Champaign.

Menn, L. (1978). *Pattern, control and contrast in beginning speech: A case study in the development of word form and word function*. Bloomington, IN: Indiana University Linguistics Club.

Menyuk, P. (1980). The role of context in misarticulations. In G. Yeni-Komshian, J. Kavanagh, & C. Ferguson (Eds.), *Child phonology: Vol. 1. Production* (pp. 211–226). New York: Academic Press.

Menyuk, P., Liebergott, J., & Schultz, M. (1986). Predicting phonological development. In B. Lindblom & R. Zetterstrom (Eds.), *Precursors of early speech* (pp. 79–93). New York: Stockton Press.

Menyuk, P., Menn, L., & Silber, R. (1979). Early strategies for the perception and production of words and sounds. In P. Fletcher & M. Garman (Eds.), *Language acquisition* (pp. 198–222). Cambridge: Cambridge University Press.

Mercer, J. R. (1973). *Labeling the mentally retarded*. Berkeley: University of California Press.

Metter, E. J. (1985). *Speech disorders: Clinical evaluation and diagnosis*. Jamaica, NY: Spectrum Publications Medical & Scientific Books.

Milisen, R. (1954). The disorder of articulation: A systematic clinical and experimental approach. *Journal of Speech and Hearing Disorders*, Monograph Supplement 4.

Miller, G., & Nicely, P. (1955). An analysis of perceptual confusions among some English consonants. *Journal of the Acoustical Society of America, 27*, 338–352.

Miller, J. F. (1988). Facilitating speech and language. In C. Tingey (Ed.), *Down syndrome. A resource book* (pp. 119–133). Boston: College-Hill Press.

Miller, J. F. (1992). Lexical development in young children with Down syndrome. In R. S. Chapman (Ed.), *Processes in language acquisition and disorder* (pp. 202–216). St. Louis, MO: Mosby Year Book.

Milloy, N. (1985). *The assessment and identification of developmental articulatory dyspraxia and its effect on phonological development*. Unpublished thesis, Leicester Polytechnic, Leicester, UK.

Milloy, N., & Morgan-Barry, R. (1990). Developmental neurological disorders. In P. Grunwell (Ed.), *Developmental speech disorders* (pp. 109–132). New York: Churchill Livingstone.

Mines, M., Hanson, B., & Shoup, J. (1978). Frequency of occurrence of phonemes in conversational English language and speech. *Language and Speech, 21*, 221–241.

Mitchell, P. R., & Kent, R. (1990). Phonetic variation in multisyllable babbling. *Journal of Child Language, 17*, 247–265.

Monnin, L. (1984). Speech sound discrimination testing and training: Why? Why not? In H. Winitz (Ed.), *Treating articulation disorders: For clinicians by clinicians* (pp. 1–20). Austin, TX: PRO-ED.

Monnin, L., & Huntington, D. (1974). Relationship of articulatory defects to speech-sound identification. *Journal of Speech and Hearing Research, 17*, 352–366.

Monsen, R. B. (1981). A usable test for the speech intelligibility of deaf talkers. *American Annals of the Deaf, 126*, 845–852.

Monsen, R. B., Moog, J. S., & Geers, A. E. (1988). *CID picture SPINE*. St. Louis, MO: Central Institute for the Deaf.

Moore, C., Yorkston, K., & Beukelman, D. R. (Eds.). (1991). *Dysarthria and apraxia of speech: Perspectives on management.* Baltimore: Paul H. Brooks.

Moore, W. M., Rosenbek, J. C., & LaPointe, L. L. (1976). Assessment of oral apraxia in brain-injured adults. In R. Brookshire (Ed.), *Clinical aphasiology: Proceedings of the conference* (pp. 64–79). Minneapolis, MN: BRK.

Moran, M., Money, S., & Leonard, L. (1984). Phonological process analysis of the speech of mentally retarded adults. *American Journal of Mental Deficiency, 89,* 304–306.

Morley, M. E. (1959). Defects of articulation. *Folia Phoniatrica, 11,* 65–124.

Morley, M. E. (1970). *Cleft palate and speech* (7th ed.). Baltimore: Williams & Wilkins.

Morley, M. E. (1972). Developmental articulatory apraxia. In M. E. Morley (Ed.), *The development and disorders of speech in childhood* (pp. 274–290). Baltimore: Williams & Wilkins.

Morley, M. E., Court, D., & Miller, H. (1954). Delayed speech and developmental aphasia. *British Medical Journal, 2,* 463–467.

Morley, M. E., & Fox, J. (1969). Disorders of articulation: Theory and therapy. *British Journal of Communication, 4,* 151–165.

Morris, H. L., Spriestersbach, D. C., & Darley, F. L. (1961). An articulation test for assessing competency of velopharyngeal closure. *Journal of Speech and Hearing Research, 4,* 48–55.

Morris, S. E. (1975). Pre-speech assessment. In S. E. Morris (Ed.), *Pre-speech and language programming for the young child with cerebral palsy.* Wauwatosa, WI: Curative Rehabilitation Center.

Morrison, J., & Shriberg, L. (1992). Articulation testing versus conversational speech sampling. *Journal of Speech and Hearing Research, 35,* 259–273.

Mosher, J. (1929). *The production of correct speech sounds.* Boston: Expression.

Moskowitz, A. (1971). *Acquisition of phonology.* Unpublished doctoral dissertation, University of California, Berkeley.

Murdoch, B. E., Porter, S., Younger, R., & Ozanne, A. (1984). Behaviors identified by South Australian clinicians as differentially diagnostic of developmental articulatory dyspraxia. *Australian Journal of Human Communication Disorders, 12,* 55–70.

Myers, F. L., & Myers, R. W. (1983). Perception of stress contrasts in semantic and non-semantic contexts by children. *Journal of Psycholinguistic Research, 12,* 327–338.

Myerson, R. F. (1978). Children's knowledge of selected aspects of sound pattern of English. In R. N. Campbell & P. T. Smith (Eds.), *Recent advances in the psychology of language* (Vol. III4, pp. 377–402). New York: Plenum Press.

Mysak, E. D. (1959). A servomodel for speech therapy. *Journal of Speech and Hearing Disorders, 24,* 144–149.

Nakazima, S. A. (1962). A comparative study of the speech developments of Japanese and American English in childhood (1): A comparison of the developments of voices at the prelinguistic period. *Studia Phonologica, 2,* 27–46.

Neary, T. (1978). *Phonetic feature systems for vowels.* Doctoral dissertation, University of Connecticut. Reproduced by Indiana University Linguistic Club.

Nelson, K. (1973). Structure and strategy in learning to talk. *Monographs of the Society of Research in Child Development, 38*(149). Chicago: University of Chicago Press.

Nelson, N. W. (1998). *Childhood language disorders in context: Infancy through adolescence* (2nd ed.). Boston: Allyn & Bacon.

Nemoy, E. M. (1954). *Speech correction through story telling units.* Magnolia, MA: Expression.

Nemoy, E. M., & Davis, S. (1937). *The correction of defective consonant sounds.* Boston: Expression.

Newcomer, P., & Hammill, D. (1988). *Test of language development-2 primary.* Austin, TX: PRO-ED.

Newman, P. W., & Creaghead, N. A. (1989). Assessment of articulatory and phonological disorders. In N. A. Creaghead, P. W. Newman, & W. A. Secord, *Assessment and remediation of articulatory and phonological disorders* (2nd ed.) (pp. 69–126). New York: Macmillan.

Nolan, M., McCartney, E., McArthur, K., & Rowson, V. (1980). A study of the hearing and receptive vocabulary of the trainees of an adult training centre. *Journal of Mental Deficiency Research, 24,* 271–286.

Noll, J. D. (1983). Diagnosis of speech and language disorders associated with acquired neuropathologies: Apraxia of speech and the dysarthrias. In I. J. Meitus & B. Weinberg (Eds.), *Diagnosis in speech-language pathology.* Baltimore: University Park Press.

Northern, J. L., & Downs, M. P. (1984). *Hearing in children* (3rd ed.). Baltimore: Williams & Wilkins.

Odell, K., McNeil, M. R., Rosenbek, J. C., & Hunter, L. (1990). Perceptual characteristics of consonant production by apraxic speakers. *Journal of Speech and Hearing Disorders, 55,* 345–359.

Oetting, J., & Horohov, J. (1997). Past tense marking by children with and without specific language impairment. *Journal of Speech and Hearing Research, 40,* 62–74.

Oetting, J., & Rice, M. (1993). Plural acquisition in children with specific language impairment. *Journal of Speech and Hearing Research, 36,* 1236–1248.

Oller, D. K. (1973). Regularities in abnormal child phonology. *Journal of Speech and Hearing Disorders, 38,* 36–47.

Oller, D. K. (1980). The emergence of the sounds of speech in infancy. In G. Yeni-Komshian, J. Kavanagh, & C. A. Ferguson (Eds.), *Child phonology: Vol. I. Production* (pp. 93–112). New York: Academic Press.

Oller, D. K., Jensen, H. T., & Lafayette, R. H. (1978). The relatedness of phonological processes of a hearing-impaired child. *Journal of Communication Disorders, 11,* 97–105.

Oller, D. K., Weiman, L. A., Doyle, W. J., & Ross, C. (1976). Infant babbling and speech. *Journal of Child Language, 3,* 1–11.

Olmsted, D. (1971). *Out of the mouth of babes: Earliest stages in language learning.* The Hague: Mouton.

Osberger, M. J. (1983). Development and evaluation of some speech training procedures for hearing-impaired children. In I. Hochberg, H. Levitt, & M. J. Osberger (Eds.), *Speech of the hearing impaired: Research, training, and personnel preparation* (pp. 333–348). Baltimore: University Park Press.

Osberger, M. J., & McGarr, N. (1982). Speech production characteristics of the hearing impaired. In N. Lass (Ed.), *Speech and language: Advances in basic science and research.* New York: Academic Press.

Owens, R. E. (1992). *Language development: An introduction* (3rd ed.). New York: Macmillan.

Owens, R. E. (1996). *Language development: An introduction* (4th ed.). Boston: Allyn & Bacon.

Owens, R. E. (1997). Mental retardation: Difference and delay. In D. K. Bernstein & E. Tiegerman-Farber (Eds.), *Language and communication disorders in children* (4th ed.) (pp. 457–523). Boston: Allyn & Bacon.

Owens, R. E., & House, L. (1984). Decision-making processes in augmentative communication. *Journal of Speech and Hearing Disorders, 49,* 18–25.

Pan, B., & Gleason, J. B. (1997). Semantic development: Learning the meanings of words. In J. Gleason (Ed.), *The development of language* (4th ed.) (pp. 122–158). Boston: Allyn & Bacon.

Panagos, J., & Prelock, P. (1982). Phonological constraints on the sentence production of language disordered children. *Journal of Speech and Hearing Research, 25,* 171–177.

Panagos, J., Quine, M., & Klich, R. (1979). Syntactic and phonological influences on children's articulation. *Journal of Speech and Hearing Research, 22,* 841–848.

Panconcelli-Calzia, G. (1924). *Experimental phonetik, Gehör und Lautwandel.* Tillägnat Hugo Pipping, Helsingfors, 429.

Parker, F. (1976). Distinctive features in speech pathology: Phonology or phonemics. *Journal of Speech and Hearing Disorders, 41,* 23–39.

Parker, F. (1994). Phonological theory. In R. Lowe (Ed.), *Phonology. Assessment and intervention applications in speech pathology* (pp. 17–34). Baltimore: Williams & Wilkins.

Parsons, C. L. (1984). A comparison of phonological processes used by developmentally verbal dyspraxic children and non-dyspraxic phonologically impaired children. *Australian Journal of Human Communication Disorders, 12,* 93–107.

Paschall, L. (1983). Development at 18 months. In J. V. Irwin & S. P. Wong (Eds.), *Phonological development in children: 18–72 months* (pp. 27–54). Carbondale, IL: Southern Illinois University Press.

Paul, R. (1989). *Outcomes of specific expressive language delay.* Paper at Symposium for Research in Child Language Disorders, Madison, WI.

Paul, R. (1991). Profiles of toddlers with slow expressive language development. *Topics in Language Disorders, 11,* 1–13.

Paul, R. (1993). Patterns of development in late talkers: Preschool years. *Journal of Childhood Communication Disorders, 15,* 7–14.

Paul, R. (1995). *Language disorders from infancy through adolescence: Assessment and intervention.* St. Louis, MO: Mosby Year Book.

Paul, R., & Jennings, P. (1992). Phonological behavior in toddlers with slow expressive language development. *Journal of Speech and Hearing Research, 35,* 99–107.

Paul, R., Looney, S., & Dahm, P. (1991). Communication and socialization skills at ages 2 and 3 in "late talking" young children. *Journal of Speech and Hearing Research, 34,* 858–865.

Paul, R., & Shriberg, L. D. (1982). Associations between phonology and syntax in speech delayed children. *Journal of Speech and Hearing Research, 25,* 536–547.

Pease, D. (1986). *The development of semantic and metalinguistic knowledge.* Unpublished doctoral dissertation, Boston University, MA.

Pendergast, K. S., Dickey, J., Selmer, J., & Soder, A. L. (1984). *PAT: Photo articulation test* (3rd ed.). Danville, IL: Interstate Press.

Perez, E. (1994). Phonological differences among speakers of Spanish-influenced English. In J. Bernthal & N. Bankson (Eds.), *Child phonology: Characteristics, assessment, and intervention with special populations* (pp. 245–254). New York: Thieme.

Peterson, H. A., & Marquardt, T. P. (1990). *Appraisal and diagnosis of speech-language disorders* (2nd ed.). Englewood Cliffs, NJ: Prentice-Hall.

Pharoah, P. O. D., Cooke, T., Rosenbloom, I., & Cooke, R. W. I. (1987). Trends in birth prevalence of cerebral palsy. *Archives of Disease in Childhood, 62,* 379–384.

Philips, B. J. W., & Bzoch, K. R. (1969). Reliability of judgements of articulation of cleft palate speakers. *Cleft Palate Journal, 6,* 24–34.

Piaget, J. (1952). *The origins of intelligence in children.* New York: International Universities Press.

Pierce, J. E., & Hanna, I. V. (1974). *The development of a phonological system in English speaking American children.* Portland: HaPi Press.

Pike, K. L. (1943). *Phonetics.* Ann Arbor, MI: University of Michigan Press.

Pollack, E., & Rees, N. (1972). Disorders of articulation: Some clinical applications of distinctive feature theory. *Journal of Speech and Hearing Disorders, 37,* 451–461.

Pollock, K. (1991). The identification of vowel errors using traditional articulation or phonological process test stimuli. *Language, Speech, and Hearing Services in Schools, 22,* 39–50.

Pollock, K., & Hall, P. K. (1991). An analysis of the vowel misarticulations of five children with developmental apraxia of speech. *Clinical Linguistics and Phonetics, 5,* 207–224.

Pollock, K., & Keiser, N. (1990). An examination of vowel errors in phonologically disordered children. *Clinical Linguistics and Phonetics, 4,* 161–178.

Pollock, K., & Schwartz, R. (1988). Structural aspects of phonological development: Case study of a disordered child. *Language, Speech, and Hearing Services in Schools, 19,* 5–16.

Pollock, K., & Swanson, L. (1986). *Analysis of vowel errors in a disordered child during training.* Paper presented at the annual convention of the American Speech-Language-Hearing Association, Detroit, MI.

Poole, I. (1934). Genetic development of articulation of consonant sounds in speech. *Elementary English Review, 11,* 159–161.

Powers, M. (1971). Clinical and educational procedures in functional disorders of articulation. In L. Travis (Ed.), *Handbook of speech pathology and audiology* (pp. 877–910). New York: Appleton-Century-Crofts.

Prather, E. M., Hedrick, D., & Kern, C. (1975). Articulation development in children aged two to four years. *Journal of Speech and Hearing Disorders, 40,* 179–191.

Pratt, C., & Grieve, R. (1983). The development of metalinguistic awareness: An introduction. In W. Tunmer, C. Pratt, & M. Herriman (Eds.), *Metalinguistic awareness in children: Theory, research and implications* (pp. 2–11). Berlin: Springer-Verlag.

Preisser, D. A, Hodson, B. W., & Paden, E. P. (1988). Developmental phonology: 18–29 months. *Journal of Speech and Hearing Disorders, 53,* 125–130.

President's Committee on Mental Retardation (PCMR). (1978). Washington, DC: PCMR Newsclipping Service.

Prince, A., & Smolensky, P. (1993). Optimality theory: Constraint interaction in generative grammar. *Technical Report No. 2 of the Rutgers Center for Cognitive Science.* New Brunswick, NJ: Rutgers University.

Prins, D. (1963). Relations among specific articulatory deviations and responses to a clinical measure of sound discrimination ability. *Journal of Speech and Hearing Disorders, 28,* 382–388.

Pulleyblank, D. (1986). Underspecification and low vowel harmony in Okpe2. *Studies in African Linguistics, 17,* 119–153.

Radziewicz, C., & Antonellis, S. (1997). Considerations and implications for habilitation of hearing impaired children. In D. K. Bernstein & E. Tiegerman (Eds.), *Language and communication disorders in children* (4th ed.) (pp. 574–603). Boston: Allyn & Bacon.

Raphael, L., & Bell-Berti, F. (1975). Tongue musculature and the feature of tension in English vowels. *Phonetica, 32,* 61–63.

Ratner, N. B. (1994). Phonological analysis of child speech. In J. Sokolov & C. Snow (Eds.), *Handbook of Research in Language Development using CHILDES* (pp. 324–372). Northvale, NJ: Erlbaum.

Read, C. (1978). Children's awareness of sounds, with emphasis on sound systems. In A. Sinclair, R. J. Jarvella, & W. J. Levelt (Eds.), *The child's conception of language* (pp. 65–82). Berlin: Springer Verlag.

Reed, V. (1994). *An introduction to children with language disorders* (2nd ed.). New York: Merrill.

Reid, J., Grieve, R., Dean, E., Donaldson, M., & Howell, J. (1993). Linguistic awareness in young children. In J. Clibbens & B. Pendleton (Eds.), *Proceedings of child language seminar* (pp. 255–274). Plymouth, UK: University of Plymouth.

Renfrew, C. (1966). Persistence of the open syllable in defective articulation. *Journal of Speech and Hearing Disorders, 31,* 370–373.

Rescorla, L. (1989). The Language Development Survey: A screening tool for delayed language in toddlers. *Journal of Speech and Hearing Disorders, 54,* 587–599.

Rescorla, L., & Ratner, N. B. (1996). Phonetic profiles in toddlers with specific expressive language impairment (SLI-E). *Journal of Speech and Hearing Research, 39,* 153–165.

Rescorla, L., & Schwartz, E. (1990). Outcome of toddlers with expressive language delay. *Applied Psycholinguistics, 11,* 393–407.

Reynolds, J. (1987). *The development of the vowel system in phonologically disordered children.* Unpublished doctoral dissertation, University of Sheffield, UK.

Reynolds, J. (1990). Abnormal vowel patterns in phonologically disordered children: Some data

and a hypothesis. *British Journal of Disorders of Communication, 25,* 115–148.

Rice, M. (1991). Children with specific language impairment: Towards a model of teachability. In N. Krasnegor (Ed.), *Biological and behavioral determinants of language development* (pp. 447–480). Hillsdale, NJ: Lawrence Erlbaum.

Rice, M. (1994). Grammatical categories of children with specific language impairments. In R. Watkins & M. Rice (Eds.), *Specific language impairment in children* (pp. 69–90). Baltimore: Brookes.

Rice, M., & Bode, J. (1993). Gaps in the verb lexicons of children with specific language impairment. *First Language, 13,* 113–131.

Rice, M., & Oetting, J. (1993). Morphological deficits of children with SLI: Evaluation of number marking and agreement. *Journal of Speech and Hearing Research, 36,* 1249–1257.

Rice, M., Wexler, K., & Cleave, P. (1995). Specific language impairment as a period of extended optional infinitive. *Journal of Speech and Hearing Research, 38,* 850–863.

Robb, M. P., & Saxman, J. H. (1990). Syllable durations of preword and early word vocalizations. *Journal of Speech and Hearing Research, 33,* 583–593.

Roberts, A. (1965). *A statistical linguistic analysis of American English.* The Hague: Mouton.

Roberts, J. E., Burchinal, M., & Footo, M. (1990). Phonological process decline from 2½ to 8 years. *Journal of Communication Disorders, 23,* 205–217.

Robin, D. A., Hall, P. K., & Jordan, L. S. (1987). *Prosodic impairment in developmental verbal apraxia.* Paper presented at the annual meeting of the American Speech-Language-Hearing Association, New Orleans, LA.

Robin, D. A., Hall, P. K., Jordan, L. S., & Gordan, A. J. (1991). *Developmentally apraxic speakers' stress production: Perceptual and acoustic analyses.* Paper presented at the annual meeting of the American Speech-Language-Hearing Association, Atlanta, GA.

Roe, K. V. (1975). Amount of infant vocalization as a function of age: Some cognitive implications. *Child Development, 46,* 936–941.

Roe, K. V. (1977). *Relationship between infant vocalizations and preschool cognitive functioning.* Paper presented at the Annual Meeting of the Washington Psychological Association, Seattle, WA.

Rosenbek, J. C. (1985). Treating apraxia of speech. In D. F. Johns (Ed.), *Clinical management of neurogenic communicative disorders* (pp. 267–312). Boston: Little, Brown.

Rosenbek, J. C., & LaPointe, L. L. (1985). The dysarthrias: Description, diagnosis and treatment. In D. F. Johns (Ed.), *Clinical management of neurogenic communicative disorders* (pp. 97–152). Boston: Little, Brown.

Rosenbek, J. C., & Wertz, R. T. (1972). A review of fifty cases of developmental apraxia of speech. *Language, Speech, and Hearing Services in Schools, 5,* 23–33.

Rosenbek, J. C., & Wertz, R. T. (1976). Workshop on speech motor disorders, Veterans Administration Hospital, Madison, WI.

Rosetti, A. (1959). *Sur la théorie de la syllable.* Gravenhage: Mouton.

Ruhlen, M. (1976). *Guide to the languages of the world.* San Diego, CA: Los Amigos Research Associates.

Saben, C., & Ingham, J. (1991). The effects of minimal pairs treatment on the speech-sound production of two children with phonologic disorders. *Journal of Speech and Hearing Research, 34,* 1023–1040.

Sagey, E. (1986). *The representation of features and relations in non-linear phonology.* Unpublished doctoral dissertation, MIT, Cambridge, MA.

Sander, E. K. (1972). When are speech sounds learned? *Journal of Speech and Hearing Disorders, 37,* 55–63.

Sapir, E. (1921). *Language: An introduction to the study of speech.* New York: Harcourt, Brace and World.

Sapir, E. (1925). Sound patterns in language. *Language, 1,* 37–51.

Saussure, F. de (1959). *A course in general linguistics* (J. Cantineau, Trans.). London: Owen. (Original work published 1916)

Scarborough, H., & Dobrich, W. (1990). Development of children with early language delay. *Journal of Speech and Hearing Research, 33,* 70–83.

Schmauch, V., Panagos, J., & Klich, R. (1978). Syntax influences the accuracy of consonant production in language-disordered children. *Journal of Communication Disorders, 11,* 315–323.

Schonweiler, R., Schonweiler, B., Schmelzeisen, R., & Ptok, M. (1995). The language and speech skills in 417 children with cleft formations. *Fortschritte in der Kieferorthopadie, 56,* 1–6.

Schprintzen, R. J., & Bardach, J. (Ed.). (1995). *Cleft palate speech management: A multidisciplinary approach.* St. Louis, MO: Mosby.

Schwartz, A., & Goldman, R. (1974). Variables influencing performance on speech discrimination tests. *Journal of Speech and Hearing Research, 17,* 25–32.

Schwartz, R. (1992a). Clinical applications of recent advances in phonological theory. *Language, Speech, and Hearing Services in Schools, 23,* 269–276.

Schwartz, R. (1992b). Nonlinear phonology as a framework for phonological acquisition. In R. Chapman (Ed.), *Processes in language acquisition and disorders* (pp. 108–124). St. Louis, MO: Mosby Year Book.

Schwartz, R., & Leonard, L. B. (1982). Do children pick and choose? An examination of phonological selection and avoidance in early lexical acquisition. *Journal of Child Language, 9,* 319–336.

Schwartz, R., Leonard, L., Folger, M., & Wilcox, M. (1980). Evidence for a synergistic view of linguistic disorders: Early phonological behavior in normal and language disordered children. *Journal of Speech and Hearing Disorders, 45,* 357–377.

Scripture, E. W. (1902). *Elements of experimental phonetics.* New York: Charles Scribner's Sons.

Scripture, E. W. (1927). Die Silbigkeit und die Silbe. *Archives fur das Studium der neueren Sprachen, CLII,* 74.

Scripture, M., & Jackson, E. (1919). *A manual of exercises for the correction of speech disorders.* Philadelphia: Davis.

Secord, W. (1981a). *C-PAC: Clinical probes of articulation consistency.* Sedona, AZ: Red Rock Education.

Secord, W. (1981b). *Eliciting sounds: Techniques for clinicians.* San Antonio: Psychological Corporation.

Secord, W. (1989). The traditional approach to treatment. In N. A. Creaghead, P. W. Newman, & W. A. Secord (Eds.), *Assessment and remediation of articulatory and phonological disorders* (2nd ed.) (pp. 129–158). New York: Macmillan.

Seymour, H., Green, L., & Hundley, R. (1991). *Phonological patterns in the conversational speech of African American children.* Paper presented at the American Speech-Language-Hearing Association national convention, Atlanta, GA.

Seymour, H., & Miller-Jones, D. (1981). Language and cognitive assessment of Black children. *Speech Language: Advances in Basic Research and Practice, 6*, 203–255.

Shane, H., & Wilbur, R. (1980). Potential for expressive signing based on motor control. *Sign Language Studies, 29*, 331–347.

Shankweiler, D., & Harris, K. (1966). An experimental approach to the problem of articulation in aphasia. *Cortex, 2*, 277–292.

Shelton, I. K., & Graves, M. M. (1985). Use of visual techniques in therapy for developmental apraxia of speech. *Language, Speech, and Hearing Services in Schools, 16*, 129–131.

Shelton, R. (1993). Grand rounds for sound system disorder. Conclusion: What was learned. *Seminars in Speech and Language, 14*, 166–178.

Sherman, D., & Geith, A. (1967). Speech sound discrimination and articulation skill. *Journal of Speech and Hearing Disorders, 10*, 277–280.

Shibamoto, J., & Olmsted, D. (1978). Lexical and syllabic patterns in phonological acquistion. *Journal of Child Language, 5*, 417–456.

Shipley, K. G. (1992). *Interviewing and counseling in communicative disorders: Principles and procedures.* New York: Merrill/Macmillan.

Shipley, K. G., & McAfee, J. G. (1992). *Assessment in speech-language pathology: A resource manual.* San Diego, CA: Singular.

Shprintzen, R. J. (1995). *Cleft palate speech management. A multidisciplinary approach.* St. Louis, MO: Mosby Year Book.

Shprintzen, R. J., Siegel-Sadewitz, V. L., Amato, J., & Goldberg, R. B. (1985). Anomalies associated with cleft lip, cleft palate, or both. *American Journal of Medical Genetics, 20*, 585–595.

Shriberg, L. D. (1975). A response evocation program for /ɝ/. *Journal of Speech and Hearing Disorders, 40*, 92–105.

Shriberg, L. D. (1980). An intervention procedure for children with persistent /r/ errors. *Language, Speech, and Hearing Services in Schools, 11*, 102–110.

Shriberg, L. D. (1991). Directions for research in developmental phonological disorders. In J. F. Miller (Ed.), *Research on child language disorders: A decade of progress* (pp. 267–276). Austin, TX: PRO-ED.

Shriberg, L. D., Aram, D. M., & Kwiatkowski, J. (1997a). Developmental apraxia of speech: I. Descriptive and theoretical perspectives. *Journal of Speech, Language, and Hearing Research, 40*, 273–285.

Shriberg, L. D., Aram, D. M., & Kwiatkowski, J. (1997b). Developmental apraxia of speech: II. Toward a diagnostic marker. *Journal of Speech, Language, and Hearing Research, 40*, 286–312.

Shriberg, L. D., Aram, D. M., & Kwiatkowski, J. (1997c). Developmental apraxia of speech: III. A subtype marked by inappropriate stress. *Journal of Speech, Language, and Hearing Research, 40*, 313–337.

Shriberg, L. D., Austin, D., Lewis, B., McSweeny, J. L., & Wilson, D. L. (1997). The percentage of consonants correct (PCC) metric: Extensions and reliability data. *Journal of Speech, Language, and Hearing Research, 40*, 708–722.

Shriberg, L. D., & Kent, R. D. (1995). *Clinical phonetics* (2nd ed.). Boston: Allyn & Bacon.

Shriberg, L. D., & Kwiatkowski, J. (1980). *Natural process analysis (NPA): A procedure for phonological analysis of continuous speech samples.* New York: Wiley.

Shriberg, L. D., & Kwiatkowski, J. (1982a). Phonological disorders II: A conceptual framework for management. *Journal of Speech and Hearing Disorders, 47*, 242–256.

Shriberg, L. D., & Kwiatkowski, J. (1982b). Phonological disorders III: A procedure for assessing severity of involvement. *Journal of Speech and Hearing Disorders, 47*, 256–270.

Shriberg, L. D., & Kwiatkowski, J. (1983). Computer-assisted natural process analysis (NPA): Recent issues and data. *Seminars in Speech and Language, 4*, 389–406.

Shriberg, L. D., & Kwiatkowski, J. (1985). Continuous speech sampling for phonologic analyses of speech-delayed children. *Journal of Speech and Hearing Disorders, 50*, 323–334.

Shriberg, L. D., & Kwiatkowski, J. (1994). Developmental phonological disorders I: A clinical profile. *Journal of Speech and Hearing Research, 37*, 1100–1126.

Shriberg, L. D., Kwiatkowski, J., Best, S., Hengst, J., & Terselic-Weber, B. (1986). Characteristics of children with phonologic disorders of unknown origin. *Journal of Speech and Hearing Disorders, 51*, 140–161.

Shriberg, L. D., Kwiatkowski, J., & Rasmussen, C. (1990). *The prosody-voice screening profile.* Tucson, AZ: Communication Builders.

Shriberg, L. D., & Lof, G. L. (1991). Reliability studies in broad and narrow transcription. *Clinical Linguistics and Phonetics, 5,* 225–179.

Shriberg, L. D., & Widder, C. J. (1990). Speech and prosody characteristics of adults with mental retardation. *Journal of Speech and Hearing Research, 33,* 627–653.

Shriner, T., Holloway, M., & Daniloff, R. (1969). The relationship between articulatory deficits and syntax in speech defective children. *Journal of Speech and Hearing Research, 12,* 319–325.

Shvachkin, N. K. (1973). The development of phonemic speech perception in early childhood. In C. A. Ferguson & D. I. Slobin (Eds.), *Studies of child language development* (pp. 91–127). New York: Holt, Rinehart & Winston.

Sievers, E. (1901). *Grundzüge der Phonetik: Zur Einführung in das Studium der indogermanischen Sprachen.* Leipzig: Breitkopf und Hartel.

Silverman, F. (1980). *Communication for the speechless.* Englewood Cliffs, NJ: Prentice-Hall.

Simon, C., & Fourcin, A. J. (1978). Cross language study of speech pattern learning. *Journal of the Acoustical Society of America, 63,* 925–935.

Sinclair, A., Jarvella, R., & Levelt, W. (Eds.). (1980). *The child's conception of language.* Berlin: Springer-Verlag.

Singh, S. (1968). *Perceptual correlates of distinctive feature systems.* Washington, DC: Howard University Press.

Singh, S. (1976). *Distinctive features: Principles and practices.* Baltimore: University Park Press.

Singh, S., & Black, J. (1966). Study of twenty-six intervocalic consonants as spoken and recognized by four language groups. *Journal of the Acoustical Society of America, 39,* 372–387.

Singh, S., & Polen, S. (1972). Use of distinctive feature model in speech pathology. *Acta Symbolica, 3,* 17–25.

Sloat, C., Taylor, S., & Hoard, J. (1978). *Introduction to phonology.* Englewood Cliffs, NJ: Prentice-Hall.

Smit, A. (1986). Ages of speech sound acquisition: Comparisons and critiques of several normative studies. *Language, Speech, and Hearing Services in Schools, 17,* 175–186.

Smit, A. B. (1993a). Phonologic error distributions in the Iowa-Nebraska Articulation Norms Project: Word-initial consonant clusters. *Journal of Speech and Hearing Research, 36,* 931–947.

Smit, A. B. (1993b). Phonologic error distributions in the Iowa-Nebraska Articulation Norms Project: Consonant singletons. *Journal of Speech and Hearing Research, 36,* 533–547.

Smit, A. B., & Bernthal, J. E. (1983). Voicing contrasts and their phonological implications in the speech of articulation-disordered children. *Journal of Speech and Hearing Research, 26,* 486–500.

Smit, A. B., Hand, L., Freilinger, J., Bernthal, J., & Bird, A. (1990). The Iowa Articulation Norms Project and its Nebraska replication. *Journal of Speech and Hearing Disorders, 55,* 779–798.

Smith, B., Marquardt, T. P., Cannito, M. P., & Davis, B. L. (1994). Vowel variability in developmental apraxia of speech. In J. A. Till, K. M. Yorkston, & D. R. Beukelman (Eds.), *Motor speech disorders* (pp. 81–89). Baltimore: Paul H. Brookes.

Smith, B. L. (1979). A phonetic analysis of consonant devoicing in children's speech. *Journal of Child Language, 6,* 19–28.

Smith, B. L., Brown-Sweeney, S., & Stoel-Gammon, C. (1989). A quantitative analysis of reduplicated and variegated babbling. *First Language, 9,* 175–189.

Smith, C. R. (1975). Residual hearing and speech production in deaf children. *Journal of Speech and Hearing Research, 18,* 795–811.

Smith, N. V. (1973). *The acquisition of phonology: A case study.* Cambridge: Cambridge University Press.

Snowling, M., Goulandris, N., & Stackhouse, J. (1994). Phonological constraints on learning to read: Evidence from single case studies of reading difficulty. In C. Hulme & M. Snowling (Eds.), *Reading development and dyslexia* (pp. 86–104). London: Whurr.

So, L., & Dodd, B. (1994). Phonologically disordered Cantonese-speaking children. *Clinical Linguistics and Phonetics, 8,* 235–255.

Sommers, R. (1969). *Factors in the effectiveness of articulation with educable retarded children.* Final report of project 7–0432. Washington, DC: U.S. Department of Health, Education and Welfare.

Sommers, R., Patterson, J., & Wildgen, P. (1988). Phonology of Down syndrome speakers, ages 13–22. *Journal of Childhood Communication Disorders, 12,* 65–91.

Sonderman, J. (1971). *An experimental study of clinical relationships between auditory discrimination and articulation skills.* Paper presented at the National Convention of the American Speech-Language-Hearing Association, San Francisco.

Sparks, R. W., Helm, N., & Albert, M. (1974). Aphasia rehabilitation resulting from Melodic Intonation Therapy. *Cortex, 10,* 303–316.

Stackhouse, J. (1982). An investigation of reading and spelling performance in speech disordered children. *British Journal of Disorders of Communication, 17,* 53–60.

Stackhouse, J. (1985). Segmentation, speech and spelling difficulties. In M. Snowling (Ed.), *Children's written language difficulties: Assessment and management* (pp. 96–115). Windsor, UK: NFER Nelson.

Stackhouse, J. (1993). Phonological disorder and lexical development: Two case studies. *Child Language Teaching and Therapy, 9,* 230–241.

Stackhouse, J. (1997). Phonological awareness: Connecting speech and literacy problems. In B. W. Hodson & M. L. Edwards (Eds.), *Perspectives in applied phonology* (pp. 157–196). Gaithersburg, MD: Aspen.

Stackhouse, J., & Snowling, M. (1983). Segmentation and spelling in children with speech disorders. In M. Edwards (Ed.), *Proceedings of XIX congress of the international association of logopedics and phoniatrics* (pp. 282–287). London: College of Speech Therapists.

Stackhouse, J., & Snowling, M. (1996). Speech, spelling and reading: Who is at risk and why? In M. Snowling & J. Stackhouse (Eds.), *Dyslexia, speech and language: A practitioner's handbook* (pp. 12–30). San Diego, CA: Singular.

Stampe, D. (1969). The acquisition of phonetic representation. *Proceedings of the Fifth Regional Meeting of the Chicago Linguistic Circle,* 443–454.

Stampe, D. (1972). On the natural history of diphthongs. *Chicago Linguistic Society* (8th Regional Meeting), 578–590.

Stampe, D. (1973). *A dissertation on natural phonology.* Unpublished doctoral dissertation, University of Chicago.

Stampe, D. (1979). *A dissertation on natural phonology.* New York: Garland.

Stark, R. (1980). Stages of speech development in the first year of life. In G. Yeni-Komshian, J. Kavanagh, & C. A. Ferguson (Eds.), *Child phonology: Vol. I. Production* (pp. 73–92). New York: Academic Press.

Stark, R. (1986). Prespeech segmental feature development. In P. Fletcher & M. Garman (Eds.), *Language acquisition. Studies in first language development* (pp. 149–173). Cambridge: Cambridge University Press.

Starr, C. D. (1993). Behavioral approaches to treating velopharyngeal closure and nasality. In K. T. Moller & C. D. Starr (Ed.), *Cleft palate: Interdisciplinary issues and treatment* (pp. 337–356). Austin, TX: PRO-ED.

Stathoppulos, E. T., & Sapienza, C. (1993). Respiratory and laryngeal measures of children during vocal intensity variation. *Journal of the Acoustical Society of America, 94,* 2531–2543.

Stemberger, J. P., & Bernhardt, B. (1997). Optimality theory. In M. Ball & R. Kent (Eds.), *The new phonologies* (pp. 211–245). San Diego, CA: Singular.

Stern, D., & Wasserman, G. (1979). *Maternal language to infants.* Paper presented at a meeting of the Society for Research in Child Development.

Stern, H. (1927). Zur Pathogenese des Sigmatismus nasalis. *Zeitschrift fur Hals-, Nasen-, Ohrenheilkunde, 18,* 585ff.

Stetson, R. H. (1936). The relation of the phoneme and the syllable. *Proceedings of the Second International Congress of Phonetic Sciences,* 245–254.

Stetson, R. H. (1951). *Motor phonetics: A study of speech movements in action.* Amsterdam: North-Holland.

Stockman, I. (1996). Phonological development and disorders in African American children. In A. Kamhi, K. Pollock, & J. Harris (Eds.), *Communication development and disorders in African American children: Research, assessment, and intervention* (pp. 117–154). Baltimore: P. H. Brookes.

Stockman, I. J., Woods, D. R., & Tishman, A. (1981). Listener agreement on phonetic segments in early infant vocalizations. *Journal of Psycholinguistic Research, 10,* 593–617.

Stoel-Gammon, C. (1985). Phonetic inventories, 15–24 months: A longitudinal study. *Journal of Speech and Hearing Research, 28,* 505–512.

Stoel-Gammon, C. (1987). Phonological skills of two-year-olds. *Language, Speech, and Hearing Services in Schools, 18,* 323–329.

Stoel-Gammon, C. (1989). Prespeech and early speech development of two late talkers. *First Language, 9,* 207–223.

Stoel-Gammon, C., & Cooper, J. A. (1984). Patterns of early lexical and phonological development. *Journal of Child Language, 11,* 247–271.

Stoel-Gammon, C., & Dunn, C. (1985). *Normal and disordered phonology in children.* Baltimore: University Park Press.

Stoel-Gammon, C., & Herrington, P. (1990). Vowel systems of normally developing and phonologically disordered children. *Clinical Linguistics and Phonetics, 4,* 145–160.

Stoel-Gammon, C., & Menn, L. (1997). Phonological development: Learning sounds and sound patterns. In J. Berko Gleason (Ed.), *The development of language* (4th ed.) (pp. 69–121). Boston: Allyn & Bacon.

Stoel-Gammon, C., & Otomo, K. (1986). Babbling development of hearing-impaired and normally hearing subjects. *Journal of Speech and Hearing Disorders, 51,* 33–41.

Subtelny, J. D. (1980). *Speech assessment and speech improvement for the hearing impaired.* Washington, DC: Alexander Graham Bell Association for the Deaf.

Sweet, H. (1877). *A handbook of phonetics.* Oxford: Clarendon Press.

Sweet, H. (1890). *Primer of phonetics.* Oxford: Oxford University Press.

Swift, E., & Rosin, P. (1990). A remediation sequence to improve speech intelligibility for students with Down syndrome. *Language, Speech, and Hearing Services in Schools, 21,* 140–146.

Tallal, P., Stark., R. E., Kallman, C., & Mellits, D. (1980). Perceptual constancy for phonemic categories: A developmental study with normal and language-impaired children. *Applied Psycholinguistics, 1,* 49–64.

Tarjan, G., Wright, S. W., Eyman, R. K., & Keeran, D. V. (1973). Natural history of mental retardation: Some aspects of epidemiology. *American Journal of Mental Deficiency, 77,* 369–379.

Tatham, M., & Morton, K. (1997). Recording and displaying speech. In M. J. Ball & C. Code (Eds.), *Instrumental clinical phonetics* (pp. 1–21). San Diego, CA: Singular.

Templin, M. (1957). *Certain language skills in children: Their development and interrelationships.* Institute of Child Welfare, Monograph 26. Minneapolis, MN: University of Minnesota Press.

Terrell, S. L., & Terrell, F. (1993). African-American cultures. In D. E. Battle (Ed.), *Communication disorders in multicultural populations* (pp. 3–37). Stoneham, MA: Butterworth-Heinemann.

Thiele, G. (1980). *Handlexikon der Medizin.* Munchen: Urban & Schwarzenberg.

Thompson, C. K. (1988). Articulation disorders in the child with neurogenic pathology. In N. J. Lass, L. V. McReynolds, J. L. Northern, & D. E. Yoder (Eds.), *Handbook of speech-language pathology and audiology* (pp. 185–217). New York: Grune & Stratton.

Thompson, L. C. (1965). *A Vietnamese grammar.* Seattle: University of Washington Press.

Tillmann, H. G. (1964). *Das phonetische Silbenproblem.* Unpublished doctoral dissertation. University of Bonn, Germany.

Toombs, M. S., Singh, S., & Hayden, M. E. (1981). Markedness of features in the articulatory substitutions of children. *Journal of Speech and Hearing Disorders, 46,* 184–191.

Travis, L., & Rasmus, B. (1931). The speech sound discrimination ability of cases with functional disorders of articulation. *Quarterly Journal of Speech, 17,* 217–226.

Trehub, S. E. (1976). The discrimination of foreign speech contrasts by infants and adults. *Child Development, 47,* 466–472.

Trost, J. E. (1981). Articulatory additions to the classical description of the speech of persons with cleft palate. *Cleft Palate Journal, 18,* 193–203.

Trost-Cardamone, J. E. (1990a). The development of speech: Assessing cleft palate misarticuations. In D. A. Kernahan & S. W. Rosenstein (Eds.), *Cleft lip and palate: A system of management* (pp. 227–235). Baltimore: Williams & Wilkins.

Trost-Cardamone, J. E. (1990b). Speech: Anatomy, physiology, and pathology. In D. A. Kernahan & S. W. Rosenstein (Eds.), *Cleft lip and palate: A system of managment* (pp. 91–103). Baltimore: Williams & Wilkins.

Trost-Cardamone, J. E., & Bernthal, J. E. (1993). Articulation assessment procedures and treatment decisions. In K. T. Moller & C. D. Starr (Eds.), *Cleft palate. Interdisciplinary issues and treatment* (p. 307ff.). Austin, TX: PRO-ED.

Trubetzkoy, N. S. (1931). Gedanken über Morphophonologie. *Travaux du Cercle Linguistique de Prague, 4,* 160 ff.

Trubetzkoy, N. S. (1939). *Grundzüge der Phonologie.* Prague: TCLP, 4.

Trubetzkoy, N. S. (1969). *Principles of Phonology.* Berkeley: University of California Press. (Original work published 1939)

Turk, A., Jusczyk, P., & Gerken, L. (1995). Do English-learning infants use syllable weight to determine stress? *Language and Speech, 38,* 143–158.

Tyler, A., & Langsdale, T. (1996). Consonant-vowel interactions in early phonological development. *First Language, 16,* 159–191.

Tyler, A., & Watterson, K. (1991). Effects of phonological versus language intervention in preschoolers with both phonological and language impairment. *Child Language Teaching and Therapy, 7,* 141–160.

United States Bureau of the Census. (1990). *Statistical abstract of the United States: 1990. The national data book* (110th ed.). Washington, DC: U.S. Department of Commerce.

Van Demark, D. R., & Hardin, M. A. (1990). Speech therapy for the child with cleft lip and palate. In J. Bardach & H. L. Morris (Eds.), *Multidisciplinary management of cleft lip and palate.* Philadelphia: W. B. Saunders.

Van Keulen, J. E., Weddington, G. T., & DeBose, C. E. (1998). *Speech, language, learning, and the African American child.* Boston: Allyn & Bacon.

Van Riper, C. (1939a). Ear training in the treatment of articulation disorders. *Journal of Speech Disorders, IV,* 141–142.

Van Riper, C. (1939b). *Speech correction. Principles and methods.* Englewood Cliffs, NJ: Prentice-Hall.

Van Riper, C. (1963). *Speech correction: Principles and methods* (4th ed.). Englewood Cliffs, NJ: Prentice-Hall.

Van Riper, C. (1978). *Speech correction. Principles and methods* (6th ed.). Englewood Cliffs, NJ: Prentice-Hall.

Van Riper, C., & Emerick, L. (1984). *Speech correction: An introduction to speech pathology and audiology* (7th ed.). Englewood Cliffs, NJ: Prentice-Hall.

Van Riper, C., & Irwin, J. (1958). *Voice and articulation.* Englewood Cliffs, NJ: Prentice-Hall.

Velleman, S. L., & Strand, K. (1994). Developmental verbal dyspraxia. In J. E. Bernthal & N. W. Bankson (Eds.), *Child phonology: Characteristics, assessment, and intervention with special populations* (pp. 110–139). New York: Thieme.

Velten, H. (1943). The growth of phonemic and lexical patterns in infant language. *Language, 19,* 281–292.

Vihman, M. M. (1984). *Individual differences in phonological development: Age one and age three.* Unpublished manuscript.

Vihman, M. M. (1992). Early syllables and the construction of phonology. In C. A. Ferguson, L. Menn, & C. Stoel-Gammon (Eds.), *Phonological development: Models, research, implications* (pp. 393–422). Timonium, MD: York Press.

Vihman, M. M. (1998). Early phonological development. In J. E. Bernthal & N. W. Bankson (Eds.), *Articulation and phonological disorders* (4th ed.) (pp. 63–112). Boston: Allyn & Bacon.

Vihman, M. M., Ferguson, C. A., & Elbert, M. (1986). Phonological development from babbling to speech: Common tendencies and individual differences. *Applied Psycholinguistics, 7,* 3–40.

Vihman, M. M., & Greenlee, M. (1987). Individual differences in phonological development: Ages one through three years. *Journal of Speech and Hearing Research, 30,* 503–521.

Vihman, M. M., Macken, M. A., Miller, R., Simmons, H., & Miller, J. (1985). From babbling to speech: A reassessment of the continuity issue. *Language, 61,* 397–445.

de Villiers, P., & de Villiers, J. (1972). Early judgements of syntactic and semantic acceptability by children. *Journal of Psycholinguistic Research, 1,* 299–310.

Voiers, W. D. (1967). *Performance evaluation of speech processing devices: Vol. 3. Diagnostic evaluation of speech intelligibility.* Bedford, MA: Air Force Research Laboratories.

Von Bremen, V. (1990). *A nonlinear phonological approach to intervention with severely phonologically disordered twins.* Unpublished master's thesis. University of British Columbia.

von Essen, O. (1979). *Allgemeine und angewandte Phonetik* (5th ed.). Berlin: Akademie-Verlag.

Waengler, H.-H. (1981). *Atlas deutscher Sprachlaute* (7th ed.). Berlin: Akademie-Verlag.

Waengler, H.-H. (1983). *Grundriss einer Phonetik des Deutschen* (4th ed.). Marburg: Elwert Verlag.

Waengler, H.-H., & Bauman-Waengler, J. A. (1980). Lautdauerverhältnisse im Sprechen von Patienten mit zentral-nervalen Störungen. In W. Kühlwein & A. Rasch (Eds.), *Sprache und Verstehen, Bd. II. Kongressberichte der 10. Jahrestagung der Gesellschaft für Angewandte Linguistik* (p. 134ff). Tübingen: Gunter Narr Verlag.

Waengler, H.-H., & Bauman-Waengler, J. A. (1984). *Phonetische Logopädie, Lieferung 2: S-Lautbildungen und ihre Störungen.* Berlin: Marhold Verlag.

Waengler, H.-H., & Bauman-Waengler, J. A. (1985). *Phonetische Logopädie, Lieferung 4.* Berlin: Marhold Verlag.

Waengler, H.-H., & Bauman-Waengler, J. A. (1987a). *Phonetische Logopädie. Die Behandlung von Kommunikationsstörungen auf phonetischer Grundlage. 2.4 Dysarthrien* (p. 562 ff.). Berlin: Marhold Verlag.

Waengler, H.-H., & Bauman-Waengler, J. A. (1987b). *Phonetische Logopädie. Die Behandlung von Kommunikationstörungen auf phonetischer Grundlage. 2.3.8. LKG-Spalten* (pp. 503ff.). Berlin: Marhold Verlag.

Waengler, H.-H., & Bauman-Waengler, J. A. (1989). *Phonological development of normal and speech/ language disordered 4-year-olds.* Paper presented at the national convention of the American Speech-Language-Hearing Association, St. Louis.

Walsh, H. (1974). On certain practical inadequacies of distinctive feature systems. *Journal of Speech and Hearing Disorders, 39,* 32–43.

Wang, W. (1990). Theoretical issues in studying Chinese dialects. *Journal of the Chinese Language Teachers Association, 25,* 1–34.

Ward, I. (1923). *Defects of speech.* New York: E. P. Dutton.

Warren, S. (1979). PERCI: A method for rating palatal efficiency. *Cleft Palate Journal, 16,* 279–285.

Washington, J. A., & Craig, H. K. (1994). Dialectal forms during discourse of poor, urban, African American preschoolers. *Journal of Speech and Hearing Research, 37,* 816–823.

Watkins, R., Rice, M., & Moltz, C. (1993). Verb use by language-impaired and normally developing children. *First Language, 13,* 133–143.

Webb, J. C., & Duckett, B. (1990). *The RULES phonological evaluation.* Vero Beach, FL: The Speech Bin.

Webster, P. E., & Plante, A. S. (1992). Effects of phonological impairment on word, syllable, and phoneme segmentation and reading. *Language, Speech, and Hearing Services in Schools, 23,* 176–182.

Weiner, F. (1979). *Phonological process analysis.* Baltimore: University Park Press.

Weiner, F. (1981). Treatment of phonological disability using the method of meaningful minimal contrast: Two case studies. *Journal of Speech and Hearing Disorders, 46,* 97–103.

Weiner, F., & Bankson, N. (1978). Teaching features. *Language, Speech, and Hearing Services in Schools, 9,* 29–34.

Weiner, F., & Ostrowski, A. (1979). Effects of listener uncertainty on articulatory inconsistency. *Journal of Speech and Hearing Disorders, 44,* 487–493.

Weiner, P. (1967). Auditory discrimination and articulation. *Journal of Speech and Hearing Disorders, 32,* 19–28.

Weinert, H. (1974). *Die Bekämpfung von Sprechfehlern.* Berlin:VEB Verlag Volk und Gesundheit.

Weismer, G. (1984). Acoustic analysis strategies for the refinement of phonological analysis. In M. Elbert, D. Dinnsen, & G. Weismer (Eds.), *Phonological theory and the misarticulating child. ASHA Monographs, 22,* 30–52. Rockville, MD: ASHA.

Weismer, G., Dinnsen, D., & Elbert, M. (1981). A study of the voicing distinction associated with omitted, word-final stops. *Journal of Speech and Hearing Disorders, 46,* 320–328.

Weiss, C. (1980). *Weiss comprehensive articulation test.* Allen, TX: DLM Teaching Resources.

Weiss, C. E. (1982). *Weiss intelligibility test.* Tigard, OR: C. C. Publicatons.

Weiss, C. E., Gordon, M. E., & Lillywhite, H. S. (1987). *Clinical management of articulatory and phonologic disorders* (2nd ed.). Boston: Williams & Wilkins.

Weiss, C. E., & Lillywhite, H. E. (1981). *Communication disorders* (2nd ed.). St. Louis, MO: C. V. Mosby.

Wellman, B. L., Case, I. M., Mengert, I. G., & Bradbury, D. E. (1931). Speech sounds of young children. *University of Iowa Studies in Child Welfare, 5,* Iowa City, IA: University of Iowa Press.

Wells, B., Stackhouse, J., & Vance, M. (1996). A specific deficit in onset-rhyme assembly in a 9-year-old child with speech and literacy difficulties. In T. W. Powell (Ed.), *Pathologies of speech and language: Contributions of clinical phonetics and linguistics.* New Orleans, LA: International Clinical Phonetics and Linguistics Association.

Wepman, J. (1973). *Wepman auditory discrimination test.* Chicago: Language Research Association.

Werker, J. F., & Tees, R. C. (1983). Developmental changes across childhood in the perception of non-native speech sounds. *Canadian Journal of Psychology, 37,* 278–286.

Wertz, R. T. (1985). Neuropathologies of speech and language. In D. F. Johns (Ed.), *Clinical management of neurogenic communicative disorders* (pp. 1–96). Boston: Little, Brown.

Wertz, R. T., LaPointe, L. L., & Rosenbek, J. C. (1984). *Apraxia of speech in adults: The disorder and its management.* Orlando, FL: Grune and Stratton.

West, R., & Ansberry, M. (1968). *The rehabilitation of speech* (4th ed.). New York: Harper & Row.

West, R., Kennedy, L., & Carr, A. (1937). *The rehabilitation of speech.* New York: Harpers.

Westlake, H., & Rutherford, D. (1961). *Speech therapy for the cerebral palsied.* Chicago: National Society for Crippled Children and Adults.

Whalen, D. H., Levitt, A. G., & Wang, Q. (1991). Intonational differences between reduplicative babbling of French- and English-learning infants. *Journal of Child Language, 18,* 501–516.

Whitehurst, G., Fischel, J., Lonigan, C., Valdez-Menchaca, M., Arnold, D., & Smith, M. (1991). Treatment of early expressive language delay: If, when, and how. *Topics in Language Disorders, 11,* 55–68.

Whitehurst, G., Smith, M., Fischel, J., Arnold, D., & Lonigan, C. (1991). The continuity of babble and speech in children with specific expressive language delay. *Journal of Speech and Hearing Research, 34,* 1121–1129.

Wickelgren, W. (1966). Distinctive features and errors in short-term memory for English consonants. *Journal of the Acoustic Society of America, 39,* 388–398.

Wilcox, K. A., Schooling, T. L., & Morris, S. R. (1991). *The preschool intelligibility measure (P-SIM).* Paper presented at the Annual Convention of the American Speech-Language-Hearing Association. Atlanta, GA.

Wilkins, J. (1668). *An essay towards a real character and a philosophical language.* London: S. Gellibrand.

Williams, F., Cairns, H. S., Cairns, C. E., & Blosser, D. F. (1970). *Analysis of production errors in the phonetic performance of school-age standard English-speaking children.* Austin, TX: University of Texas.

Williams, G., & McReynolds, L. (1975). The relationship between discrimination and articulation training in children with misarticulations. *Journal of Speech and Hearing Research, 18,* 401–412.

Williams, R. L., & Wolfram, W. (1977). Social dialects: Differences versus disorders. In K. Jeter (Ed.), *Bilingual language learning system.* Rockville, MD: American Speech-Language-Hearing Association.

Winitz, H. (1969). *Articulation acquisition and behavior.* New York: Appleton-Century-Crofts.

Winitz, H. (1975). *From syllable to conversation.* Baltimore: University Park Press.

Winitz, H. (1984). Auditory considerations in articulation training. In H. Winitz (Ed.), *Treating articulation disorders: For clinicians by clinicians.* Baltimore: University Park Press.

Winitz, H. (1989). Auditory considerations in treatment. In N. Creaghead, P. Newman, & W. Secord (Eds.), *Assessment and remediation of articulatory and phonological disorders* (2nd ed.) (pp. 243–264). New York: Macmillan.

Winitz, H., & Irwin, O. C. (1958). Syllabic and phonetic structure of infants' early words. *Journal of Speech and Hearing Research, 1,* 250–256.

Winitz, H., Sanders, R., & Kort, J. (1981). Comprehension and production of the /əz/ plural allomorph. *Journal of Psycholinguistic Research, 10,* 259–271.

Winteler, J. (1876). *Die Kerenzer Mundart des Kantons Glarus in ihren Grundzügen dargestellt.* Leipzig: C. F. Winter'sche Verlagsbuchhandlung.

Wise, C. M. (1958). *Introduction to phonetics.* Englewood Cliffs, NJ: Prentice-Hall.

Witzell, M. A. (1995). Communicative impairment associated with clefting. In R. J. Schprintzen & J. Bardach (Eds.), *Cleft palate speech management: A multidisciplinary approach.* St. Louis, MO: Mosby.

Wode, H. (1980). Grammatical intonation in child language. In L. R. Waugh & C. H. van Schooneveld (Eds.), *The melody of language: Intonation and prosody* (pp. 331–345). New York: Academic Press.

Wolfram, W. (1986). Language variation in the United States. In O. Taylor (Ed.), *Treatment of communication disorders in culturally and linguistically diverse populations* (pp. 73–116). San Diego, CA: College-Hill Press.

Wolfram, W. (1994). The phonology of a sociocultural variety: The case of African American Vernacular English. In J. Bernthal & N. Bankson (Eds.), *Child phonology: Characteristics, assessment, and intervention with special populations* (pp. 227–244). New York: Thieme.

Wolk, L. (1986). Markedness analysis of consonant error productions in apraxia of speech. *Journal of Communication Disorders, 19,* 133–160.

Yavaş, M. (1998). *Phonology development and disorders.* San Diego, CA: Singular.

Yorkston, K. M., & Beukelman, D. R. (1981). Communication efficiency of dysarthric speakers as measured by sentence intelligibility and speaking rate. *Journal of Speech and Hearing Disorders, 46,* 296–301.

Yorkston, K. M., & Beukelman, D. R. (Eds.). (1988). *Recent advances in clinical dysarthria.* Boston: Little, Brown.

Yorkston, K. M., Beukelman, D. R., & Bell, K. R. (1988). *Clinical management of dysarthric speakers.* Boston: College-Hill Press.

Yoss, K. A., & Darley, F. L. (1974a). Developmental apraxia of speech in children with defective articulation. *Journal of Speech and Hearing Research, 17,* 399–416.

Yoss, K. A., & Darley, F. L. (1974b). Therapy in developmental apraxia of speech. *Language, Speech, and Hearing Services in Schools, 5,* 23–31.

Young, E. H., & Hawk, S. S. (1955). *Moto-kinesthetic speech training.* Palo Alto, CA: Stanford University Press.

Zemlin, W. R. (1988). *Speech and hearing science: Anatomy and physiology* (3rd ed.). Englewood Cliffs, NJ: Prentice-Hall.

Zlatin, M. A., & Koenigsknecht, R. A. (1975). Development of the voicing contrast: Perception of stop consonants. *Journal of Speech and Hearing Research, 18,* 541–543.